Bhutani's

Color Atlas of

SEXUALLY TRANSMITTED INFECTIONS

Bhutani's
Color Atlas of
SEXUALLY TRANSMITTED INFECTIONS

Second Edition

Editors

Neena Khanna MD
Professor
Department of Dermatology and Venereology
All India Institute of Medical Sciences
New Delhi, India

Sushruta Kathuria MD
Dermatologist
Supreme Court of India
New Delhi, India

JAYPEE

JAYPEE BROTHERS MEDICAL PUBLISHERS
The Health Sciences Publisher
New Delhi | London

Jaypee Brothers Medical Publishers (P) Ltd

Headquarters
EMCA House, 23/23-B
Ansari Road, Daryaganj
New Delhi 110 002, India
Landline: +91-11-23272143,
+91-11-23272703
+91-11-23282021, +91-11-23245672
e-mail: jaypee@jaypeebrothers.com

Corporate Office
4838/24, Ansari Road, Daryaganj
New Delhi 110 002, India
Phone: +91-11-43574357
Fax: +91-11-43574314
e-mail: jaypee@jaypeebrothers.com

Overseas Office
JP Medical Ltd.
83, Victoria Street, London
SW1H 0HW (UK)
Phone: +44-20 3170 8910
e-mail: info@jpmedpub.com

EU GPSR Authorised Representative
Logos Europe, 9 rue Nicolas Poussin
17000, La Rochelle, France
Phone: +33 (0) 6 67 93 73 78
e-mail: contact@logoseurope.eu

Website: www.jaypeebrothers.com
Website: www.jaypeedigital.com

Inquiries for bulk sales may be solicited at: jaypee@jaypeebrothers.com

Bhutani's Color Atlas of Sexually Transmitted Infections

First Edition: 1986
Second Edition: 2013

Reprint: **2026**

ISBN 978-93-5090-453-4

Printed in India

Preface to the Second Edition

The profile of sexually transmitted diseases (oops infections!) has changed dramatically from the time, the first edition of the atlas was brought out by Professor LK Bhutani as an add-on to his immensely popular *Colour Atlas of Sexually Transmitted Diseases*. Several batches of postgraduate students were initiated into the field of 'venereology' by the colorful (in the era of black and white) book.

With the advent of HIV pandemic, sexually transmitted infections (STIs) have gained a new academic lease of life and have also changed their profile. The atlas is a pictorial journey of STIs from the past (rare photographs of tertiary syphilis) to the present (protean cutaneous manifestations of HIV). Though keeping the tradition of 'LKBism' (inimitable crisp style), an effort has been made to make the atlas more than just a visual treat, by incorporating diagnostic techniques (with several pictures clicked at the bench) and treatment. To make the atlas comprehensive, a section has been added on anatomy of genital tract and syndromic management.

Neena Khanna
Sushruta Kathuria

Preface to the First Edition

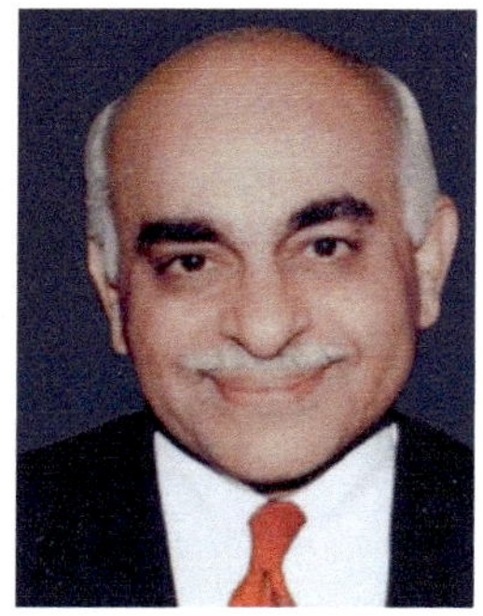

Sexually transmitted diseases (STD) are defined as a group of infectious diseases in which sexual transmission is epidemiologically important. The term has supplanted the erstwhile designation of venereal diseases (VD), which conventionally had included syphilis, gonorrhea, chancroid, lymphogranuloma venereum and granuloma inguinale. STD is a broader concept and includes several additional diseases—non-gonococcal urethritis and nonspecific genital infections, genital herpes, venereal warts, pediculosis pubis and in certain situations conditions like scabies, cytomegalovirus and hepatitis B virus infections, trichomoniasis, candidiasis, and the most dreaded of them all—acquired immunodeficiency syndrome (AIDS).

Sexuality is a basic human (and animal) instinct. Sexually transmitted diseases have thus been with mankind since antiquity. Several factors, in the recent past, seem to have influenced pattern(s), incidence and prevalence of STD. The introduction of chemotherapeutic agents and antibiotics in the treatment of STD caused a dramatic and precipitous decline in the incidence and morbidity of these infections. The diseases that used to cause profound and protracted suffering could simply be 'cured' with a 'single-shot' therapy. Fear, doubt and anxiety were all too quickly replaced by confidence and a (partly justified) sense of security.

The post-war era witnessed a laxity in sexual standards in the Western world. Several factors contributed to this change. The influence of religion waned; young people became economically independent and lived individually and separately; the family fabric disintegrated. Cinema, television and other mass media played on the sexual and erotic impulses; once 'infamous' pornographic literature enjoyed social acceptability—even respectability. Sex is no longer taboo.

The 'counter-culture' of the 1960s caused sociocultural upheavals. The uninhibited approach to sex encouraged freer heterosexual, homosexual or bisexual relationships—more particularly among the teenagers. Heterosexual relationships became promiscuous also due to easy accessibility to oral and conventional contraceptives thus removing the fear of unwanted pregnancies. The monogamous relationships—marital or extramarital—became less stable. Polygamous relationships, often casual and brief, brought acquisition and spread of sexually transmitted diseases. Chastity ceased to be a cherished virtue; sex experience as a preliminary to marriage almost became a norm. High divorce rate, broken homes, collapse of the traditional family structure caused a rupture in the accepted human relationships and drove parents and children alike into the wilderness—seeking affection and often finding (sexual) gratification and sexually transmitted diseases. The use of drugs and alcohol coupled with communal living aggravated matters further. The effects were noticed in an upswing of gonorrhea, non-gonococcal urethritis, genital herpes and genital warts. Genital herpes caused widespread scare and anxiety accentuated by its possible relationship to cervical cancer and neonatal infections. Non-gonococcal infections caused persistent and/or recurrent discomfort.

Changes in patterns of sexuality brought into sharper focus conditions like gonococcal pharyngitis, gonococcal proctitis and AIDS. AIDS emerged almost as a direct consequence of homosexual contact. This viral (HTLV-III/LAV) infection caused a specific depletion of T-helper/inducer cells with consequent immunodeficiency. Kaposi's sarcoma and opportunistic bacterial, viral and fungal infections in the lungs, brain, skin and other organs caused a high morbidity and mortality.

The picture for sexually transmitted diseases looks bright! Permissiveness is spreading in the developing world too (with the possible exception of the Islamic countries where the influence of religion is strong), as indeed is the use of drugs and alcohol. There is a very real danger that most countries will show an upward trend in the incidence of STD as urbanization and economic improvement occurs.

The book may seem to have an understandable bias towards the so-called tropical sexually transmitted diseases. Ease of travel and widespread migration have increased the intermingling of populations, and consequently many diseases are no longer restricted within geographical regions. The conceptual division between tropical and non-tropical sexually transmitted diseases thus seems to be less relevant today than in the past.

The Utopia of 'STD-Zero' does not appear on the horizon!

LK Bhutani

Acknowledgments

It is a proud albeit emotional time for us to be revising after a gap of almost three decades, a color atlas on sexually transmitted diseases, the first edition of which initiated many of us into the field of venereology. We are indeed indebted to Dr (Mrs) Bhutani for reposing faith in us and believing that we could carry out the task of bringing out the atlas. And had it not been her unflinching encouragement, the work would not have fructified.

The present work would not have been possible without the exceptional contribution of the Residents of the Department (at AIIMS), who thoroughly fine-tooth combed the original manuscript and metamorphosed it to the present shape. We would especially like the thank Drs Riti, Priyanka, Aanchal, Neetu, Rajeshwari, Sunil and Vishal, for prompt and detailed response, whenever and wherever needed.

We are grateful to Drs Ramam, Lalit Dhar, Benu Dhawan and Saurabh Singh, for allowing us to use photographs from their large collection. So also my gratitude to my faculty colleagues (many of who were Dr Bhutani's students), for letting us photograph their 'in-patients'.

Several 'pairs of hard working hands' and 'pairs of astute eyes' assisted us (almost) meet the deadlines. My office colleagues Tanu and Meenu helped endlessly at word processing the manuscript.

We would be failing in our duty if we did not thank the *behind the scene* people. Anil and Sanjeev who put up with sharing our time with the laptop. Chandni, Abhishek and Siya who did not get quality time with one of their parents.

My acknowledgments to Shri Jitendar P Vij (Group Chairman), Mr Ankit Vij (Managing Director), Mr Tarun Duneja (Director-Publishing), Mrs Samina Khan (PA to Director-Publishing), Mr KK Raman (Production Manager), Mr Sunil Kumar Dogra (Production Executive), Mr Neelambar Pant (Production Coordinator), Mr Manoj Pahuja (Senior Graphic Designer), Mr Varun Rana (Typesetter), Mr Himanshu Sharma (Proofreader) and other staff of M/s Jaypee Brothers Medical Publishers (P) Ltd, New Delhi, India, for their immense patience to bring out the book.

Contents

Section 1: Epidemiology

Section 2: Bacterial Sexually Transmitted Infections

Section 4: Miscellaneous

Section 5: Annexures

1 SECTION

EPIDEMIOLOGY

Chapter 1

Epidemiology of Sexually Transmitted Infections

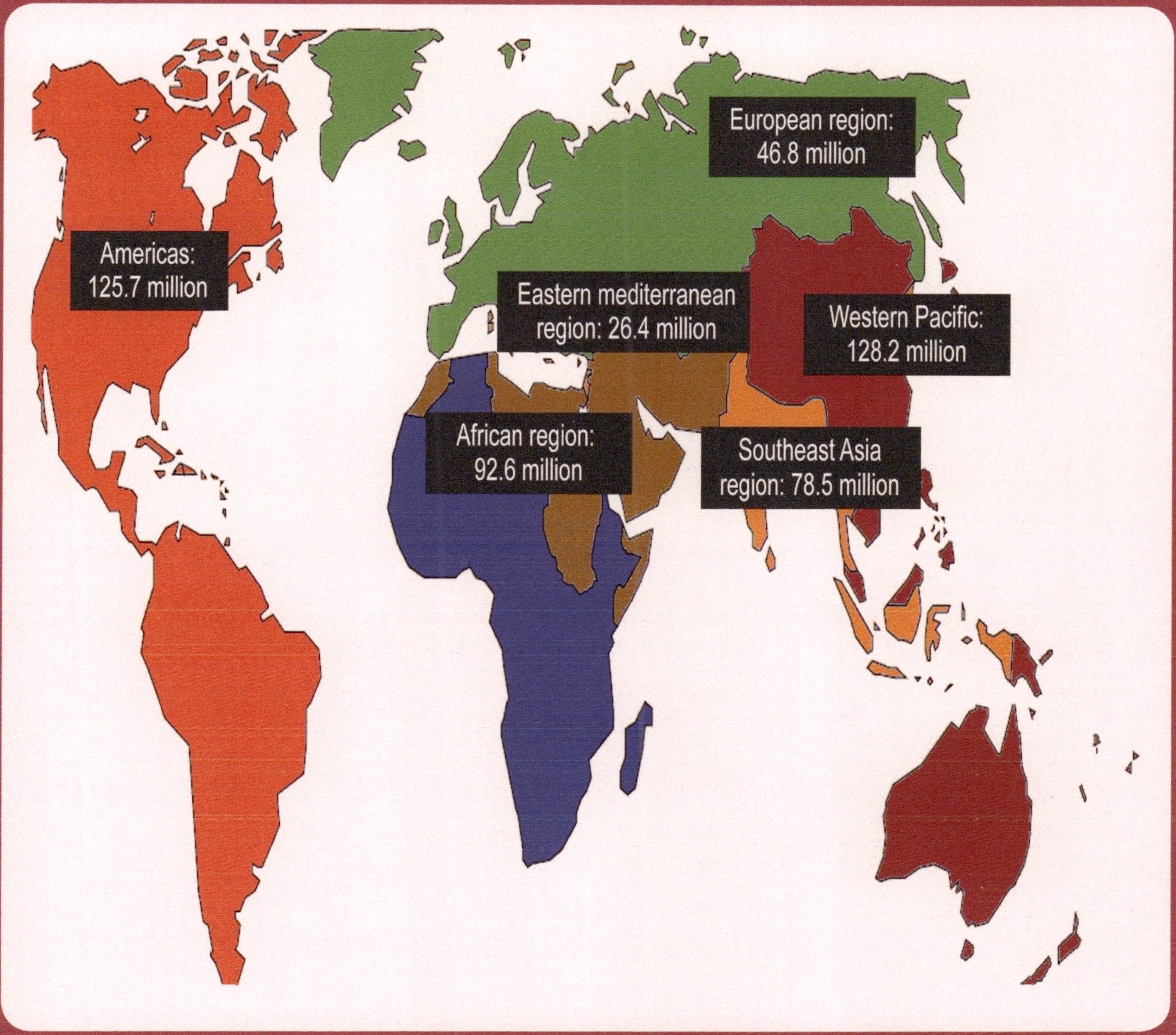

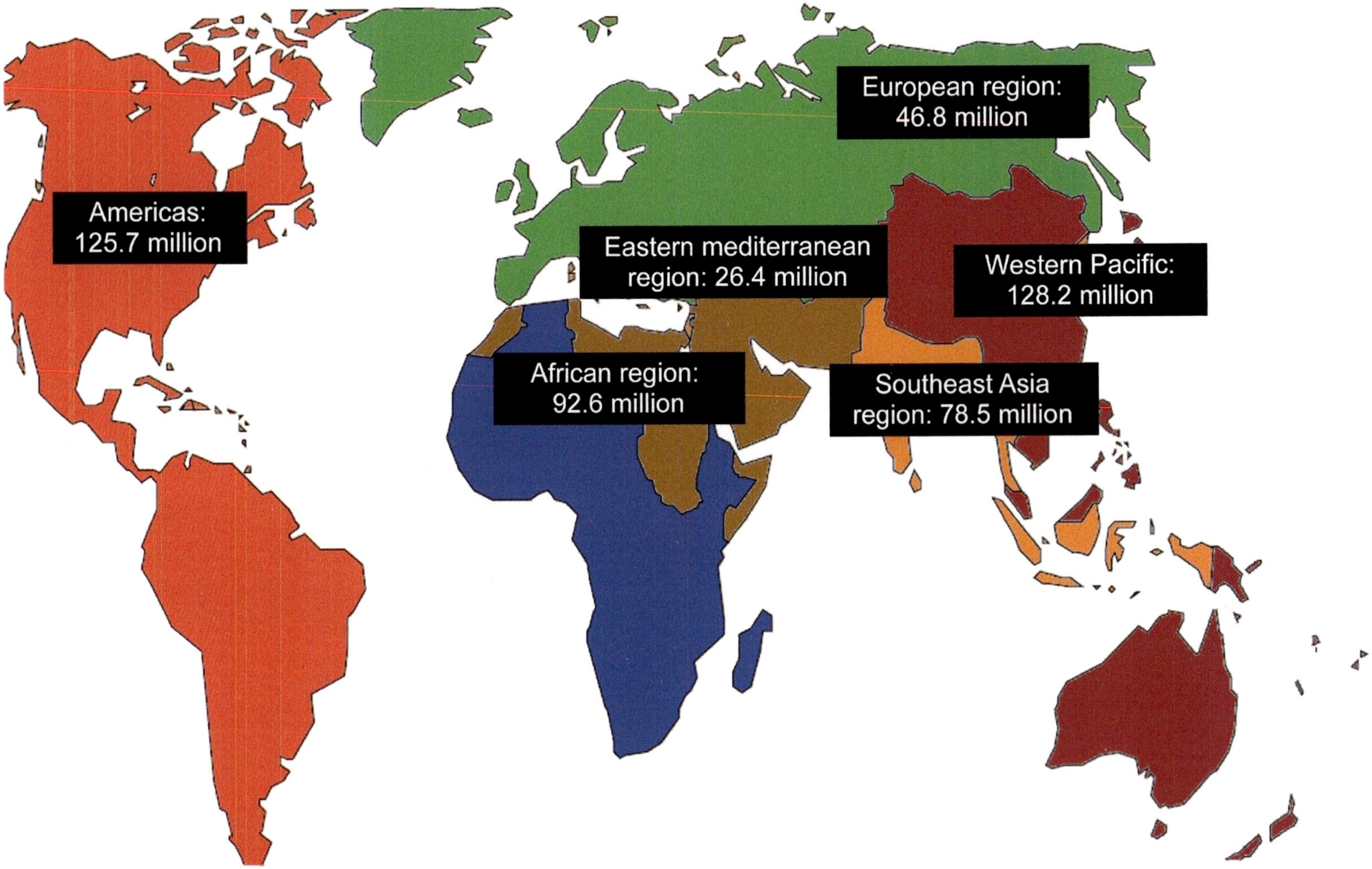

Estimated incidence of selected curable STIs (*C. trachomatis, N. gonorrhoeae*, syphilis and trichomoniasis) 2008 (WHO, 2008)

DEFINITIONS

Sexually Transmitted Infections (STIs)

Invasion by and multiplication of an organism (*e.g.* bacteria/virus/protozoan) that is usually (more than half the time) passed from one person to another during sexual intercourse or intimate bodily contact. STI may be symptomatic or asymptomatic.

Sexually Transmitted Diseases (STDs)

Symptomatic pathology secondary to an infection that is usually (more than half the time) passed from one person to another during sexual intercourse or intimate bodily contact. STI a broader term, all STDs are STIs, but not all STIs are STDs.

Epidemiology

Is study of disease frequency, distribution and determinants of health-related states and events in populations and its application to control health populations.

Incidence

Defined as number of new cases of specific disease occuring in a defined population during a specified period of time. Is given by the formula:

$$\frac{\text{Number of new cases of disease during a given time period} \times 1000}{\text{Population at risk}}$$

Prevalence

Defined as all current cases (old and new) existing at a given point in time or over a period of time in a given population. It is expressed as a percentage. Or as the number of cases per 10,000 or 100,000 people.

Point Prevalence

Defined as number of all current cases (old and new) of a disease at one point of time in a given population. Is given by the formula:

$$\frac{\text{Number of all current cases (old and new) of a disease at one point of time} \times 100}{\text{Population at risk at same point of time}}$$

Period Prevalence

Frequency of all current cases (old and new) of a disease during a defined period of time (*e.g.* annual prevalence) in relation to a defined population. Is given by the formula:

$$\frac{\text{Number of existing cases (old and new) of a specified disease during a given period of time interval} \times 100}{\text{Estimated mid-interval population at risk}}$$

Person-Years

Product of number of years times the number of members of a population who have been affected by a disease. Is used in large prospective studies where the time spent by each patient in study differs as it incorporates both variables (number of people in study and time each person spends in study). Person years and person months are used in studies that analyze their data using Kaplan Meier curves.

GLOBAL INCIDENCE AND PREVALENCE OF STIs

- According to 2008 WHO estimates, globally 499 million new infections with curable sexually transmitted infections (syphilis, gonorrhoea, chlamydia and trichomoniasis) occur annually in adults aged 15-49 years (Table 1.1, 1.2).
- Estimate higher than 2005 estimates. Apparent increase attributable to increasing number of youths entering sexually active population each year, social changes conducive to spread of STIs, greater emphasis on drug resistance. And better diagnostic facilities.
- In developing countries, STIs and their complications top five diseases for which adults seek health care.

Table 1.1: Global incidence for curable STIs for 2005 and 2008 (millions of cases)

	2005	2008	% change
Chlamydia trachomatis	101.5	105.7	4.1
Neisseria gonorrhoeae	87.7	106.1	21.0
Syphilis	10.6	10.6	0
Trichomonas vaginalis	248.5	276.4	11.2
Total	448.3	498.9	11.3

- STIs main preventable cause of infertility, particularly in women. Untreated chlamydial infection → symptomatic pelvic inflammatory disease (PID) in 10–40% of women→ infertility in 30–40%. Women with PID, 6 – 10 times more likely to develop an ectopic (tubal) pregnancy. And 40 – 50% of ectopic pregnancies attributable to PID.
- Untreated early syphilis in pregnant women → 40% perinatal mortality (still birth 25%; neonatal death 14%).
- Untreated gonococcal infection → 35% perinatal morbidity (spontaneous abortions and premature deliveries; 35%, perinatal deaths, 10%).
- Ophthalmia neonatorum in 50% of infants born to mothers with gonorrhea. And in 30% of those born to mothers with untreated chlamydial infection. Leads to blindness, if not treated early.

- In United States, annual incidence of HPV infection 5.5 million.
- In some parts (e.g. Pacific region), 1 in 3 women attending antenatal clinic, has STI (chlamydia and trichomonas being commonest).

SCENARIO IN INDIA

- Most data available from institution based publications. Prevalence and incidence derived from population based surveys very sparse. A countrywide Rapid Assessment Survey (RAS) indicates 12% of females and 6% of males attend primary health care facility with complaints related to STI/RTI. The 2002 ICMR multicenter community prevalence study of STI/RTI has shown that 5–6% of sexually active adult population suffer from STI/RTI.
- Incidence of viral STIs increasing while that of bacterial STIs decreasing. Probably attributable to curability of bacterial STDs (due to specific therapy, and rampant 'mis' use of antibiotics) and relative 'incurability' of viral STDs.
- Absolute numbers of patients with STDs attending hospitals is decreasing, consequent to better peripheral health services. And also safer sexual practices.

STI SYNDROMES

Although many different pathogens cause STIs, some display similar or overlapping signs and symptoms. Some of these signs and symptoms are easily recognizable and consistent, giving what is known as a syndrome that indicates presence of one or a number of pathogens.

The main syndromes of common STIs are:

- Urethral discharge.
- Genital ulcers.
- Inguinal swelling.
- Scrotal swelling.
- Vaginal discharge.
- Lower abdominal pain, in females.
- Oral and anal STIs.

Table 1.2: Global estimates (2008) for curable STIs in adults between 15 and 49 years in different parts of the world

	In millions	S-E Asia		W Pacific region		E Mediterranean	
		P (F/M) %	I (F/M) /1,000	P (F/M) %	I (F/M) /1,000	P (F/M) %	I (F/M) /1,000
Chlamydia	105.7	1.1/0.6	9.2/6.2	4.3/3.4	38.4/42.5	1.1/0.9	9.8/10.9
Gonorrhea	106.1	0.8/1.2	16.2/37.0	1.5/1.3	34.9/49.9	0.3/0.3	8.1/11.6
Trichomoniasis	276.4	5.6/0.6	40.3/50.1	5.7/0.6	45.6/47.0	8.0/0.8	64.0/66.1
Syphilis	10.6	1.3/1.3	3.2/3.1	0.1/0.1	0.5/0.5	0.5/0.5	0.1/0.1

	In millions	European region		Africa		Americas	
		P (F/M) %	I (F/M) /1,000	P (F/M) %	I (F/M) /1,000	P (F/M) %	I (F/M) /1,000
Chlamydia	105.7	3.9/3.8	37.1/54.2	2.6/2.1	22.3/20.9	7.6/2.9	72.6/38.2
Gonorrhea	106.1	0.3/0.2	8.3/7.0	2.3/2.0	49.7/60.3	0.8/0.7	18.5/27.6
Trichomonas	276.4	5.8/0.6	51.7/48.4	20.2/2.0	146.0/164.8	22.0/2.2	177.7/180.6
Syphilis	10.6	0.1/0.1	0.6/0.6	3.5/3.9	8.5/9.4	1.3/1.5	5.3/6.4

Abbreviations: P: Prevalence, I: Incidence, F: Females, M: Males

2 SECTION

BACTERIAL SEXUALLY TRANSMITTED INFECTIONS

CHAPTER 2

Syphilis

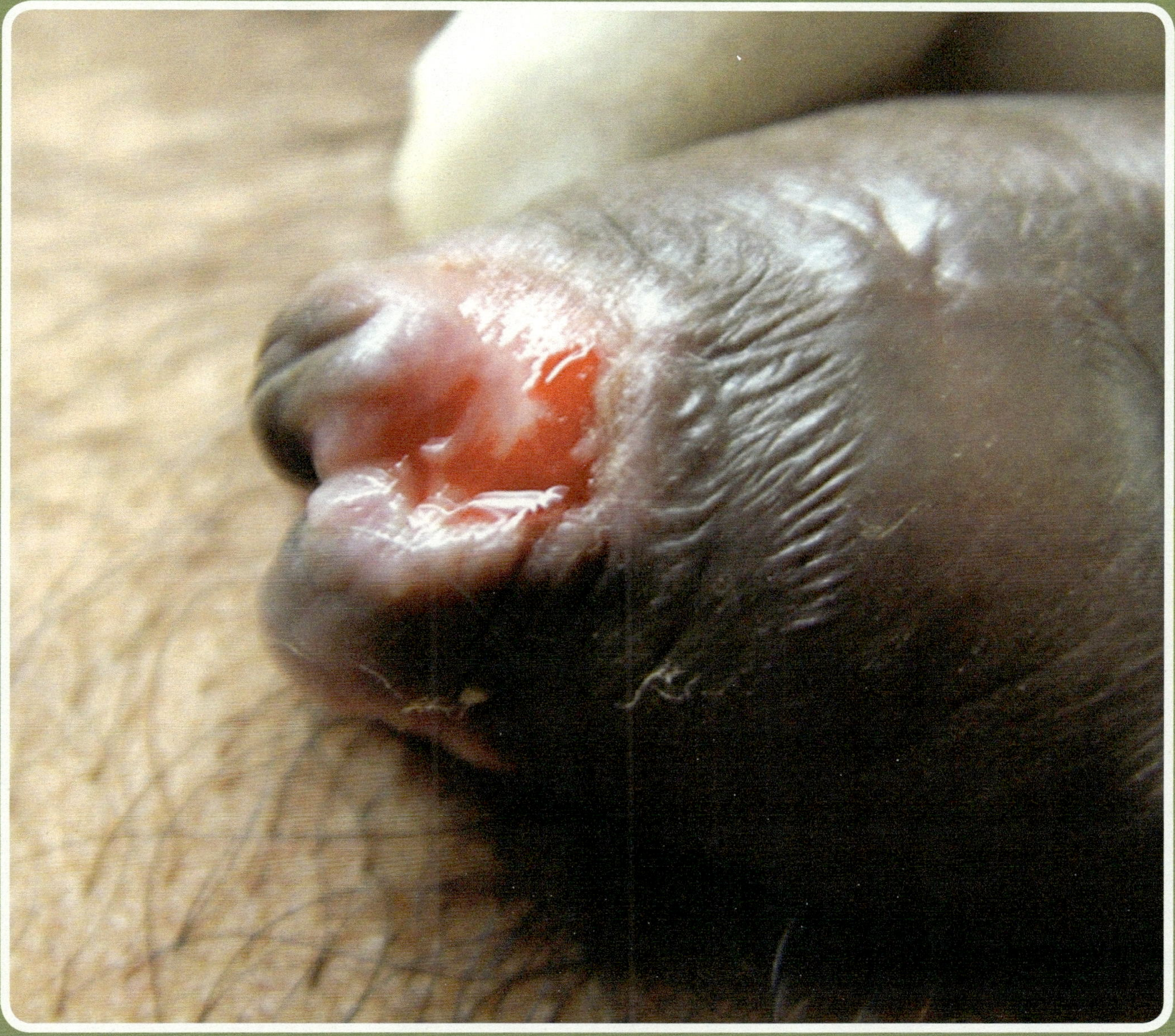

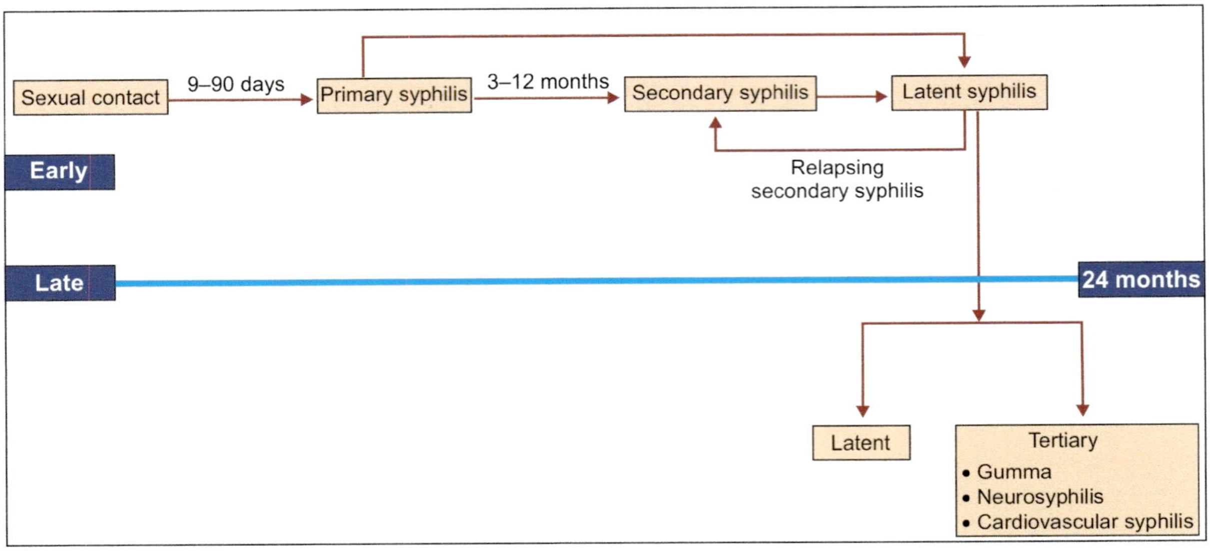

Course of syphilis

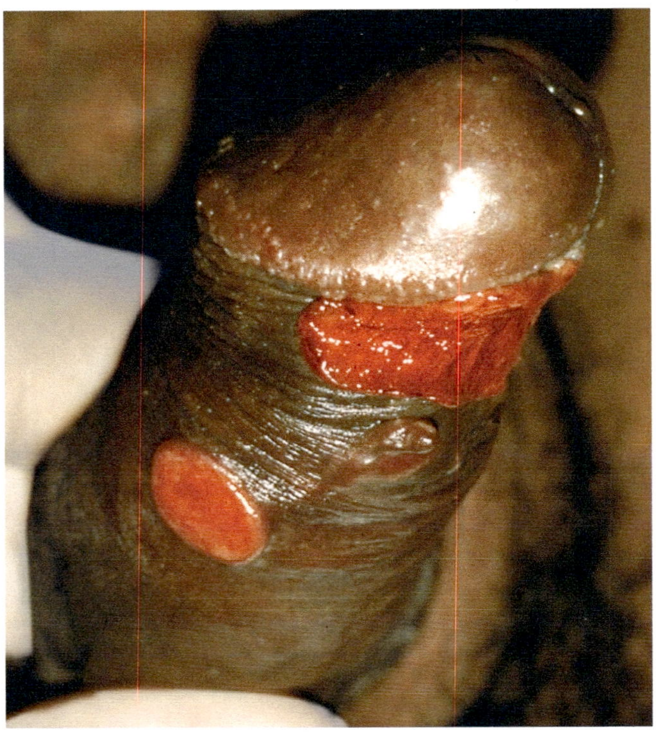

Syphilis: Chancre. Indurated ulcer with clean floor. On horizontal pressure, exudes serum which is teaming with *T. pallidum*.

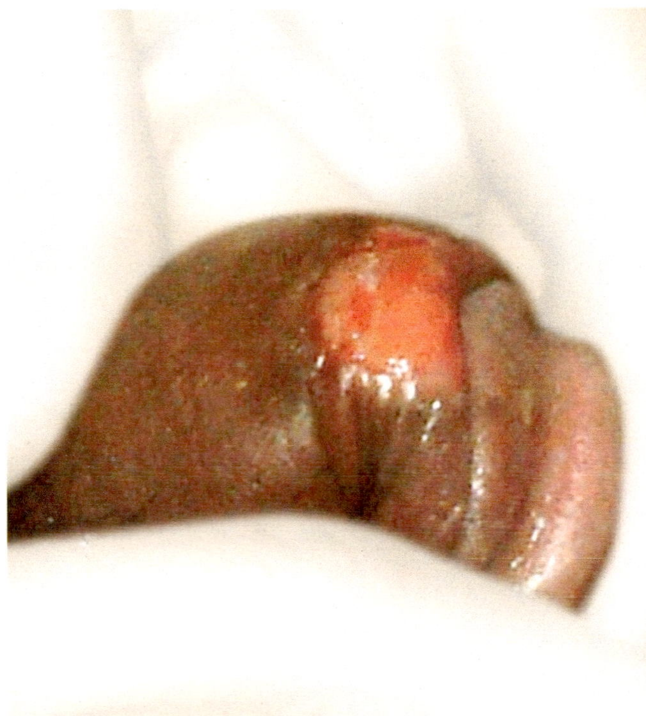

Syphilis: Chancre. Indurated ulcer on prepuce, visible after retracting the prepuce. Due to induration, when prepuce retracted, it typically flips back (dory flap sign).

ETIOLOGY

Etiological Agent

Caused by a spirochete—*Treponema pallidum*:

- ***Structure:*** Delicate, uniformly spiralled, 8-16 μm organism.
- ***Visualization:*** Not visualized using ordinary microscope. Live viewed using dark ground illumination microscope (DGI/DGM). Not seen in routine hematoxylin-eosin sections but take up silver and immunofluorescent stains.
- ***Movements:*** 'To and fro', compression, cork screw-like. And angulating characteristic.
- ***Culture:*** Pathogenic strain cannot be cultured on artificial media. Multiplies in rabbit's testicles (Nichol's strain).

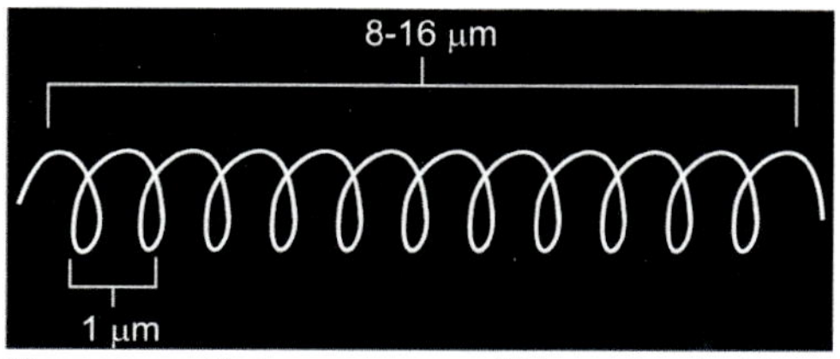

Structure of *Treponema pallidum:* A spiral bacteria with 8-16 regular close coils of ~1μm

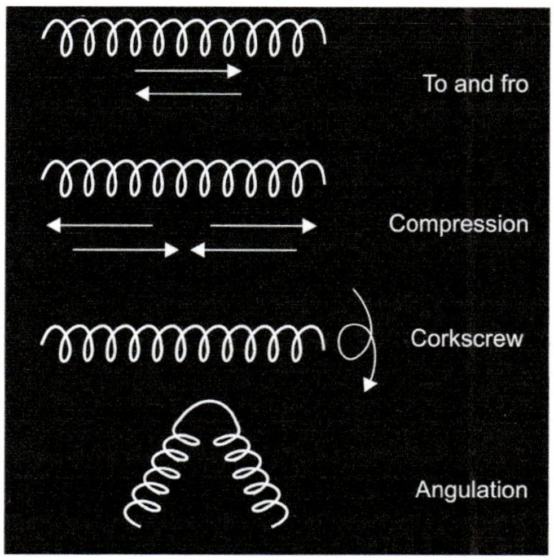

Movements of *T. pallidum*

Transmission

- ***Sexual:*** Mostly. Sexual contact with early infectious (cutaneous or mucosal) lesions. Survives only briefly outside body; thus, transmission almost always requires direct contact with infectious lesions. Discontinuity in skin surface promotes entry of treponemes. Condoms protective.
- ***Non-sexual:*** Rarely. Transplacentally. Or through blood products.

EPIDEMIOLOGY

Geographic Distribution

- Most infections in sub-Saharan Africa and South Asia.
- Preceding prevalence of 70s and 80s in USA and Europe re-emerged in HIV era. Two-thirds of new cases in MSMs with high rate of HIV co-infection.

Demographic Distribution

- Found mainly in people aged 15-39 years. Congenital infection rare.
- Men present with primary stage (women asymptomatic). Women present with secondary stage. Or asymptomatic, with chance positive serology.

CLINICAL FEATURES

Incubation Period

Variable, 9-90 days (average 2-3 weeks).

Stages

Clinically manifests in distinct or overlapping stages–primary, secondary, latent and tertiary. Also classified as early (primary, secondary and early latent) and late (late latent and tertiary) syphilis, early being less than 2 years from time of infection. Though disease systemic from onset, infectivity confined to early syphilis, as treponemes scanty in late stages.

Primary Syphilis

Consists of primary lesion (syphilitic or primary chancre) and regional lymphadenopathy.

Chancre

Morphology

- ***Typical (Hunterian) chancre:*** Solitary, painless (unless secondarily infected), indurated, non-tender, non-bleeding papule/plaque with an erythematous halo. Ulcerates superficially. Has a clean floor which exudes serum on pressure. Heals spontaneously in 3-8 weeks, leaving a small macule or superficial scar.
- ***Atypical chancre:*** May be multiple. Or painful/tender. Or soft. Often HIV coinfection. Or mixed infection.

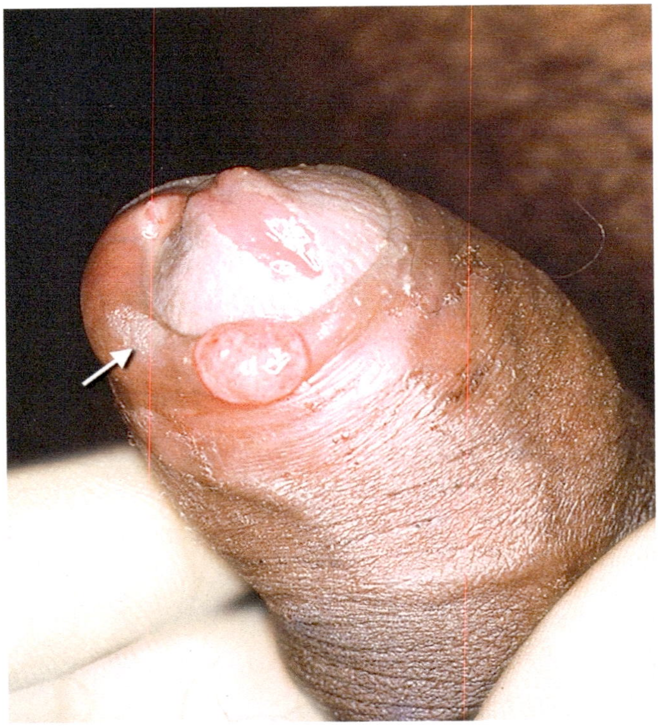

Syphilis: Chancre redux. Indurated, raised ulcer with clean floor, occurring at site of a healed primary (marked). Type of relapse.

Syphilis: Secondary syphilis. Roseolar syphilide. Symmetrical, asymptomatic macular lesions on trunk.

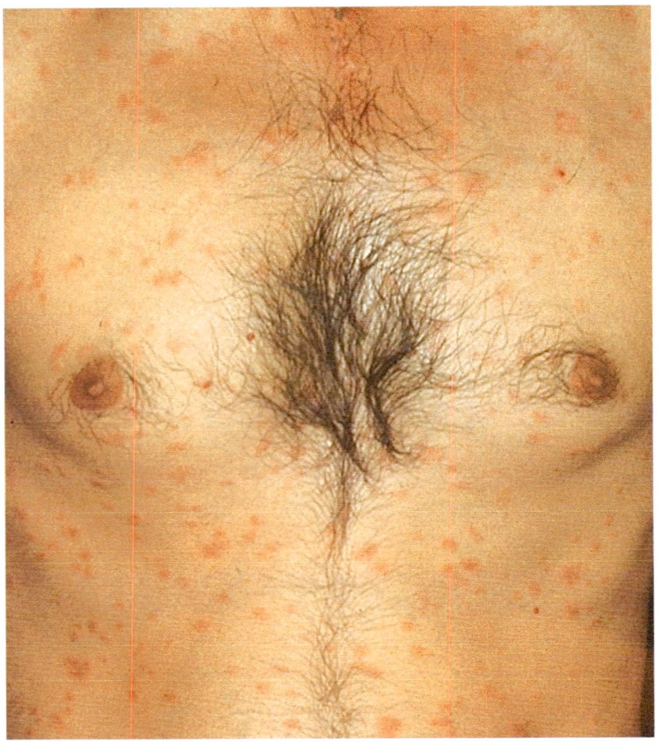

Syphilis: Secondary syphilis. Papular syphilide. Symmetrical, multiple erythematous, mildly scaly papules and oval plaques. Trunk, a characteristic site.

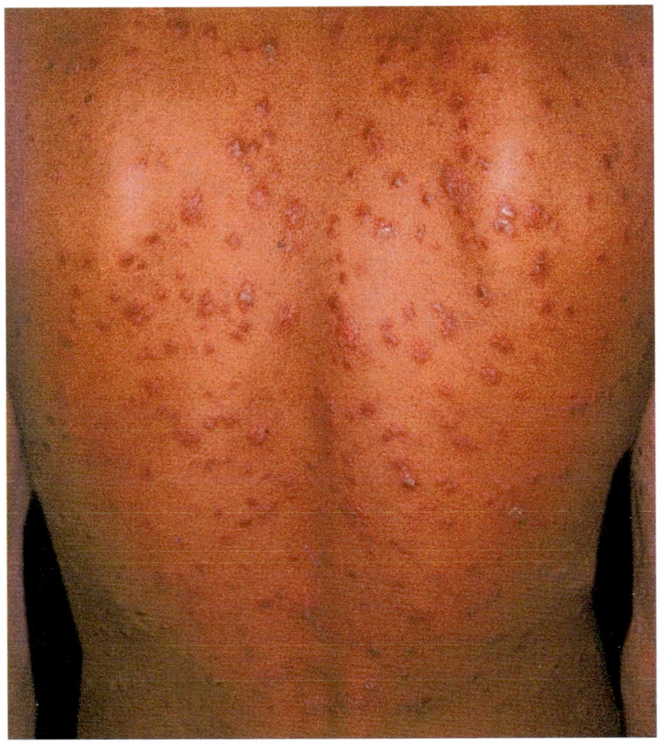

Syphilis: Secondary syphilis. Generalized symmetrical involvement on back with multiple erythematous small, scaly plaques.

❖ ***Chancre redux:*** Relapse at site of previous chancre.

Sites

❖ ***Anogenital:*** In males, glans, coronal sulcus, prepuce. Or shaft of penis, scrotum. In females, cervix, vagina (so asymptomatic). Or labia (where often seen as kissing lesions on opposing skin surfaces). In MSM, anus.
❖ ***Extragenital:*** Less common. Lips, breasts, tips of fingers.

Lymphadenopathy

Regional (so inguinal), generally unilateral. Small, shotty, non-tender, discrete and non-adherent; overlying skin normal. Subsides spontaneously without residue.

Secondary Stage

Generalized infection. Manifests as cutaneous and mucosal lesions, lymphadenopathy and extracutaneous disease. May superimpose on a healing primary lesion (in 25% of patients). Or may follow several weeks later. Or occurs *de novo* without primary stage (syphilis *dé emb lee*) especially in women.

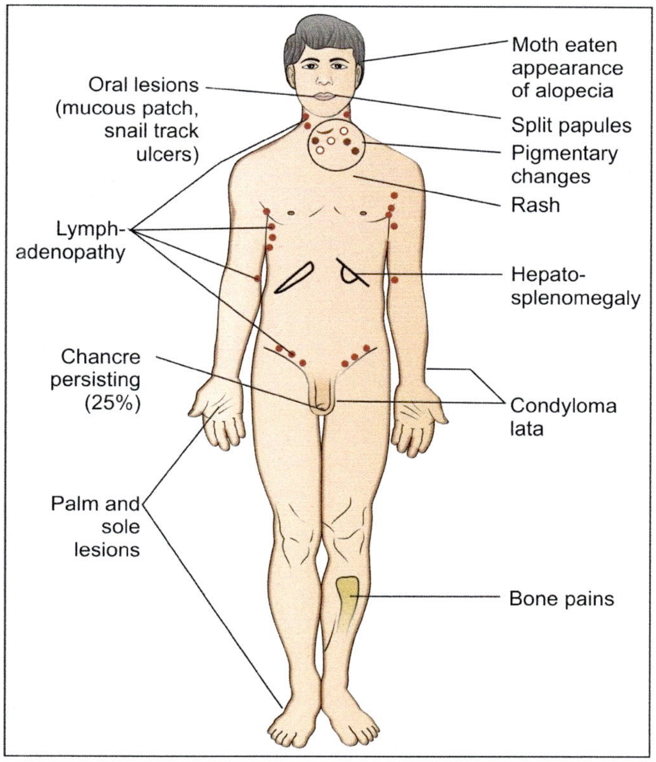

Clinical manifestations of secondary syphilis

Cutaneous lesions

Morphology

Asymptomatic, generalized rash with variable morphology, but never vesicular.

❖ ***Early lesions:*** Several erythematous macules (roseolar syphilide) evolving to papules (papular syphilide) and papulonodules (nodular syphilide). Lesions sometimes lichenoid–these and follicular lesions itchy. And rarely pustules (malignant lues).
❖ ***Late lesions:*** Fewer plaques and nodules (nodular/granulomatous syphilide). Often surmounted with scales, sometimes conspicuous (so psoriasiform syphilide). Heal without residue. Or with hypo-or hyperpigmentation (leucoderma colli of Venus).
❖ ***Other lesions:*** Palmar and plantar hyperpigmented (usually copper-colored) macules. Or scaly papules. Both characteristic.

Distribution

Lesions mostly on trunk and proximal extremities. Early lesions, numerous and distributed bilaterally symmetrically. Late lesions, fewer and distributed asymmetrically.

Mucosal lesions

Highly infectious. Anogenital and oral mucosae involved.

❖ ***Anogenital lesions:*** Asymptomatic, indurated, moist, flat papules or nodules, known as condylomata lata. Often eroded/macerated/vegetating. Perianal area, vulva, glans penis and penoscrotal fold.
❖ ***Oral lesions:*** Moist papules (similar to genital ones); often divide at angles of mouth and nasolabial folds to form split papules. And mucous patches: oval or circinate, asymptomatic, flat-topped gray-white patches with red halo. Confluence may result in serpiginous configuration (snail track ulcers). Palate, tonsils, buccal mucosa, gums, tongue or larynx.

Hair

Patchy, irregular, non-cicatricial alopecia (moth-eaten appearance) in occipital area.

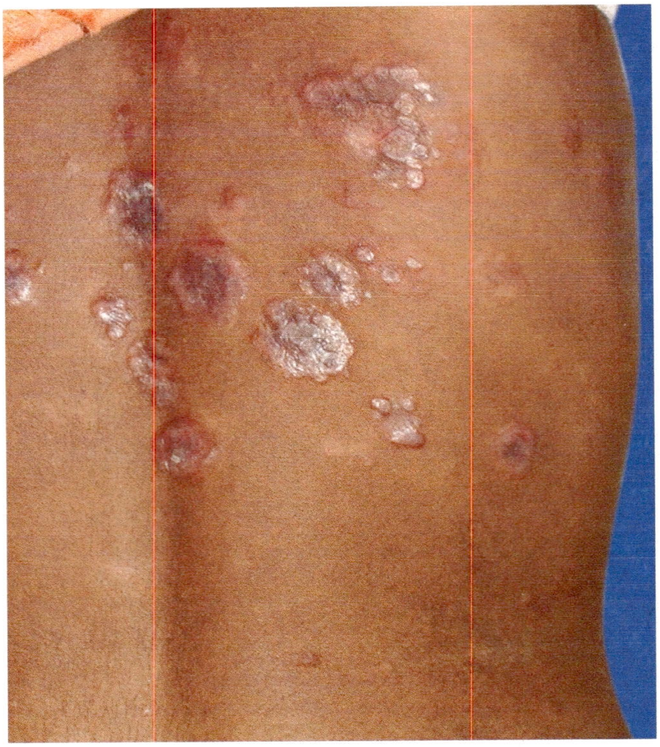

Syphilis: Secondary syphilis. Annular, violaceous, discrete plaques on back. Pressing plaques with pin-head causes pain on releasing the pin (Buschke-Ollendorf sign).

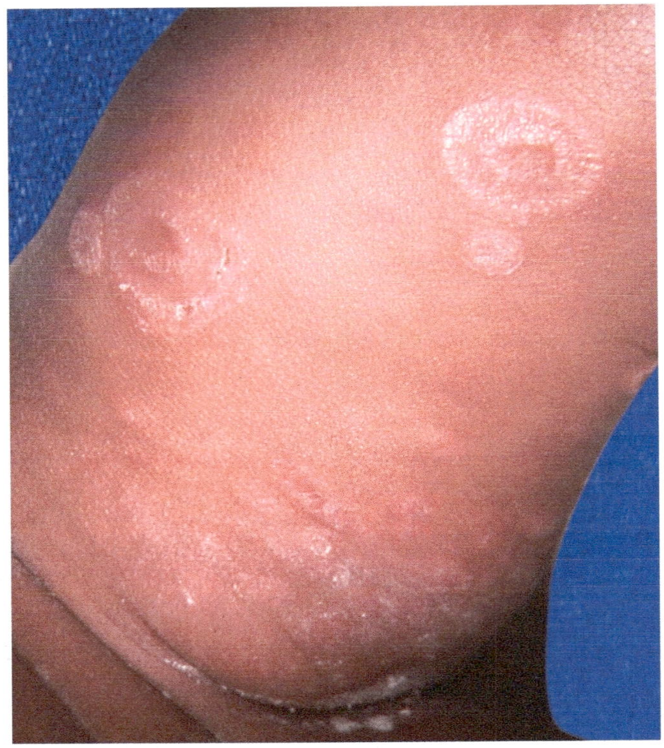

Syphilis: Secondary syphilis. Annular variant. Annular erythematous scaly plaques. Lesions are typically seen on trunk.

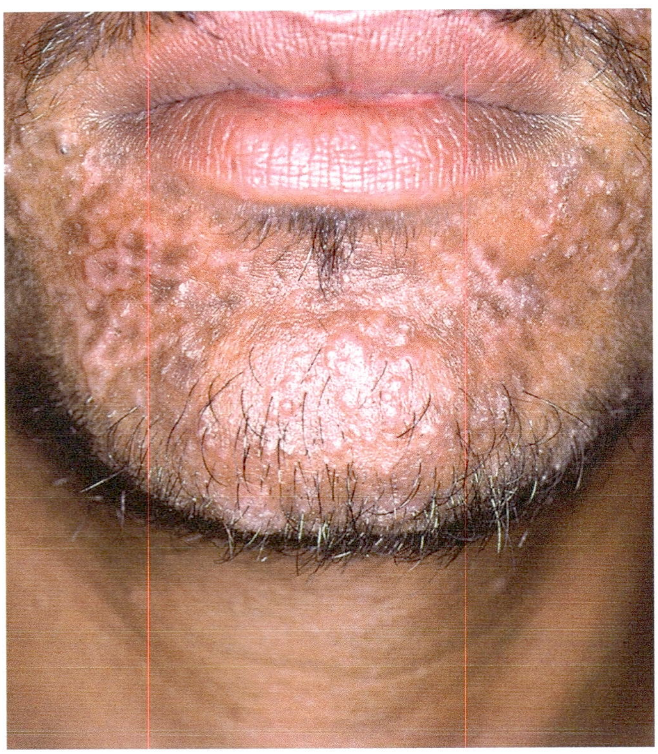

Syphilis: Secondary syphilis. Small, annular erythematous plaques on chin and perioral area.

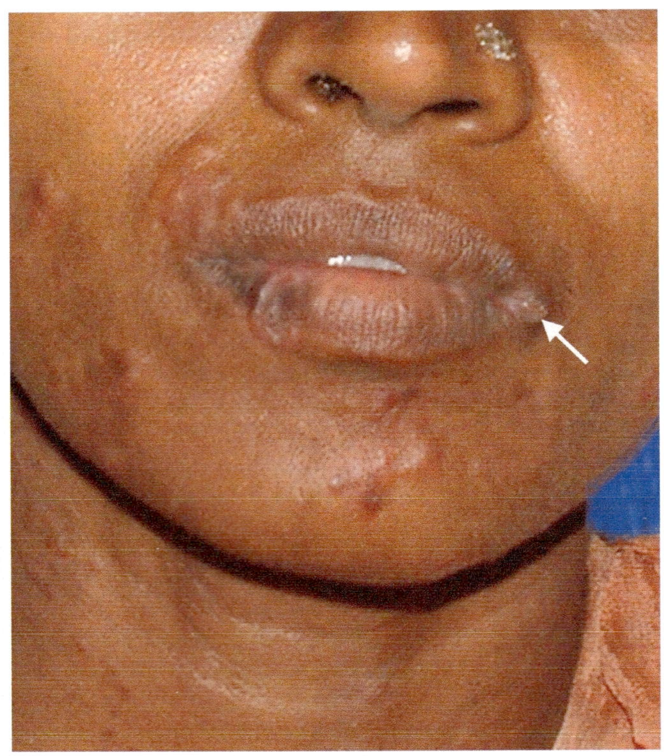

Syphilis: Secondary syphilis. Multiple well-defined, annular plaques on face and lips. Note split papules at angle of mouth.

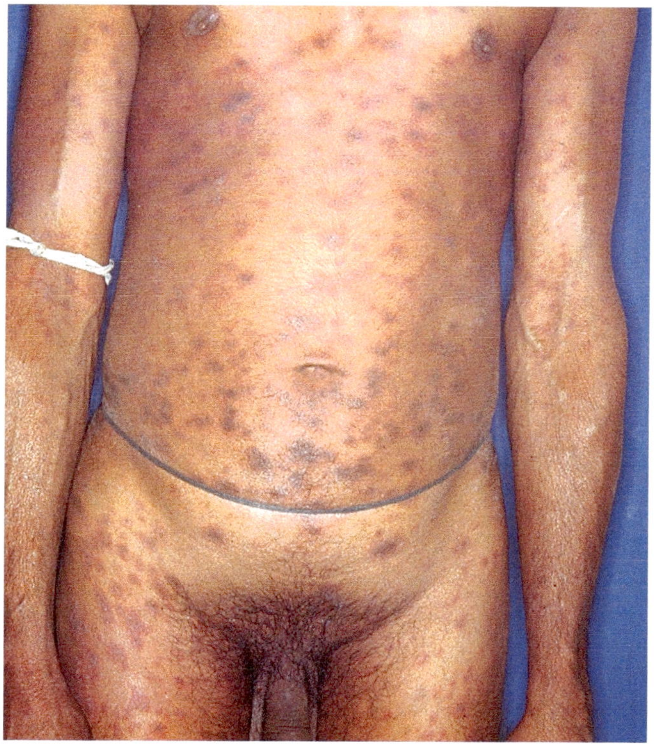

Syphilis: Secondary syphilis. Lichenoid variant. Symmetrical violaceous papules and plaques on trunk.

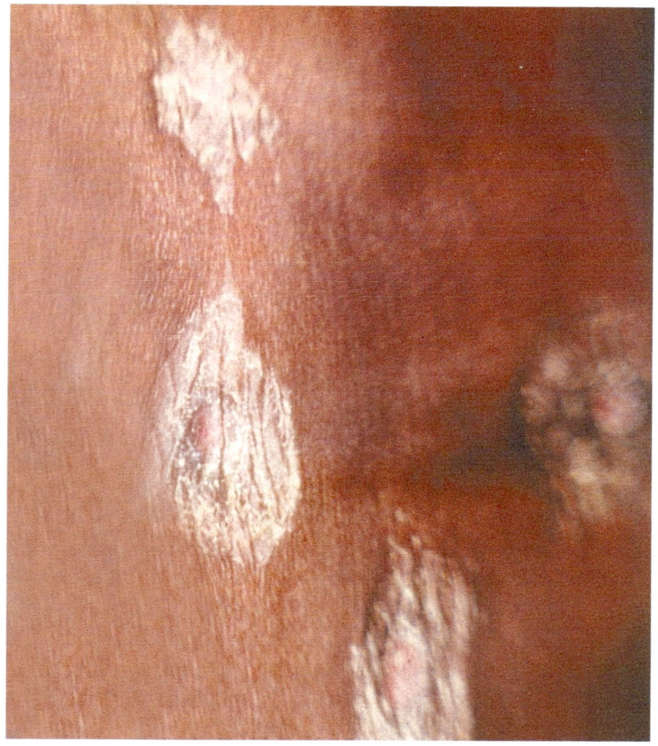

Syphilis: Secondary syphilis. Psoriasiform variant. Well-defined, erythematous plaques with thick, psoriasiform scales.

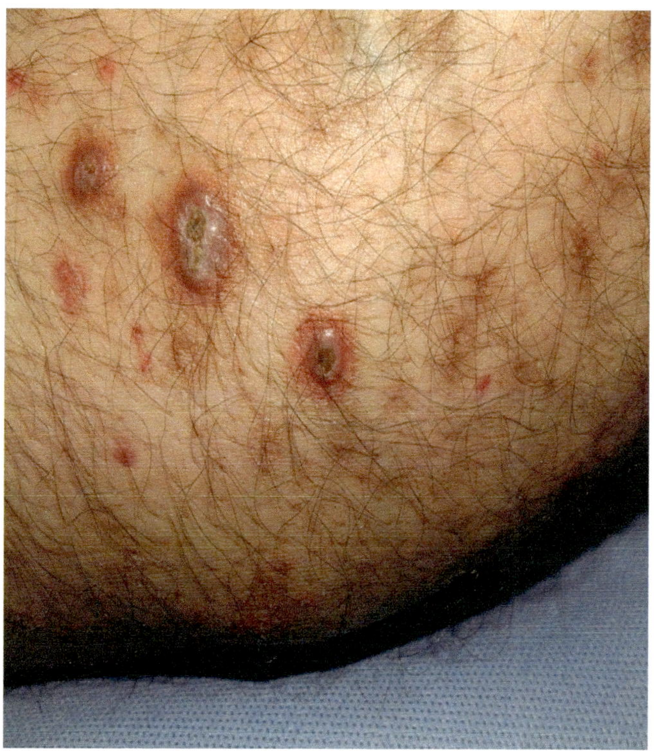

Syphilis: Secondary syphilis. Lues maligna or malignant secondary syphilis characterized by an explosive widespread eruption of papulopustular lesions which rapidly evolve into necrotic sharply marginated ulcers with hemorrhagic crusts.

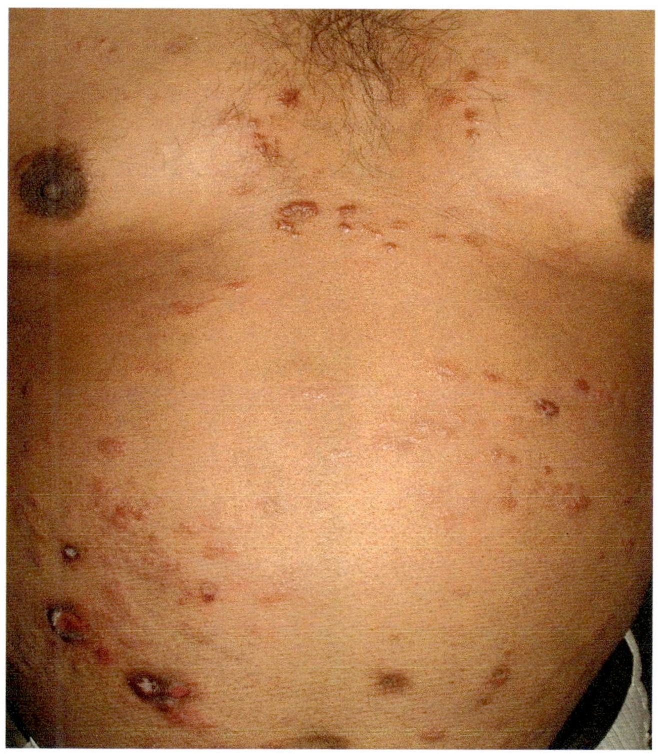

Syphilis: Secondary syphilis. Granulomatous variant. Few asymmetrically distributed nodules on trunk.

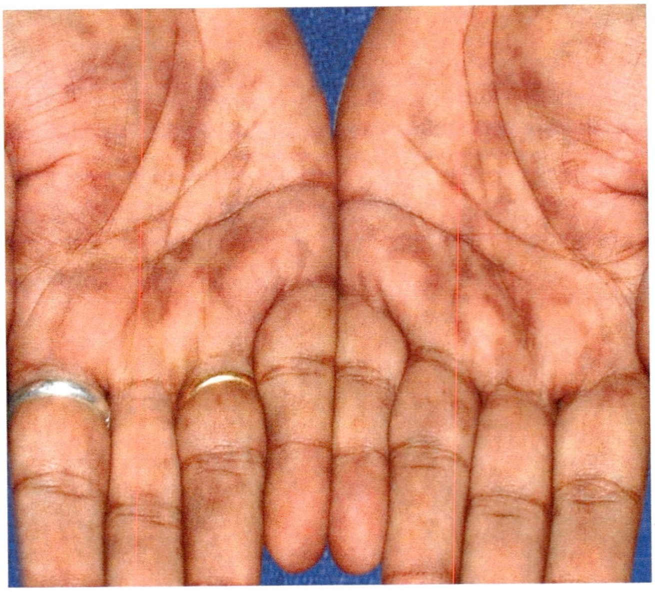

Syphilis: Secondary syphilis. Brown (coppery), mildly scaly plaques, present bilaterally, symmetrically, on palms. Presence of such lesions with even a nondescript truncal rash examination of mucosae and perianal areas and warrants performance of a serological test for syphilis.

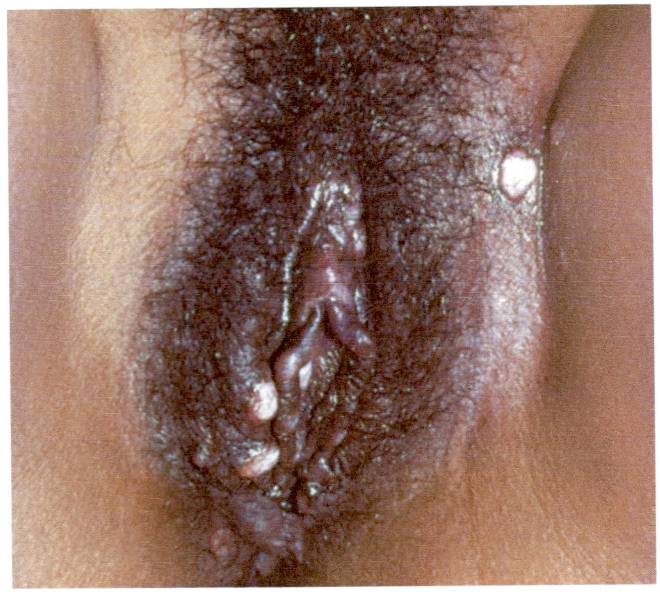

Syphilis: Secondary syphilis. Condyloma lata. Moist plaques with smooth well-defined margins on labia.

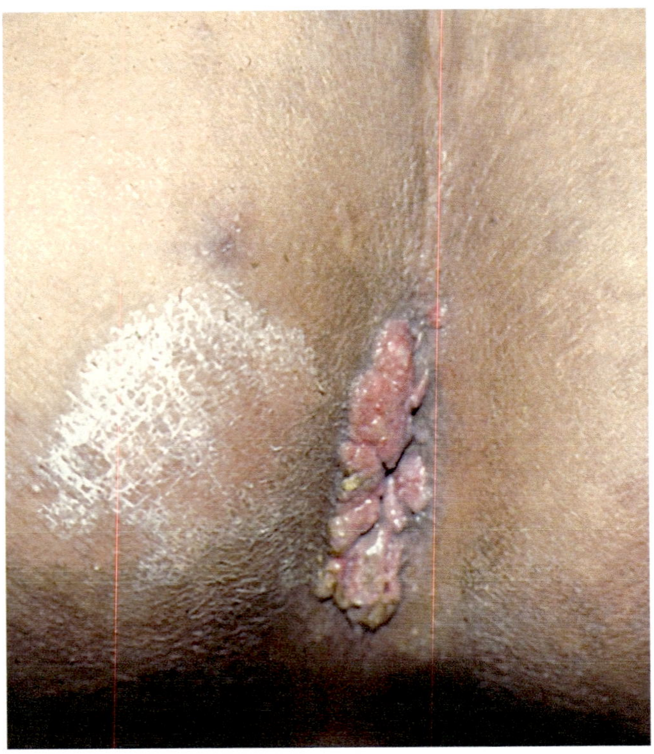

Syphilis: Secondary syphilis. Condyloma lata. Perianal area showing coalescent moist plaques. Incidentally, tinea cruris present on adjacent buttock.

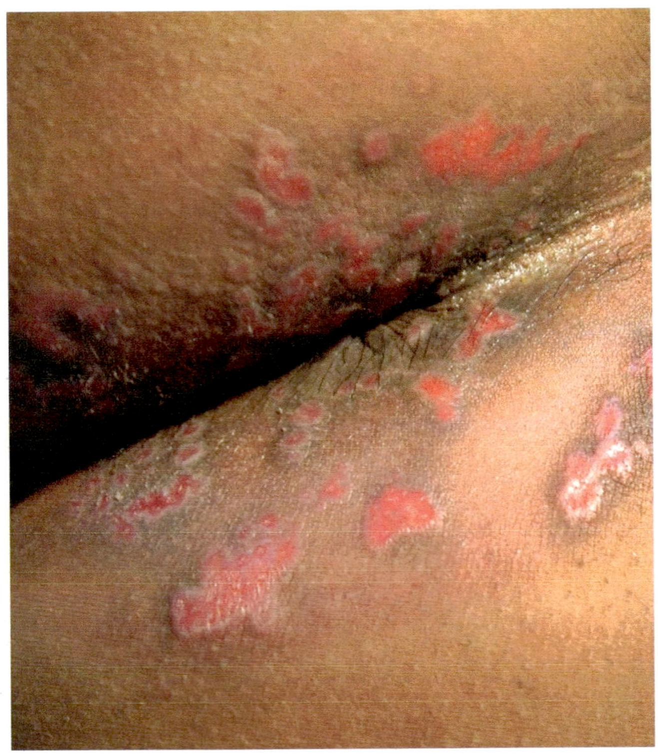

Syphilis: Secondary stage. Condyloma lata. Eroded indurated moist papules in perianal area. Lesions often resolve spontaneously.

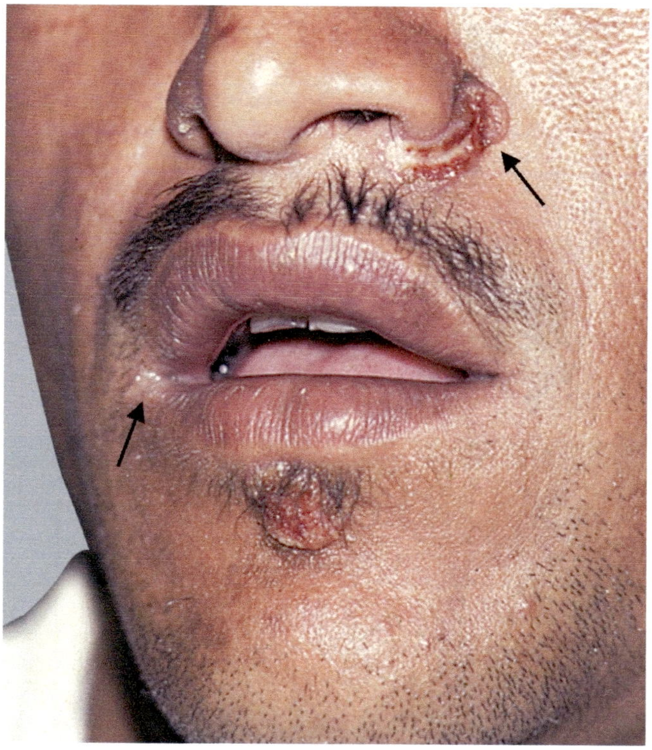

Syphilis: Secondary syphilis. Split papules at angle of mouth and nasolabial folds. Lesions are indurated, moist papules with a fissure.

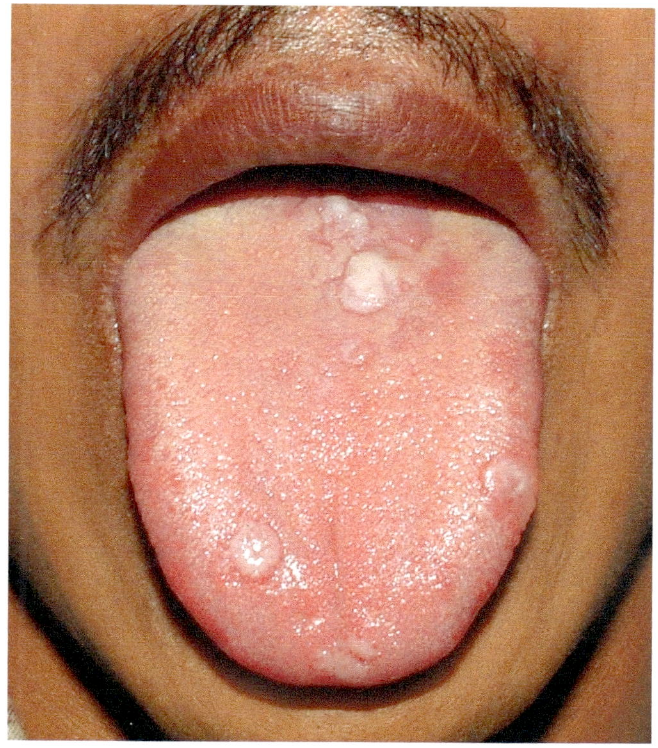

Syphilis: Secondary stage. Grayish discoid plaques on tongue.

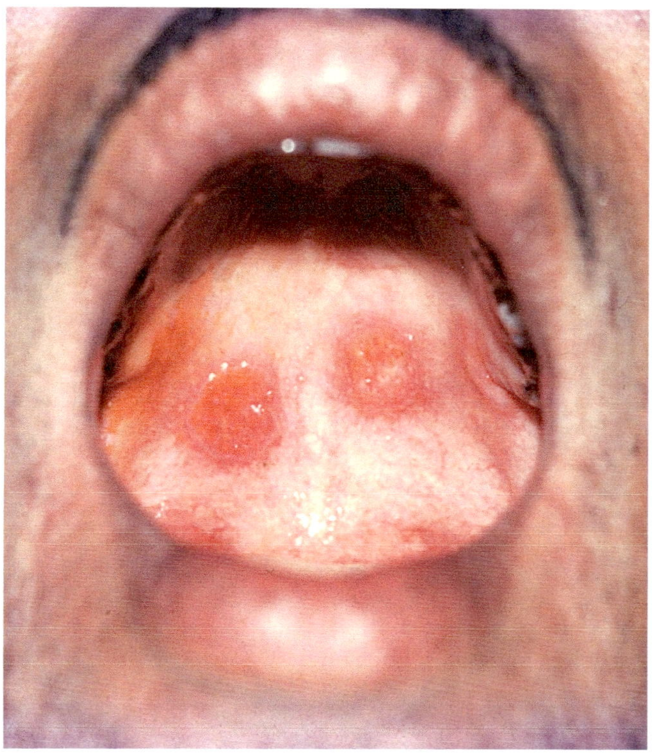

Syphilis: Secondary syphilis. Mucous patches. Well-defined discoid lesions on palate.

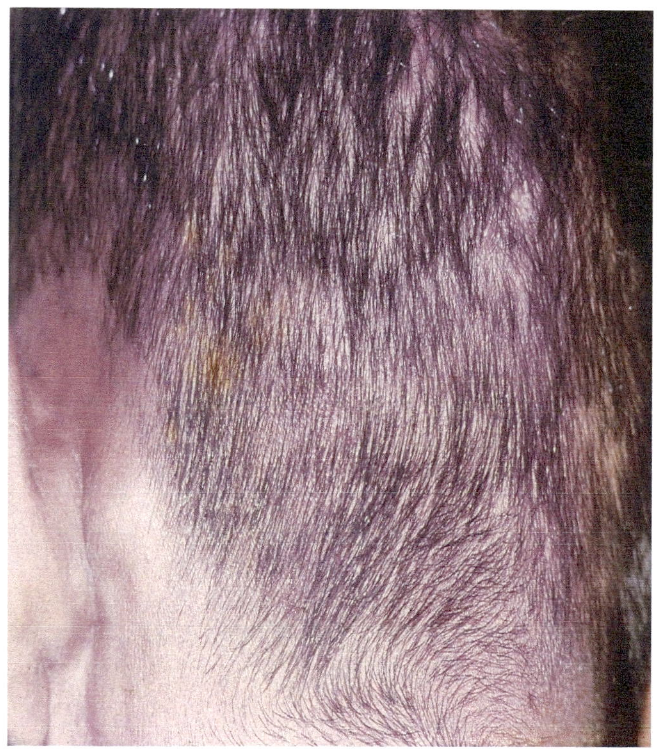

Syphilis: Secondary syphilis. Non-scarring alopecia on scalp with 'moth-eaten appearance'.

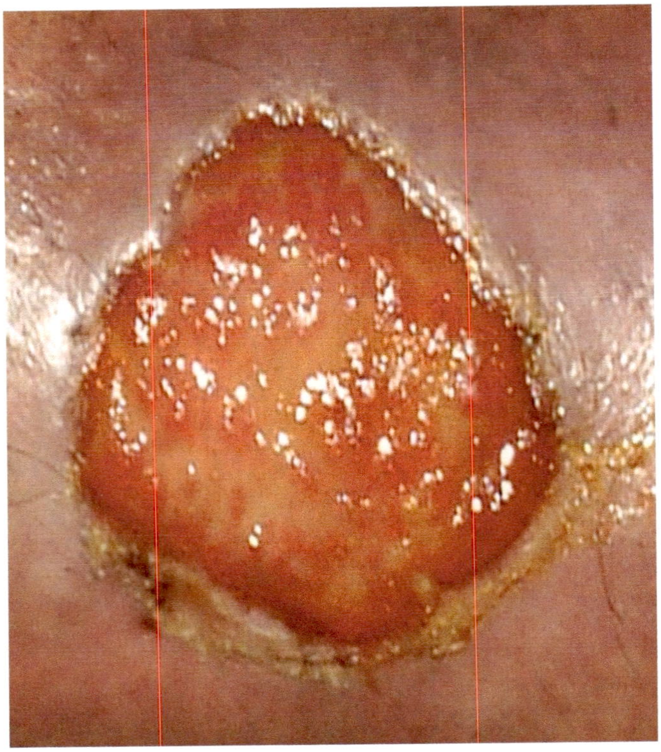

Syphilis: Tertiary syphilis. Gumma showing well-defined ulcer with wash leather floor.

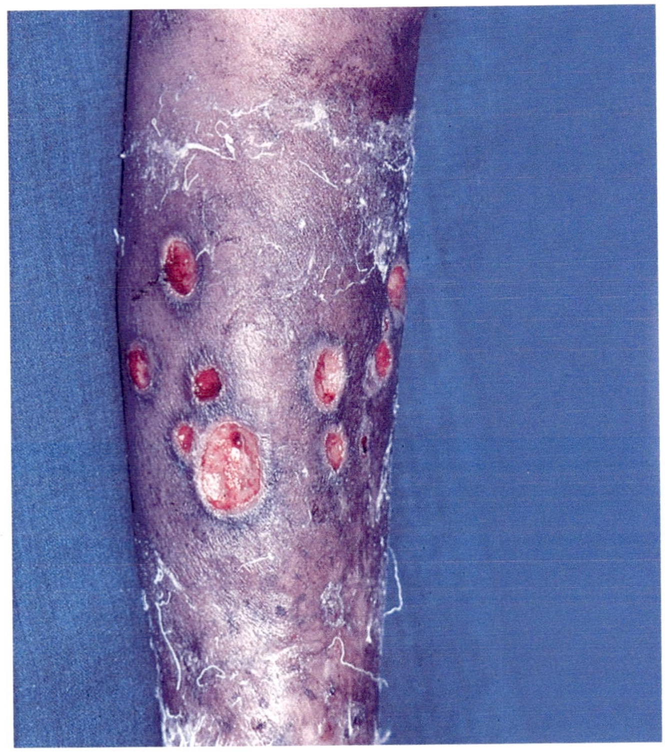

Syphilis: Tertiary syphilis. Multiple gummata on the shins; a common site.

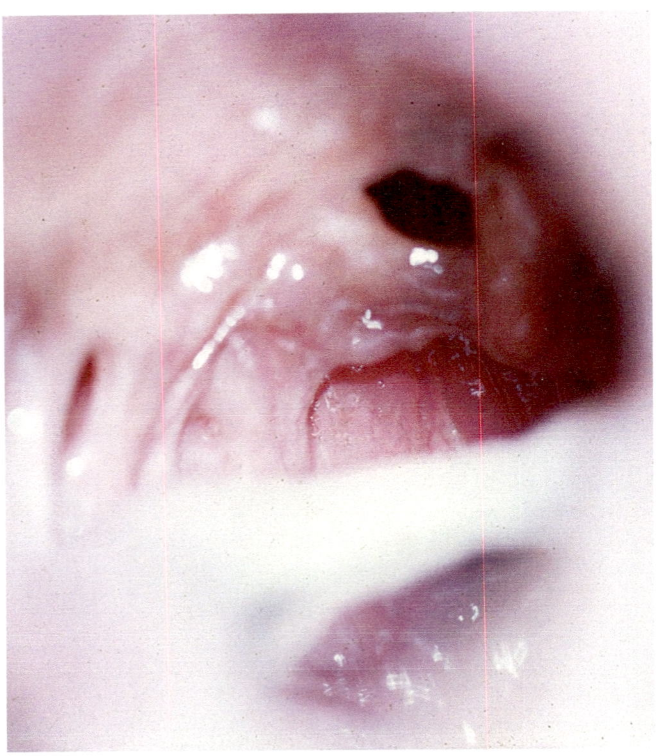

Syphilis: Tertiary syphilis. Palatal perforation seen in late syphilis.

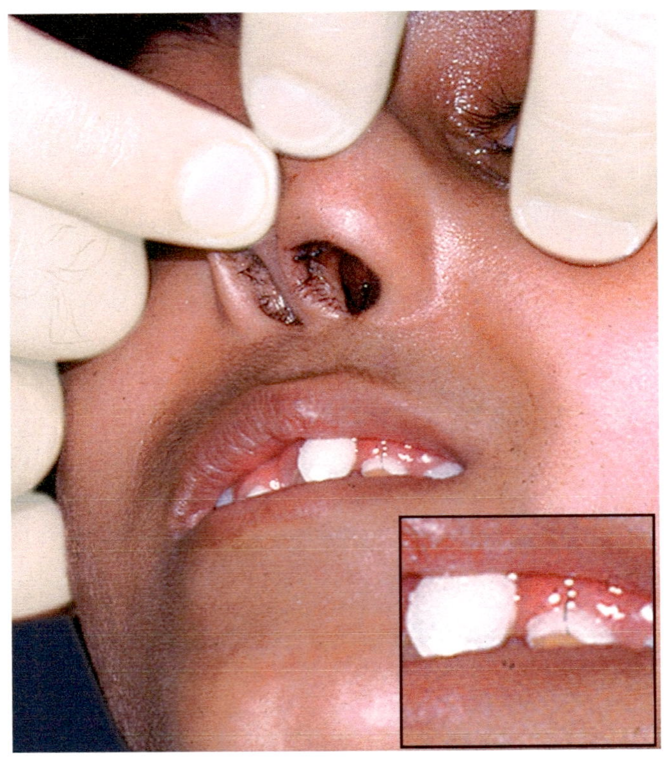

Syphilis: Tertiary syphilis. Perforation of nasal septa seen in late syphilis. Note notched incisors.

Lymphadenopathy

Asymptomatic, generalized, discrete, firm, mobile non-tender. Epitrochlear, posterior cervical and suboccipital of greater diagnostic importance.

Systemic involvement

Constitutional symptoms frequent. Ocular involvement. Less frequent hepatosplenomegaly, meningitis, bone or joint pains rare.

Latent syphilis

No clinical or laboratory evidence of syphilis except a reactive syphilitic serology in blood. Any abnormality,[1] including reactive syphilitic serology in CSF or any other evidence of syphilis precludes diagnosis of latent stage.

Latent syphilis acquired within preceding year is early latent syphilis (infectious, but easier to treat). All others labelled either late latent syphilis (non-infectious, but difficult to treat) or latent syphilis of unknown duration. May resolve spontaneously, last interminably, or evolve into tertiary syphilis.

A serologically positive patient, to be diagnosed as having early latent syphilis if within a year preceding evaluation has:

- Documented seroconversion. Or ≥ 4 fold increase in titer of a non treponemal test.
- Unequivocal symptoms/signs of primary or secondary syphilis.
- Sex partner documented with primary, secondary or early latent syphilis.
- Only possible exposure within the previous 12 months.

Tertiary Syphilis

Rare, even in less developed world. Classified as benign (cutaneous, mucosal or osseous), cardiovascular and neurosyphilis. Noninfectious. Therapy prevents progression but does not reverse damage already caused. Characteristic lesion—localized gumma. Or diffuse gummatous infiltrate—a destructive granulomatous reaction.

Benign tertiary syphilis

Involves subcutaneous tissue and skin. And submucosal tissue and mucous membranes. And bones.

- ***Skin lesions:*** Generally secondary to subcutaneous or bony lesions. Asymmetrical, indurated and painless lesions. Starts as a subcutaneous nodule which involves overlying skin by contiguity; breaks down to form punched out ulcers with vertical edges. Heals in the center with an atrophic tissue-paper scar and spreads peripherally. Dull red wash-leather floor. Common sites: Sternoclavicular joints, presternal region, shins, scalp.
- ***Mucosal lesions:*** Primary lesion submucosal. Spreads deep to affect bone and superficially to involve mucosa. Affects soft or hard palate or nasal septum causing perforation—clean, punched out ulcer. Uvula partially or completely destroyed. Laryngeal gummata cause ulcers which heal with scarring manifesting as hoarseness. Diffuse gummatous infiltration of the tongue—chronic superficial interstitial glossitis—dull red, swollen, bald and furrowed tongue with leukoplakic plaques.
- ***Bones:*** Periosteitis: long bones; laying down of new bone as in tibia—so called 'sabre-tibia'; osteitis: destructive lesions in flat bones—skull, palate, nasal septum or clavicle.

Neurosyphilis

- Rare.
- Clinically manifests in late (and only rarely in early) syphilis. May involve meninges, blood vessels or parenchyma of brain or spinal cord. Overlapping involvement of different components frequent.
- ***Manifestations:*** Tabes dorsalis, dementia paralytica, optic atrophy; pupillary abnormalities (Argyll-Robertson pupil). Presentation modified or masked by chance antibiotic therapy (happenstance).

Cardiovascular syphilis

- Rare.
- Lesions largely confined to aorta (ascending or arch), aortic ring, cusps of aortic valve, ostia of coronary arteries.
- ***Manifestations:*** Aortitis, aneurysm of aorta, aortic incompetence. Symptoms depend on type and site of pathology.

Congenital Syphilis (Prenatal Syphilis)

- Rare.
- Syphilis acquired *in utero* through transplacental transmission from a syphilitic mother.
- Early syphilitic mother more infective. And infection rare before 16 weeks of gestation.
- About a third of pregnancies escape infection, another third abort or are stillborn and a third get congenital syphilis.

[1]Apart from cutaneous examination, all patients with latent syphilis should have careful examination of all accessible mucosal surfaces (i.e. oral cavity, perineum in women, underneath the foreskin in uncircumcised men and perianal area).

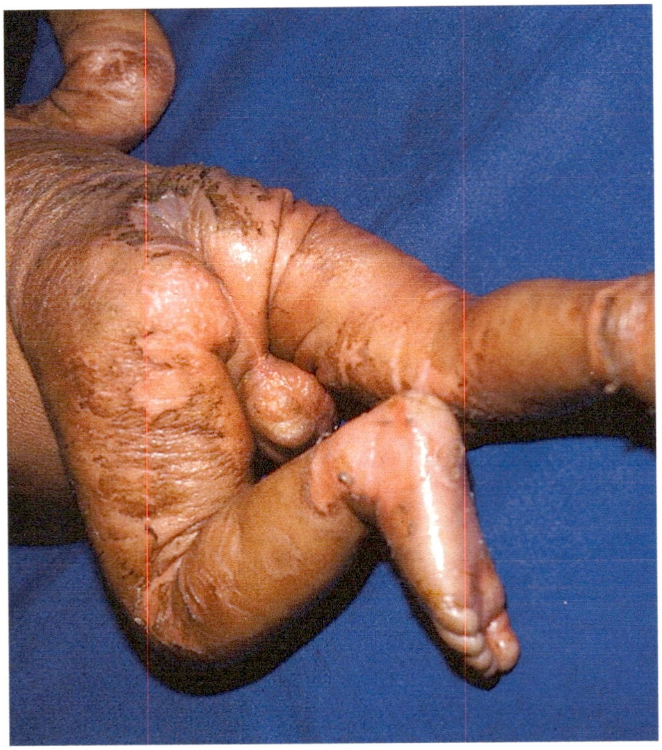

Syphilis: Congenital syphilis. Child born with erythematous scaly plaques. Erosions due to preceding bullae.

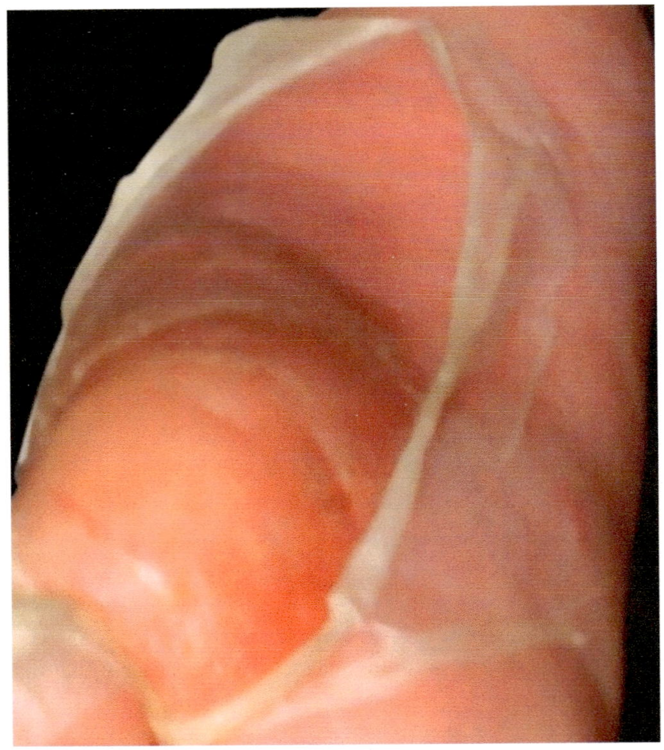

Syphilis: Congenital syphilis. Bullous lesions (usually on normal skin) presenting at birth or soon thereafter (pemphigus syphiliticus).

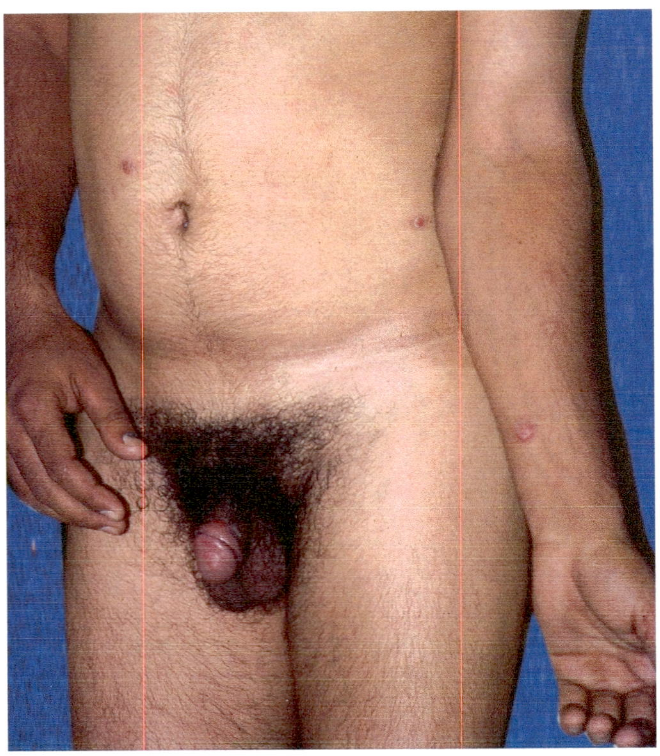

Syphilis: Congenital syphilis. Child born with congenital syphilis develops cubitus varus as he grows older due to periostitis.

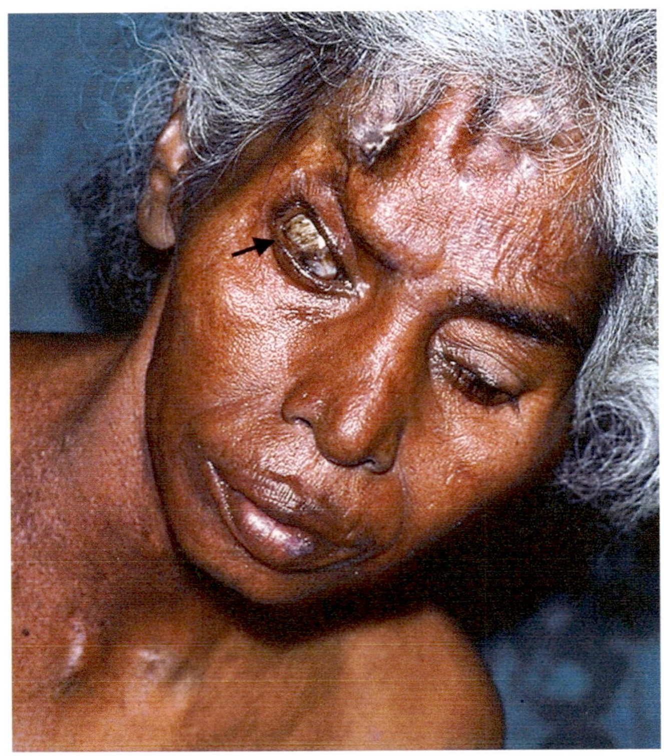

Syphilis: Late congenital syphilis. Interstitial keratitis and healed gummata on forehead.

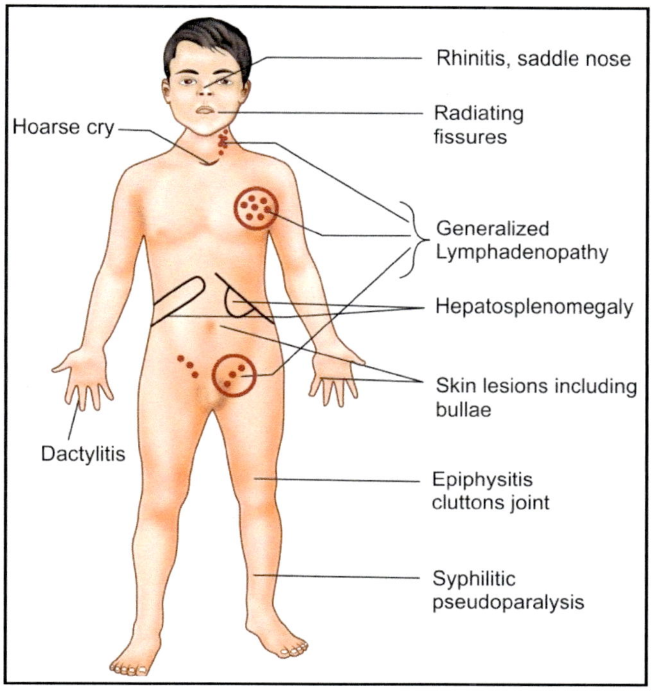

Congenital syphilis

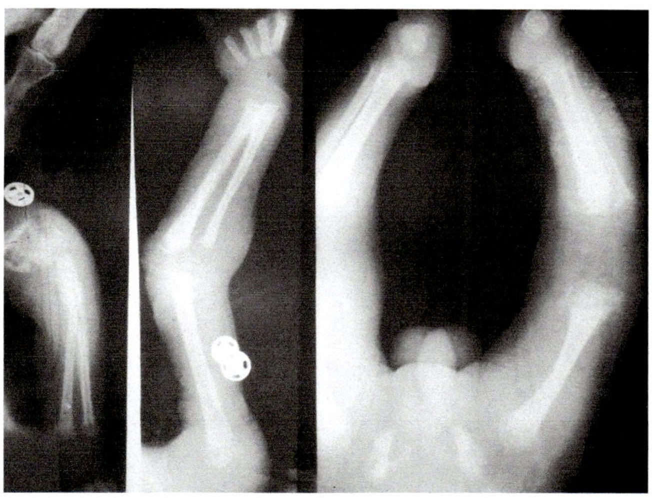

Syphilis: Congenital syphilis. Periostitis of long bones.

Clinical features

Two stages recognized:

- ***Early congenital syphilis:*** Similar to secondary stage of acquired syphilis[2]–cutaneous lesions (all types including vesicobullous lesions *cf*, acquired secondary syphilis) and mucosal; lymphadenopathy, hepatosplenomegaly, osseous (osteochondritis. Or periostitis) changes, leading to parrot pseudoparalysis.

[2]In congenital syphilis, no primary stage.

- ***Late congenital syphilis:*** Similar to late stage of acquired syphilis but cardiovascular involvement rare. Triad of ocular involvement (interstitial keratitis), eighth nerve deafness and abnormalities of permanent dentition (notched incisors and mulberry molars) comprise Hutchinson's triad. Palatal or nasal septal perforation, collapse of nose, periostitis with laying down of new bone clinically appearing as anterior bowing of tibia—sabre tibia. Cutaneous and mucosal lesions rare in this stage.

HIV AND SYPHILIS

- ***Effect of syphilis on HIV:*** Amplified transmission of HIV in presence of chancre, mucosal lesions and condyloma lata.
- ***Effect of HIV on syphilis:***
  - Usually manifestation and course of syphilis in HIV unaltered, especially if no immune depletion. So also serological and therapeutic response.
  - Less frequently atypical features. Include:
    - Chancre: Slow healing of chancre, multiple chancres, phagedenic lesions and large painful ulcers.
    - Secondary syphilis: Leus maligna.
    - Neurosyphilis: Rapid progress to neurosyphilis even in secondary stage. More frequent occurrence.
    - Serology: Aberrant response. So other tests (DGM, biopsy) needed.

DIAGNOSTIC TESTS

Clinical picture too capricious to be entirely dependable. Diagnosis almost always needs to be supported with laboratory evidence. All patients with suspected syphilis (or any STI) should be screened for HIV and hepatitis B infections.

Detection of *T. pallidum*

Are tests for definite diagnosis.

- ***Sample collected:*** Early lesions-primary and secondary stage. Chancre, condylomata lata high yield lesions. Also oral mucosa (with caution, as saprophytic treponemes present) and lymphnodes. Three consecutive daily examinations negative before lesion declared non-syphilitic; scrupulous avoidance of systemic or topical antibiotics/antiseptics before test.

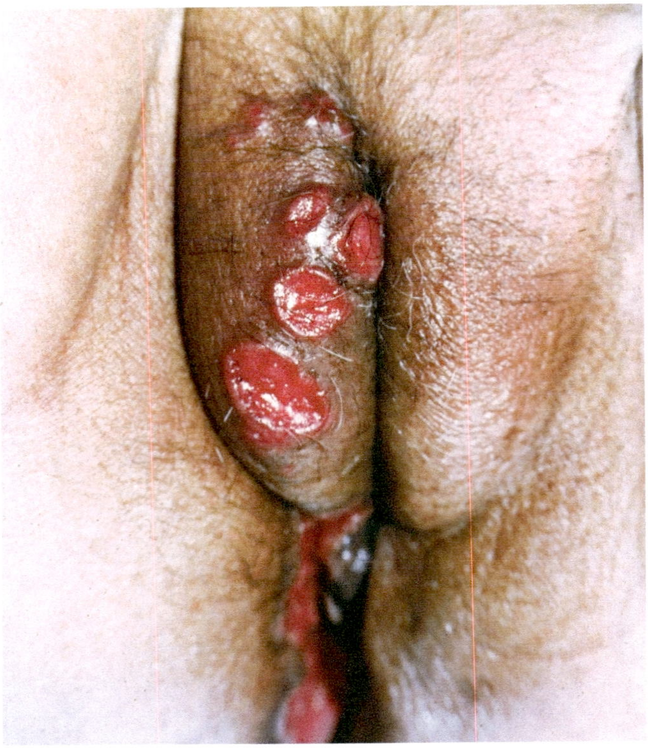

Syphilis in HIV positive patient: Multiple chancres. Many raised indurated ulcers with regular margins and clean base.

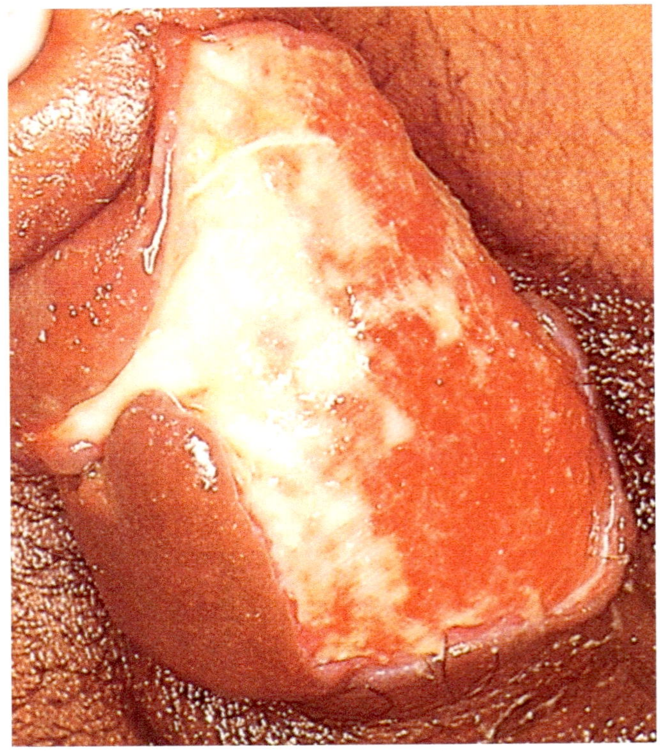

Syphilis in HIV positive patient: Large phagedenic indurated ulcer teaming with *T. pallidum*.

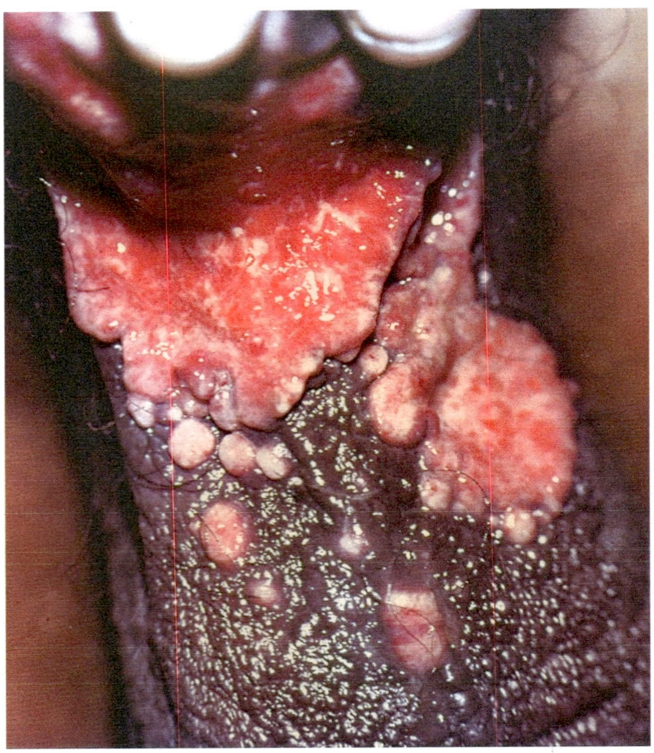

Syphilis: Secondary syphilis. Condyloma lata. Involvement of scrotum with moist velvety plaques with smooth margins.

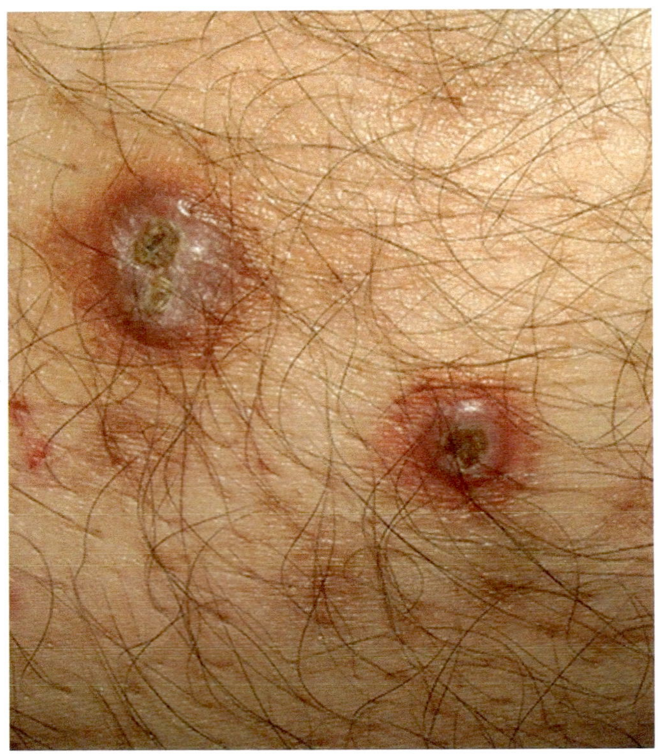

Syphilis: Secondary syphilis. Leus maligna or malignant secondary syphilis characterized by an explosive widespread eruption of papulopustular lesions which rapidly evolve into necrotic sharply marginated ulcer with hemorrhagic crusts.

- ***Dark ground microscopy (DGM):*** Visible as delicate regularly coiled organisms showing 'to and fro', compression, corkscrew and angulation (almost graceful!) movements.
- ***Direct fluorescent antibody (DFA) test:*** Appear as apple green spirocheates.
- ***Polymerase chain reaction (PCR):*** Very sensitive and specific. Also multiplex PCR for *T. pallidum*, *Hemophilus ducreyi* and herpes simplex virus (pathogens for genital ulcer disease). Useful in background of HIV infection and in mixed infections.

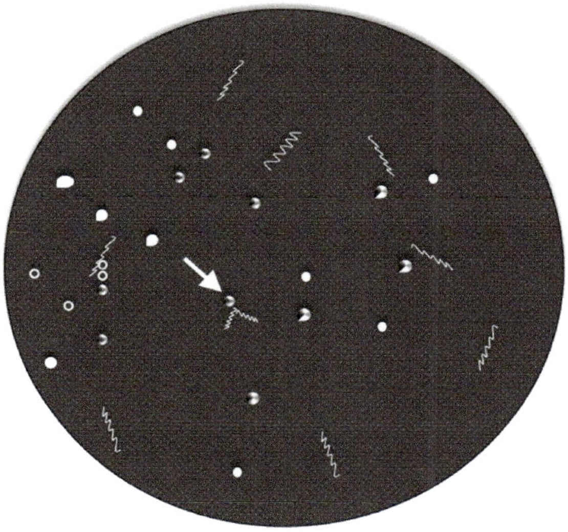

Dark ground microscopy: *T. pallidum* appear as slender, coiled organisms showing corkscrew, to-and-fro and angulation (marked) movement.

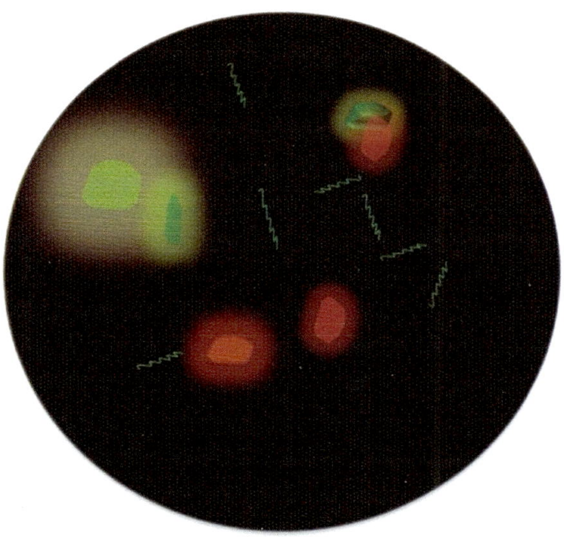

Direct fluorescent antibody test: *T. pallidum* appear as apple green spiral organism.

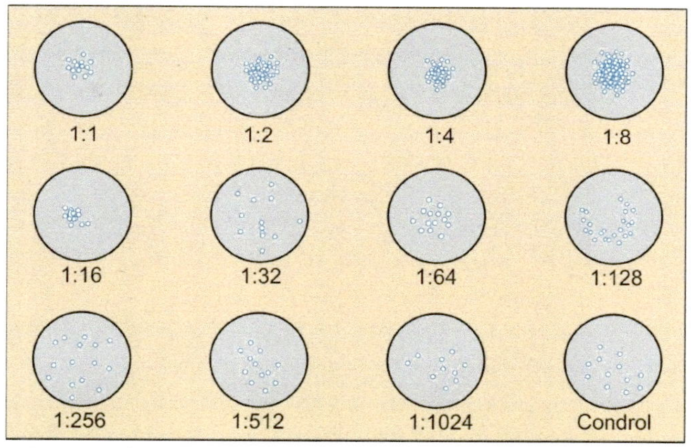

VDRL: Qualitative slide microflocculation test. The highest dilution which gives a positive test is the titer of VDRL. The titer in this case is 1:16.

Serological Tests for Syphilis (STS)

STS demonstrate presence of circulating antibodies. Are tests for presumptive diagnosis and are of 2 types:

- ***Non treponemal tests:***
  - Most frequently used serological tests.
  - Commonly used—Venereal Disease Research Laboratory (VDRL) test and its modification, Rapid Plasma Reagin (RPR). Both employ flocculation techniques.
  - High sensitivity (no false negatives), so good screening tests.
  - Not specific, as employ nonspecific antigen (cardiolipin-lecithin) to detect non-specific antibodies (reagins).
  - May be reactive in absence of syphilis. Biological false positivity (BFP) seen in unrelated conditions (e.g. lepromatous leprosy, malaria, systemic lupus erythematosus, infectious mononucleosis, pregnancy); so not confirmatory.
  - Quantitative tests useful (for assessment of progression/regression of disease) as titers correlate with disease activity. Occasionally positivity persists (usually at low titers for life), despite adequate treatment (serofast state).
- ***Treponemal tests:***
  - Detect specific anti-treponemal antibodies. Commonly used tests—Fluorescent treponemal antibody-absorption (FTA-ABS) test and

Treponema pallidum hemagglutination (TPHA) test. Recently treponemal enzyme immuno assay (EIAs) introduced. Very sensitive. And specific. Also TP IgM test which detects early infection. *Treponema pallidum immobilisation* (TPI) test, most specific but cumbersome and expensive. So not commonly used.
- Highly specific (i.e. fewer false positives), so confirmatory for diagnosis.
- Do not revert unless disease treated early, so not good for evaluating response.

Both tests important—treponemal tests for confirmation of diagnosis and non treponemal for screening and evaluating response to therapy. Recent recommendation for doing initial EIA. If positive, do non treponemal test in titers for evaluating response to treatment at follow-up.

Biopsy

- Indications for documentation. And for diagnosis primary stage (if DGM not available and serological tests negative), and tertiary syphilis (if serological tests are not helpful). And in syphilis in HIV. When DGM not available and STS aberrant.
- ***Histopathology:*** 2 basic changes.
  - Perivascular infiltration with lymphocytes and plasma cells.
  - Intimal proliferation in both arteries and veins (endarteritis obliterans).
- Treponemes demonstrated by silver stain. Or fluorescent staining.

CSF Evaluation

- ***Indications:*** To rule out neurosyphilis patients with syphilis and any of following should have CSF examined:
  - Neurologic or ophthalmic signs or symptoms.
  - Evidence of active tertiary syphilis (e.g. aortitis, gumma).
  - Treatment failure.[3]
  - HIV infection (especially if CD4 count < 350) with late latent syphilis or syphilis of unknown duration.
- Test done CSF serology (VDRL, FTA ABS) microscopy (for cells), and biochemistry (glucose, protein).

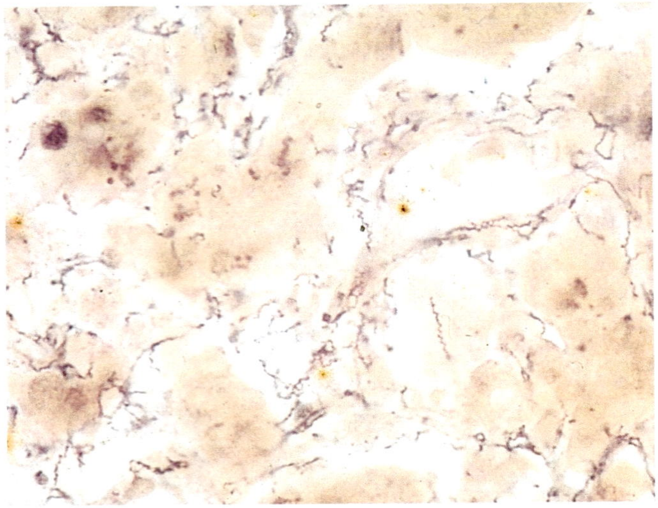

Syphilis: Histopathology of liver showing multiple treponemes stained with silver stain.

DIAGNOSTIC ALGORITHMS

Primary Syphilis

- ***Demonstration of T. pallidum:*** Definitive diagnosis. Demonstration of *T. pallidum* from chancre or lymph node by DGM or DFA test.
- ***Serology:*** STS undependable in primary stage. Negative in early lesions (< 4 weeks). Treponemal tests first to become positive. (EIA→, FTA (Abs)→ TPHA→VDRL).

Secondary Syphilis

- ***Demonstration of T. pallidum:*** By DGM or DFA test. From cutaneous/mucosal lesions or lymph nodes. Oral mucosal lesions often falsely positive, due to commensal treponemes.
- ***Serology:*** STS invariably positive. If negative but clinical suspicion strong, exclude prozone phenomenon — negative serological test due to high antibody titer; repeat test after dilution.

Latent Syphilis

- ***Demonstration of T. pallidum:*** Not possible, as no lesions.

[3]Treatment failure: VDRL titer not decreasing. Or remaining at same titer. Or increasing titer after adequate treatment.

- ***Serology:*** Only STS reactive in blood alone. Non treponemal serologic titers usually higher during early latent syphilis than late latent syphilis—but not sacrosanct. No other laboratory evidence (including CSF serology) of syphilis positive.

Tertiary Syphilis

- ***Demonstration of T. pallidum:*** Not helpful, because lesions paucibacillary.
- ***Serology:*** Treponemal tests (FTA-ABS and low titer of TPHA) are positive. Non treponemal tests (VDRL) also positive but not always. Clinical and radiological evaluation and CSF examination done in appropriate situations.

In HIV-infected

- ***Demonstration of T. pallidum:*** In early lesions: (DGM/DFA).
- ***Serology:*** For majority of HIV-infected patients, STS accurate and reliable both for diagnosis of syphilis, as also for assessing response to treatment. In some STS aberrant—i.e. unusually high, unusually low, fluctuating titers, prozone phenomena. For such patients, if serological tests discordant, other tests (biopsy and direct microscopy) required.

Neurosyphilis

- No single test highly specific and sensitive to diagnose neurosyphilis.
- Diagnosis generally based on combination of reactive STS, CSF cell count and reactive VDRL/FTA-(Abs) in cerebrospinal fluid with or without clinical manifestations.
- VDRL-CSF highly specific, i.e. when reactive (in absence of contamination of CSF with blood) diagnostic of neurosyphilis. But not sensitive (sometimes nonreactive in presence of neurosyphilis). Also poor correlation with therapy.
- CSF FTA-Abs less specific (i.e. more false-positive results) for neurosyphilis than VDRL-CSF, but highly sensitive (i.e. very few false negatives, so a negative CSF FTA-ABS test excludes neurosyphilis).
- CSF leukocyte count elevated (> 5 WBC/mm^3). And a sensitive measure of therapeutic efficacy.
- Other tests both insensitive and nonspecific.

Congenital Syphilis

In mother

Effective prevention of congenital syphilis depends on detection and treatment of infection in pregnant women.

- ***Demonstration of T. pallidum:*** If lesions present.
- ***Serology:*** Antepartum screening for syphilis by non treponemal antibody routinely done; sometimes treponemal antibody testing also done, but non treponemal tests with titers preferred. Serologic screening of pregnant women done:
  - At 1st prenatal visit.
  - Repeated in populations with high prevalence of syphilis, at 28-32 weeks and at delivery.
  - Any woman with delivery of stillborn infant > 20 weeks' gestation.
- Seropositive pregnant women considered infected unless clear documentation of adequate treatment with declining sequential antibody titers. Serofast low antibody titers do not warrant treatment but persistent higher titer antibody tests require treatment.

In Neonate

- Routine serological screening of newborn sera/ umbilical cord blood not recommended. Testing mother's serum preferred.
- Interpretation of STS in neonates difficult due to transplacental transfer of maternal IgG antibodies to fetus.
- Infants born to seropositive mothers should be evaluated:
  - Clinically, for congenital syphilis (e.g. nonimmune hydrops, jaundice, hepatosplenomegaly, rhinitis, skin rash and pseudoparalysis of an extremity).
  - By DFM examination or DFA staining of suspicious lesions or body fluids. Serologically, by using quantitative non treponemal tests (RPR or VDRL) performed on infant's serum (not cord blood).[4] Treponemal tests on newborn not necessary.
  - Pathologically, examining placenta or umbilical cord.
- Treatment decision based on:
  - Presence of syphilis in mother.
  - Inadequacy of maternal treatment.
  - Presence of clinical/laboratory/radiographic evidence of syphilis in infant.

[4]Cord blood may be contaminated with maternal blood, giving false positive.

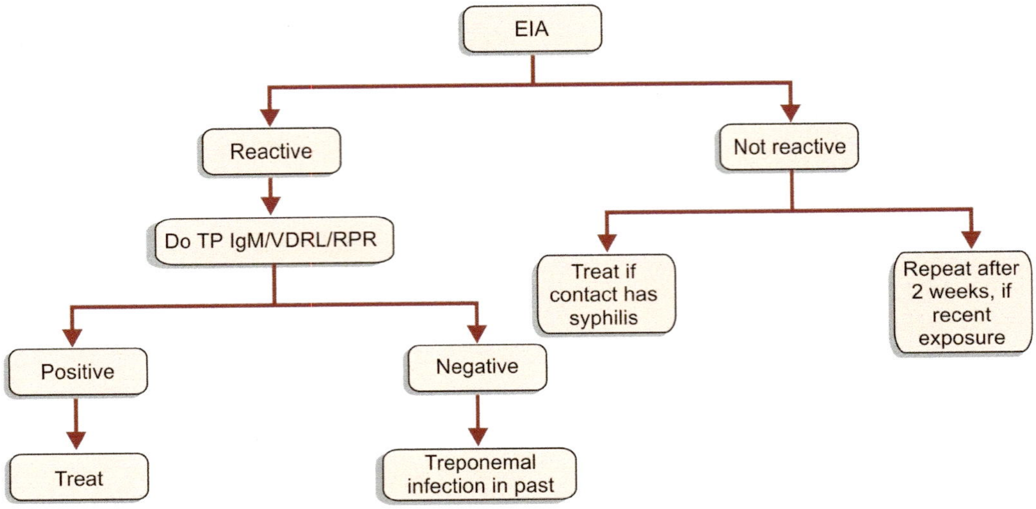

Recent recommendation for serological testing of syphilis

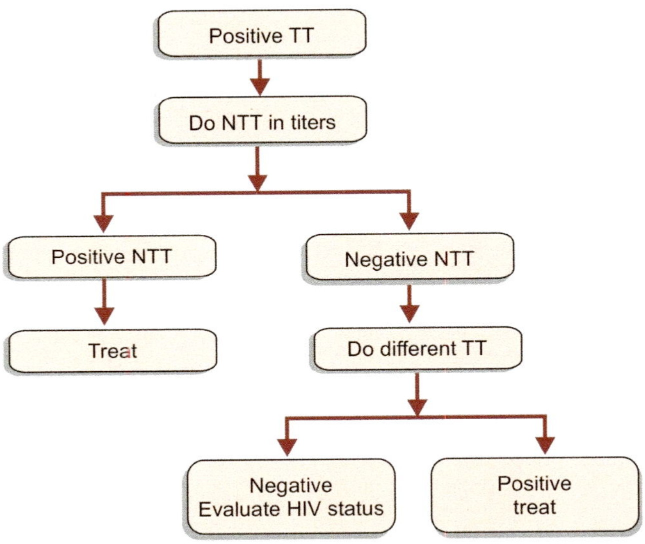

NTT: non-treponemal test, TT: treponemal test

For patients who have a positive treponemal test in resource limited settings

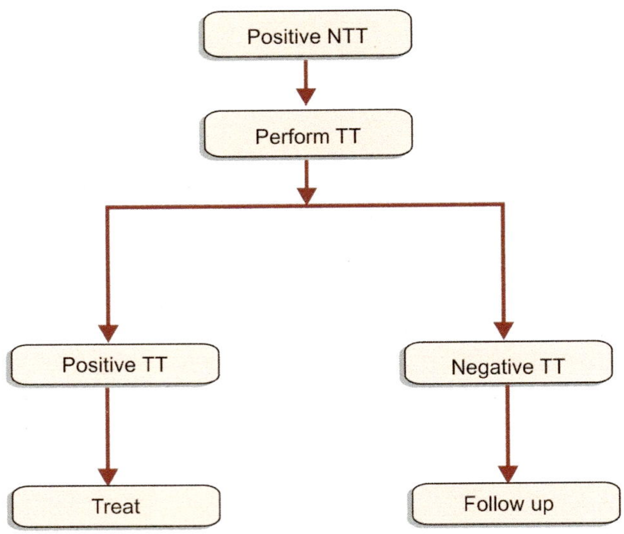

NTT: non-treponemal test, TT: treponemal test

For patients who have a positive non treponemal test in resource limited settings

- Comparison of maternal (at delivery) and infant non treponemal serologic titers.

TREATMENT

Early Syphilis

Drug regimens (same in CDC 2010, WHO 2003, NACO 2007 guidelines).

- ***1st line of treatment:*** Benzathine penicillin, 2.4 million units, intramuscularly (after testing for sensitivity) in a single session. Because of volume involved, dose divided into 2 injections given at 2 separate sites (usually both buttocks).
- ***In penicillin-sensitive individuals:*** Doxycyline, 100 mg twice daily (preferably on an empty stomach) × 14 days.
- ***In penicillin-sensitive pregnant women:*** Desensitize.

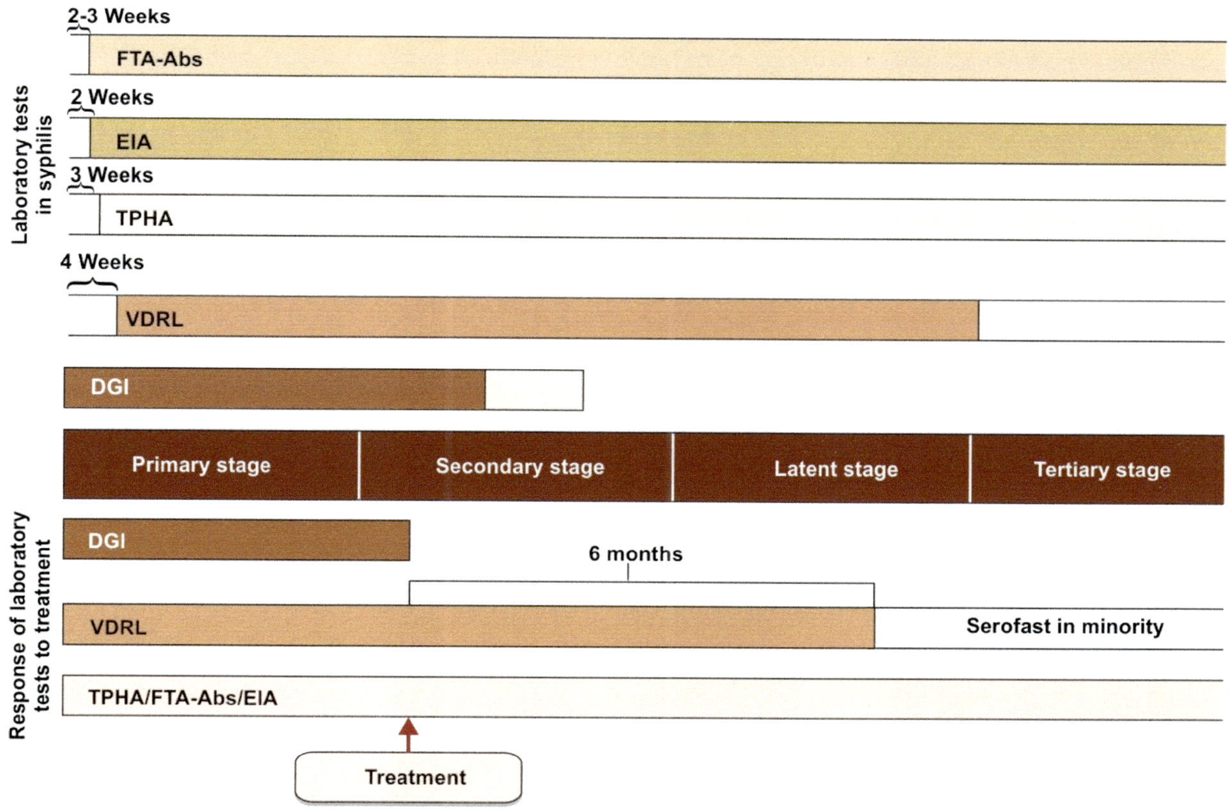

Sensitivity of diagnostic tests for syphilis and response to treatment

- ***In penicillin-sensitive pregnant women who cannot be desensitized:*** Erythromycin stearate (never estolate, as hepatotoxic), 2 g daily (in 4 divided doses) x 14 days.

Late Syphilis

Latent syphilis

- ***Positive treponemal STS with positive non treponemal STS:***
  - *1st line of treatment:* benzathine penicillin, 2.4 million units, intramuscularly divided in both buttocks, given weekly for 3 weeks.
  - *In penicillin-sensitive individuals:* doxycyline, 100 mg twice daily (preferably on an empty stomach) × 14 days.
- ***Positive treponemal STS with negative non treponemal STS:***
  - Rule out whether specific treatment (for syphilis) taken. If taken without any history of re-exposure, further treatment not required.[5]
  - If treatment not taken, do another non treponemal STS based on different antigen:
    - If positive → treat patient.
    - If negative → no treatment required.

Late syphilis without CNS involvement

- ***1st line of treatment:*** Benzathine penicillin, 2.4 mega units, intramuscularly divided in both buttocks given weekly for 3 weeks.
- ***In penicillin-sensitive individuals:*** Doxycyline, 100 mg twice a day (preferably on an empty stomach) x 28 days.

[5] Treponemal tests remain positive despite adequate treatment.

- ***In penicillin-sensitive pregnant women:*** Desensitize.
- ***In penicillin-sensitive pregnant women, who cannot be desensitized:*** Erythromycin stearate (never estolate, as hepatotoxic), 2 g (in 4 divided doses) × 28 days.

Neurosyphilis

- ***1st line of treatment:*** Aqueous crystalline penicillin G 18-24 million units daily, intravenous in divided doses every 4 hours. Or continuous infusion. For 10-14 days. Or procaine penicillin G 2.4 million units intramuscular once daily with probenicid 500 mg 4 times daily, both for 10-14 days.
- ***In penicillin-sensitive individuals:*** Ceftriaxone 2 g daily for 10-14 days after sensitivity testing.[6] Consider desensitization, if sensitive to ceftriaxone.

Syphilis in Pregnancy

- ***1st line of therapy:*** Penicillin effective for preventing maternal-fetal transmission. And also for treating fetal infection. Optimal penicillin regimens not defined but regimen appropriate for stage of syphilis recommended.
- ***In penicillin-sensitive women:*** Desensitize (as no proven alternative to penicillin available for maternal syphilis).
- ***In penicillin sensitive pregnant women who cannot be desensitized:*** Erythromycin stearate (never estolate) 2 g daily (in 4 doses) × 14 days (early syphilis)–28 days (late syphilis). However erythromycin not ideal, as does not reliably cure infected fetus.
- ***Other management considerations:***
  - *In early syphilis:* 2nd dose of benzathine penicillin 2.4 million units 1 week after 1st dose sometimes recommended.
  - *In 2nd half of pregnancy:* management facilitated by sonographic evaluation of fetus (for hepatomegaly, ascites, hydrops) and placenta (for thickening). Sonographic signs predictive of higher risk for fetal treatment failure, but optimal regimen not defined. Women treated for syphilis in 2nd half of pregnancy at risk for premature labor and/or fetal distress, due to Jarisch-Herxheimer reaction, so careful monitoring for uterine contractions or decreased fetal movements. Still birth a rare complication of treatment.
  - *Missed doses:* not acceptable in pregnant patients. If any dose missed, repeat full course.

Syphilis in HIV Positive Patients

- ***Primary and secondary syphilis:*** Benzathine penicillin G, 2.4 million units IM as a single dose. Some recommend additional doses of benzathine penicillin G administered at 1 week intervals for 3 weeks (as recommended for late syphilis).
- ***Latent syphilis:*** Patients with late latent syphilis or syphilis of unknown duration and a normal CSF examination treated with benzathine penicillin G, at weekly doses of 2.4 million units for 3 weeks.
- ***Tertiary syphilis:*** Treatment as HIV negative.
- ***Other treatment considerations:*** CSF evaluation in all stages recommended by some, before initiation of therapy. If CSF abnormalities present, treat as neurosyphilis.

Jarisch-Herxheimer Reaction (JHR)

- Associated with specific treponemicidal therapy. Obscure mechanism.
- ***Early syphilis:*** More frequent. Flare-up of local lesions within a day of instituting penicillin (as also other treponemicidal) therapy and variable constitutional symptoms.
- ***Late syphilis:*** Flare-up of local lesions; theoretically more dangerous.
- ***Treatment:*** Symptomatic. Debatable use of steroids in late syphilis.

SURVEILLANCE/FOLLOW-UP

Follow-up in Early Syphilis

- ***Response:*** Clinical healing within a few days of treatment, serological negativity within a few months.
- ***Follow-up:*** Clinical and serological (quantitative with non treponemal tests) evaluation at:
  - 3 months.
  - 6 months (expect a 4 fold decline in serological titers).
  - 24 months (expect seronegativity in most).
  - Further follow-up, if seropositivity persists.

[6]Ceftriaxone sensitivity: Always test for ceftriaxone sensitivity in patients with penicillin sensitivity because of cross reactivity.

Follow-up in Late Syphilis

- Response slow and sequelae common.
- Clinical, serological, CSF and radiological evaluation of heart in follow-up:
  - Follow-up as for early syphilis.
  - Repeat serology yearly till negativity or near negativity; ideally for entire life.

Retreatment

Retreatment required in following circumstances:

- Signs or symptoms of syphilis develop.
- Non treponemal test titers increase 4 fold.
- An initial high titer (> 1:32) fails to decline 4 fold (2 dilutions) within 24 months of therapy.
- If patient seropositive at 24 months. Evaluate CSF.
  - *If normal:* re-treat for latent syphilis.
  - *If abnormal:* treat for neurosyphilis.

Management of Sex Partners

- Sexual transmission possible only in presence of mucocutaneous syphilitic lesions (so uncommon after 1st year of infection).
- All at-risk sexual partners of patients with syphilis (of any stage) need evaluation clinically and serologically and treatment if required:
  - For sex partners of patients with primary, secondary or early latent syphilis:[7]
    - For exposure within 90 days preceding diagnosis, even if seronegative, partners treated presumptively.
    - For exposure > 90 days preceding diagnosis:
      - If serological test negative: no treatment.
      - If test not available treat.
  - Long-term sex partners of patients with latent/late syphilis evaluated clinically and serologically for syphilis and treated accordingly.

[7]Patients with syphilis of unknown duration but with high non treponemal serologic test titers (i.e. > 1:32) assumed to have early syphilis.

CHAPTER 3

Chancroid

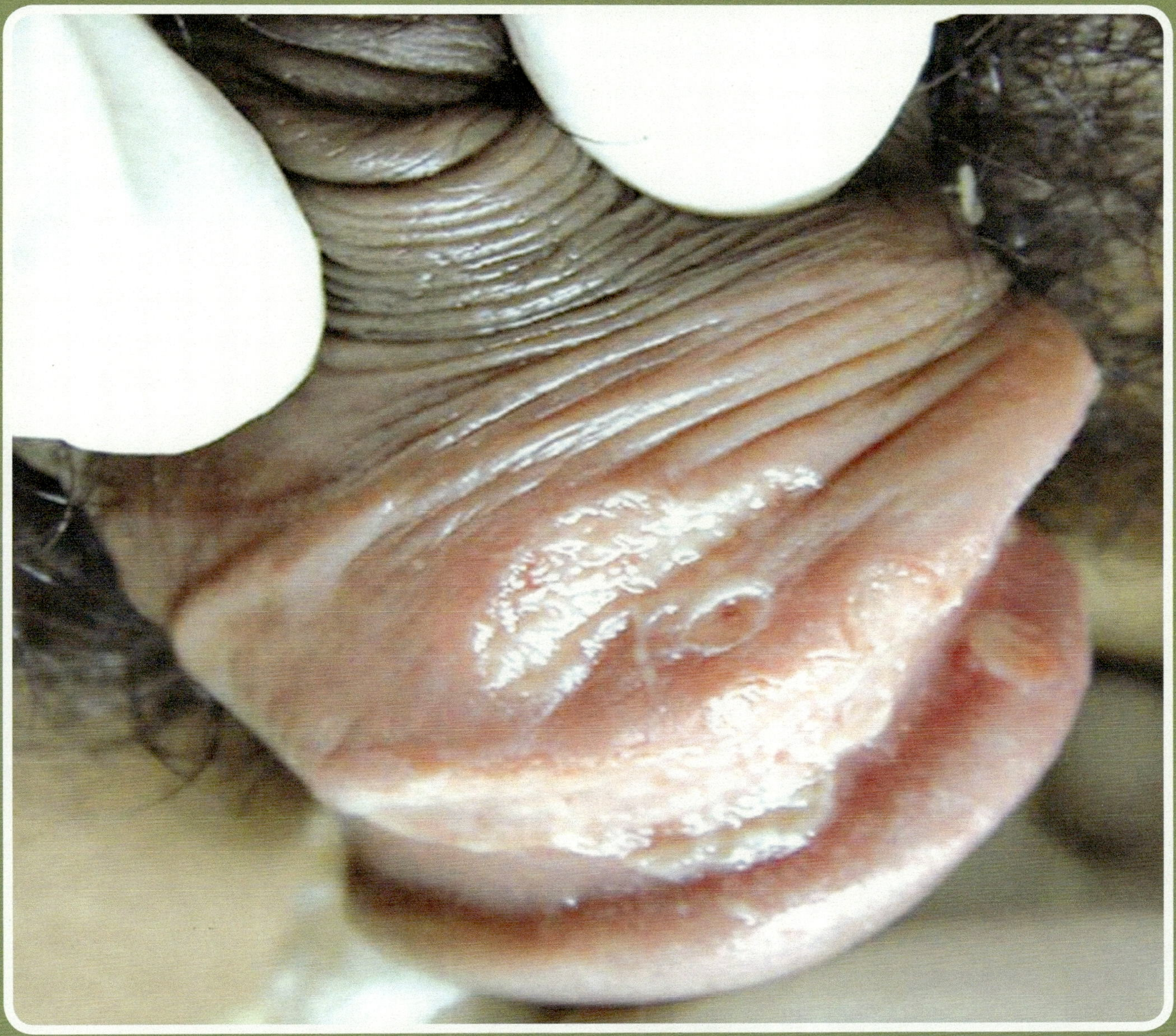

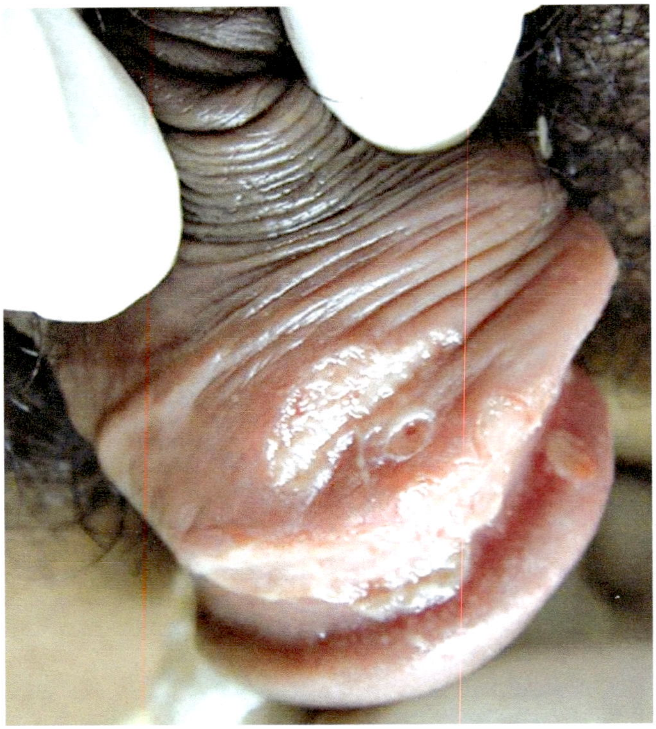

Chancroid: Dwarf variant. Multiple, small, shallow, painful ulcers with dirty floor on inner aspect of prepuce.

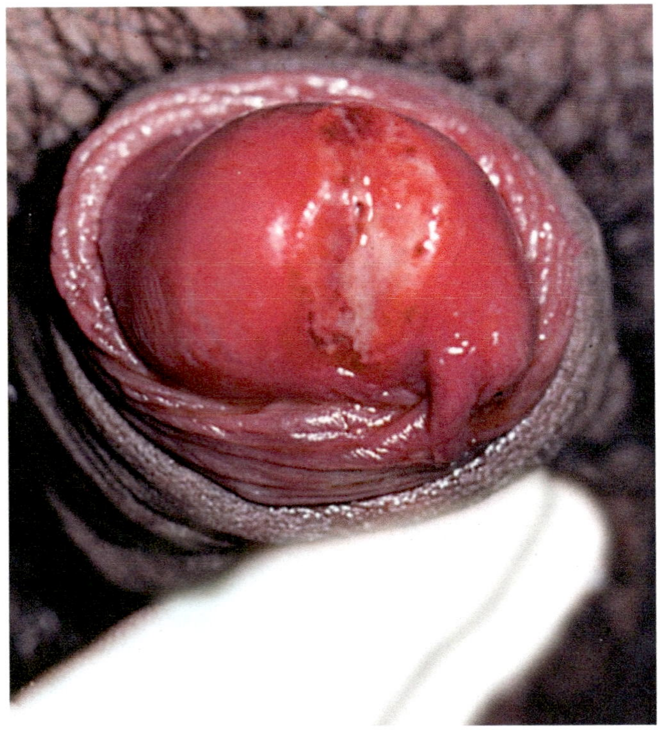

Chancroid: Giant variant. Urethral meatus involved with a large ulcer with irregular margins, necrotic slough on floor, and a non-indurated base.

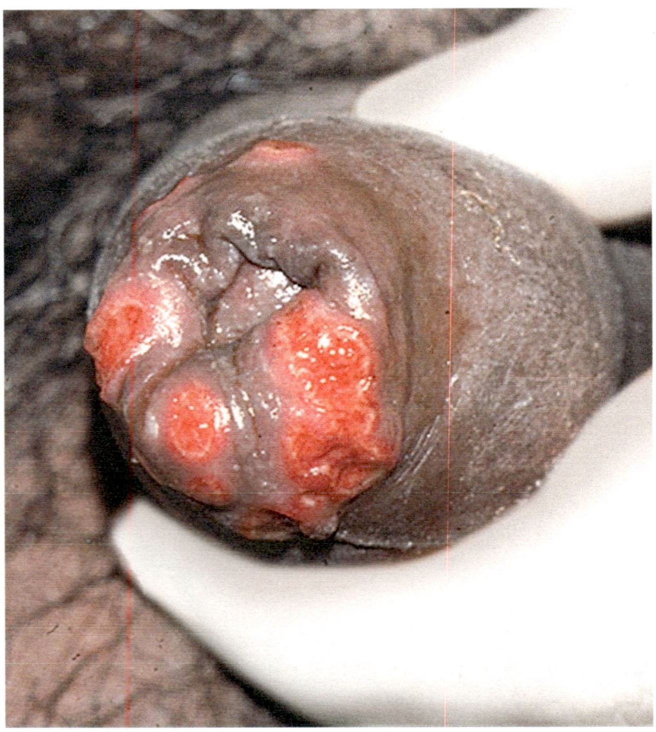

Chancroid: Involvement of prepuce with multiple, well-defined, small ulcers forming a rosette. Ulcers have irregular margins and necrotic material on floor. Patient is developing a phimosis.

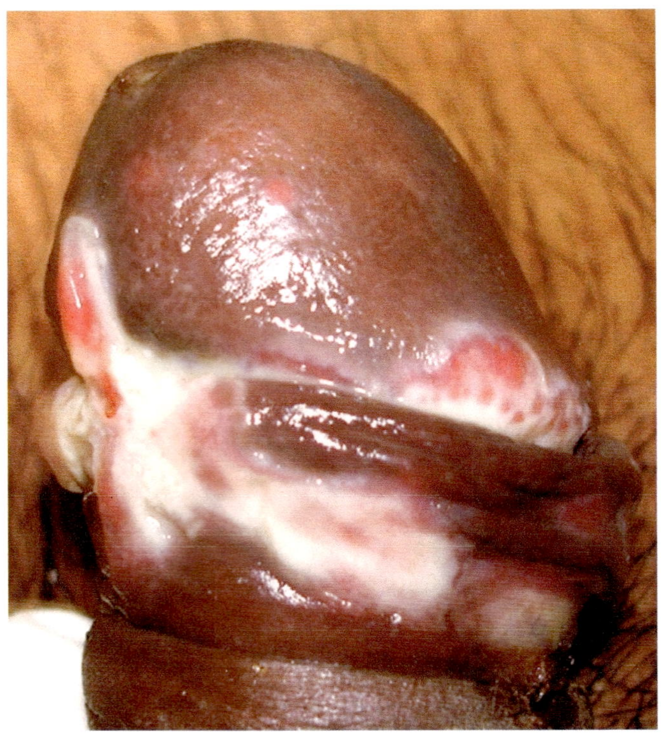

Chancroid: Extensive involvement of glans and inner surface of prepuce with multiple ulcers covered with necrotic slough.

Also known as soft sore; soft chancre; ulcus molle.

ETIOLOGY

Etiological Agent

- *Haemophilus ducreyi.*
- Gram-negative short rods with rounded ends (coccobacillus). Found in clumps or short chains of 5-20 bacilli—"school of fish" appearance. Intracellular and extracellular distribution.
- *Fastidious organism:* Cultured with difficulty on blood-containing media.

Transmission

- Sexually transmitted.

EPIDEMIOLOGY

Geographic Distribution

- Worldwide distribution but prevalence declining. Rare in developed countries. Now, also uncommon in India.
- Reported from South East Asia, Africa, South America.
- Regarded as disease of socially under-privileged with poor personal hygiene.

Demographic Distribution

- Prevalence 10 times higher in men, probably because infection mostly 'asymptomatic' in women.
- Commercial sex workers act as carriers.

CLINICAL FEATURES

Incubation Period

1-8 days.

Morphology

- ***Initial lesion:*** Erythematous macule or papule. Rapidly evolves (often through a vesicle) to a pustule which ruptures to form ulcer.
- ***Ulcer:*** Shallow, undermined edge painful, tender, sharply circumscribed. Dirty (slough-covered) easily-bleeding floor. Non-indurated with ragged edges.
- Multiple lesions due to auto-inoculation; so in different stages of evolution. Form 'rosette' on prepuce resulting in phimosis. Or serpiginous ulcer on coronal sulcus.

Sites

- ***Sites of most intimate contact and trauma during sex act affected:*** Prepuce, glans penis, coronal sulcus, frenulum in males; fourchette, labia, cervix in females.
- Rarely perianal region, thighs, scrotum.

Lymphadenopathy

- Occurs (10-40%) within a week of ulcer.
- Often unilateral, sometimes bilateral.
- Painful and tender; suppurate to form a unilocular abscess (bubo); adheres to the overlying skin which becomes inflamed.
- Bubo may rupture through skin to form a sinus with its mouth resembling chancroidal ulcer.

Variants

Several variants described

- ***Dwarf chancroid:*** Small herpetiform ulcers.
- ***Giant chancroid:*** Usually single large ulcer.
- ***Follicular chancroid:*** On hair bearing areas.
- ***Phagedenic chancroid:*** Leads to destruction of genitalia.

COMPLICATIONS

- Phimosis. Or paraphimosis.
- Suppurative balanoposthitis.
- Secondary bacterial infection with *Borrelia vincentii* and *Fusobacterium fusiformis* causing destructive phagedenic lesions.

HIV AND CHANCROID

- ***Effect of chancroid on HIV:*** Chancroidal ulcers facilitate transmission of HIV ten fold.
- ***Effect of HIV on chancroid:***
  - Ulcers of chancroid (may be) atypical (more in number, larger, extragenital lesions).
  - Reduced response of chancroid to therapy, so single dose regimens avoided.

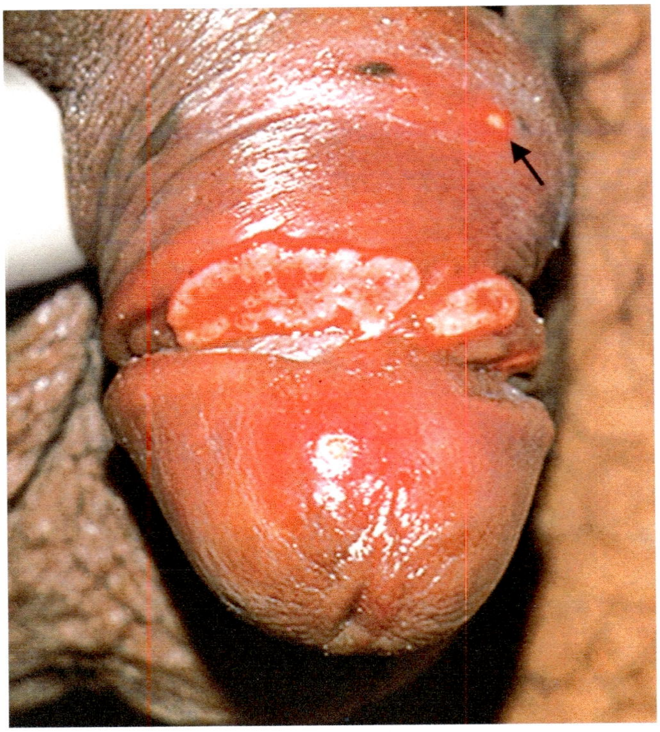

Chancroid: Multiple ulcers with ragged margins and necrotic slough. Small lesion on prepuce—lesions in different stages of evolution on coronal sulcus and glans penis.

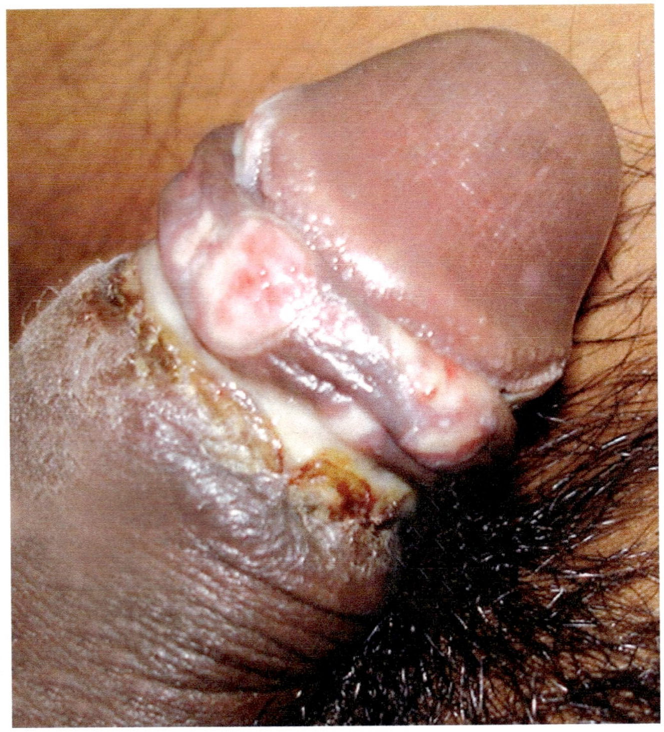

Chancroid: Multiple painful ulcers on coronal sulcus with necrotic slough.

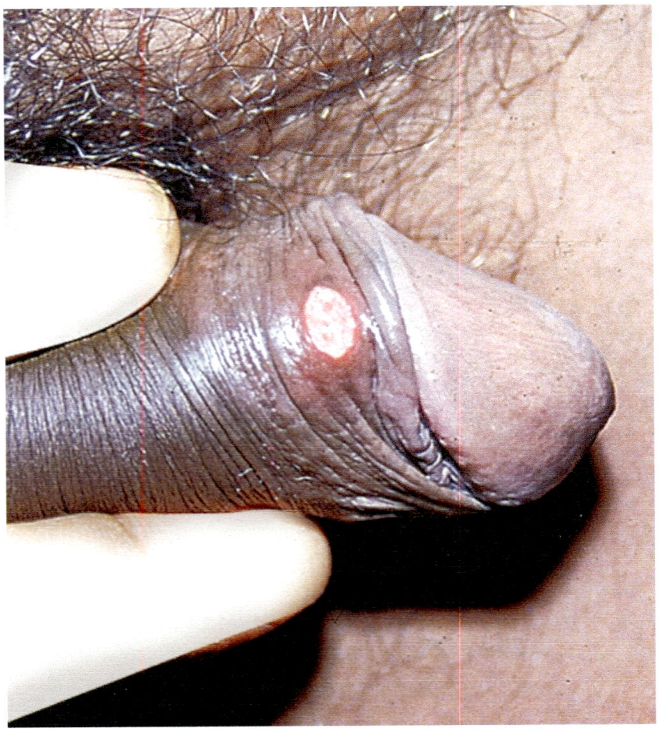

Chancroid: Single ulcer can occur occasionally. Non-indurated base and necrotic material on floor suggests that it is chancroid and not chancre.

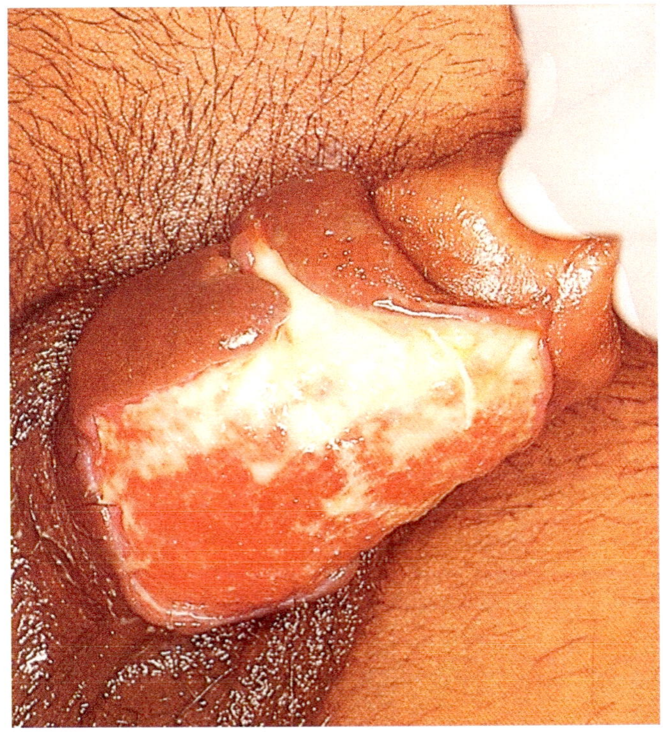

Chancroid: Phagedenic variant: most of the shaft of penis involved.

DIAGNOSIS

Based on Clinical Features

- Combination of painful genital ulcer.
- And tender suppurative inguinal adenopathy suggests diagnosis of chancroid.

Probable diagnosis of chancroid made if **all** following criteria met:
- Presence of one or more painful genital ulcers.
- Clinical presentation, appearance of genital ulcers and, if present, regional lymphadenopathy typical for chancroid.
- No evidence of *T. pallidum* infection by darkfield examination of ulcer exudate. Or by serologic test for syphilis performed at least 7 days after onset of ulcers.
- Negative HSV test performed on ulcer exudate.

Laboratory Investigations

Isolation and Identification of Organism

- ***Direct:***
  - *Gram stain of smear from ulcer or bubo:* gram negative coccobacilli in typical school of fish or rail road arrangement. Not sensitive.
  - *Antigen detection by immunofluorescence:* very sensitive, but less specific.
- ***Culture:*** Difficult. Fastidious organism requiring expensive supplements. Commonly used media include Mueller-Hinton, chocolate agar with vancomycin, Gonococcal agar with 2% bovine hemoglobin and 5% fetal calf serum. Colonies yellow/waxy, opaque, of different sizes. Can be slided on plate. Confirmed by Gram staining and biochemical tests.
- ***Polymerase chain reaction (PCR):*** Though not FDA approved, several CLIA approved PCR tests available. Multiplex PCR for *H. ducreyi, T. pallidum* and *HSV–1,2* commercially available with excellent sensitivity and specificity.

Other Tests

- ***Serological tests:*** Complement fixation test of limited value due to cross reactivity with other bacteria.
- ***Ito-Reenstierna's skin test:*** Intradermal innoculation of heat-killed *H. ducreyi*. Limited value and obselete.

TREATMENT

Specific Treatment

- Treatment guidelines depend on sensitivity pattern (Table 3.1).
- Often managed syndromically (genital ulcer syndrome).

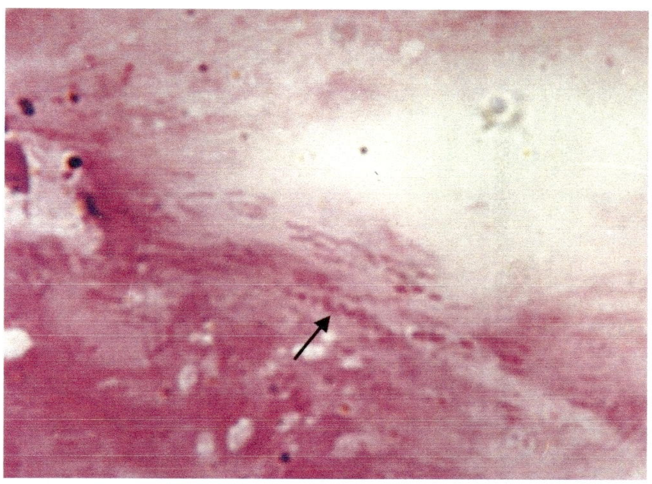

Chancroid: Gram stained smear of ulcer exudate showing Gram negative bacilli in parallel chains, the so called "school of fish" appearance (100x).

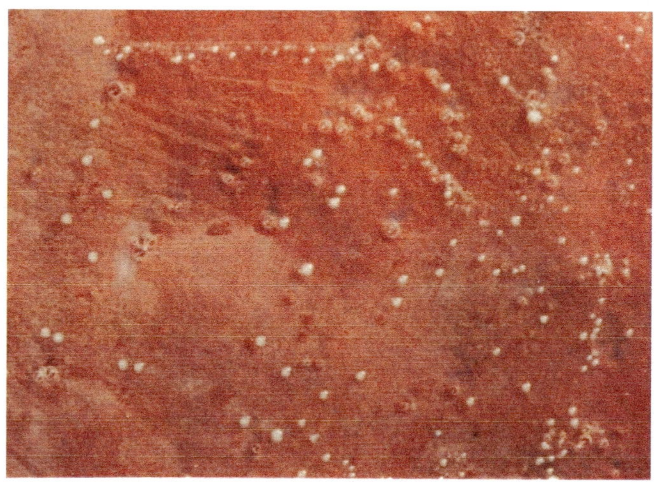

Chancroid: Culture: Close up view of *H. ducreyi* colonies which are yellowish, waxy (opaque) and of variable size. Colonies can be slided on plates.

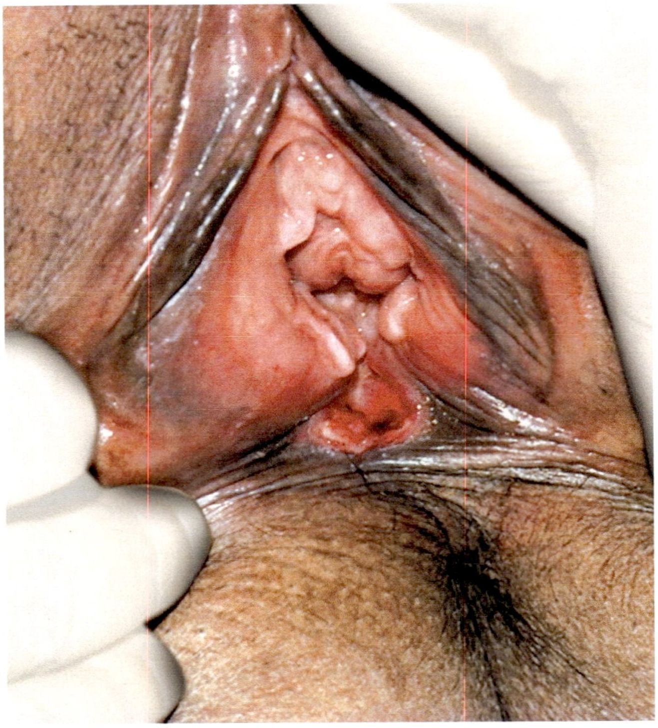

Chancroid: Ulcers with ragged erythematous margins present on vaginal introitus.

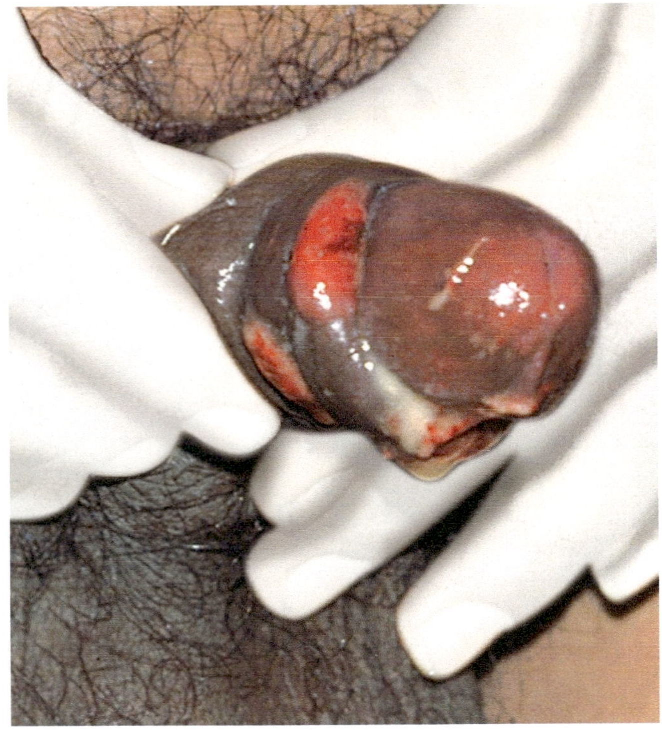

Chancroid: Multiple deep, soft ulcers with necrotic slough on floor.

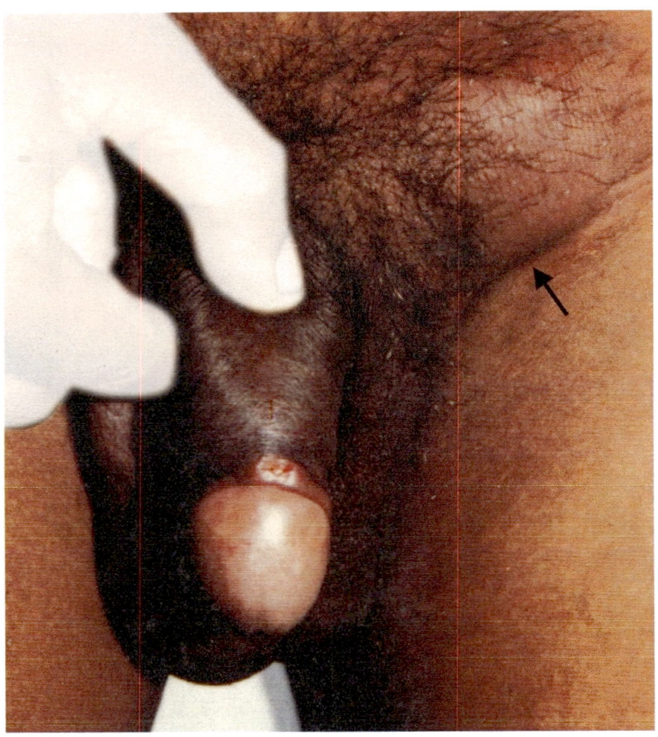

Chancroid: Single, irregular, necrotic ulcer on prepuce with grossly enlarged and inflammed left inguinal lymphadenopathy.

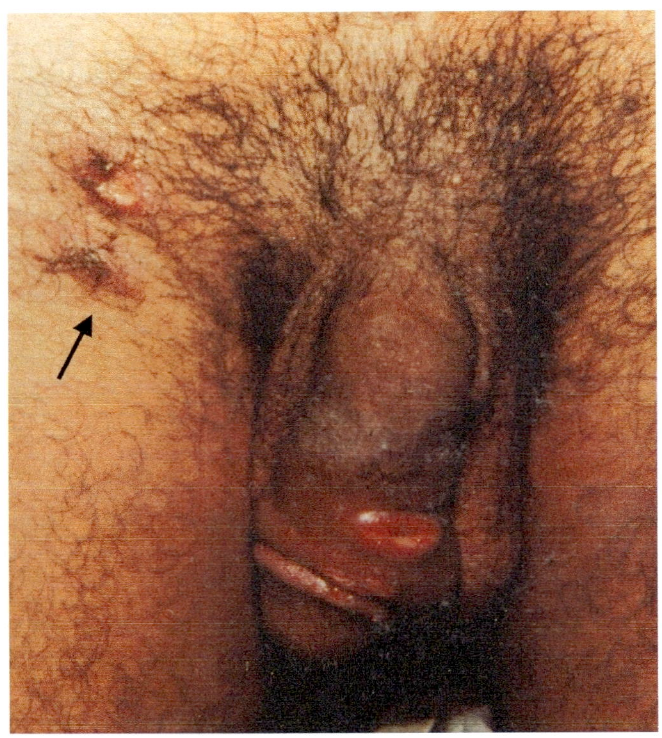

Chancroid: Multiple soft dirty ulcers on sulcus and penile shaft along with suppurating right inguinal buboes.

General Measures

- Clean lesions with normal saline.
- If phimosis and balanoposthitis, irrigate sub-preputial sac. And if severe, slit prepuce along the dorsum (dorsal slit).
- Aspiration (sometimes 2-3 times) from non dependent area of the fluctuant bubo may be done. Or incision and drainage from non dependent area.

Partner Management

Treat partner (symptomatic and asymptomatic) who have had sexual contact with patient in preceding 10 days.

Pregnant Woman

Azithromycin 1 gm single oral dose. Ciprofloxacin avoided.

In HIV Infected

- Treatment failure and slower response.
- Avoid regimens with single dose. Erythromycin 1.5 gm daily × 7 days or till healing of all ulcers preferred, which ever later.

Follow-up

- Re-examine 3-7 days after treatment for healing of ulcers. Spontaneous (without treatment) healing may take 2 weeks.
- Healing of lymph nodes is slower.

Other Considerations

- Rule out HIV, HBV and syphilis at first visit.
- If negative, retest for syphilis and HIV 3 months after initial visit.

Table 3.1: Recommended treatment guidelines for chancroid

CDC 2010	WHO 2003	NACO 2007
• Azithromycin 1 gm SOD* OR • Ceftriaxone 250 mg IM stat OR • Ciprofloxacin 500 mg bid × 3 days OR • Erythromycin base 500 mg tid × 7 days	• Ciprofloxacin 500 mg bid × 3 days OR • Azithromycin 1 gm SOD* OR • Erythromycin base 500 mg qid × 7 days	• Azithromycin 1 gm SOD* OR • Ciprofloxacin 500 mg bid × 3 days

*SOD: Single oral dose

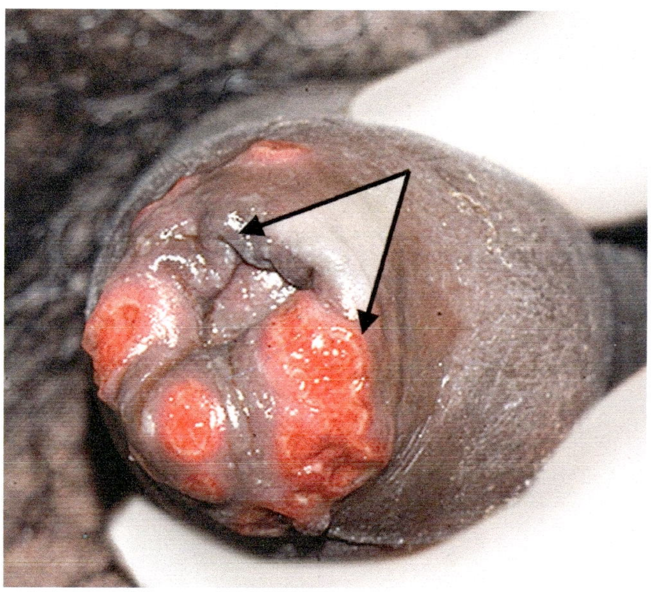

Chancroid with phimosis: Treated with local hygiene, dorsal slit (marked) and specific antibiotics.

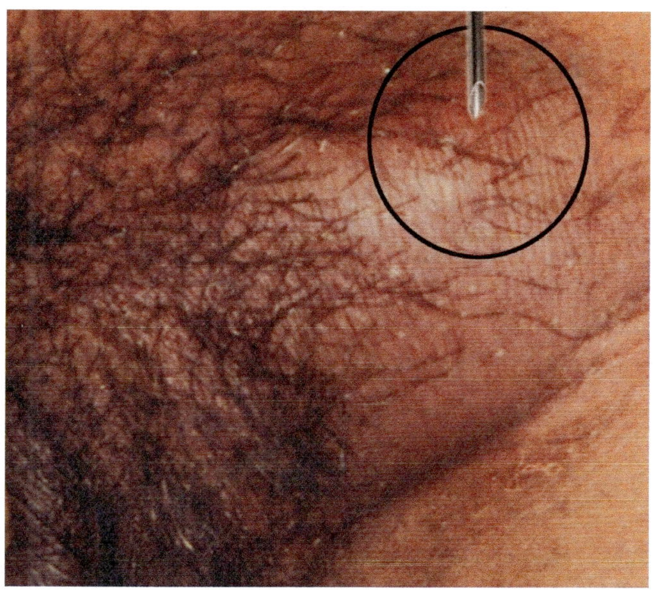

Chancroid with bubo: Aspirated from nondependent (marked) area with wide bored (gauge 18) needle.

Chapter 4

Lymphogranuloma Venereum

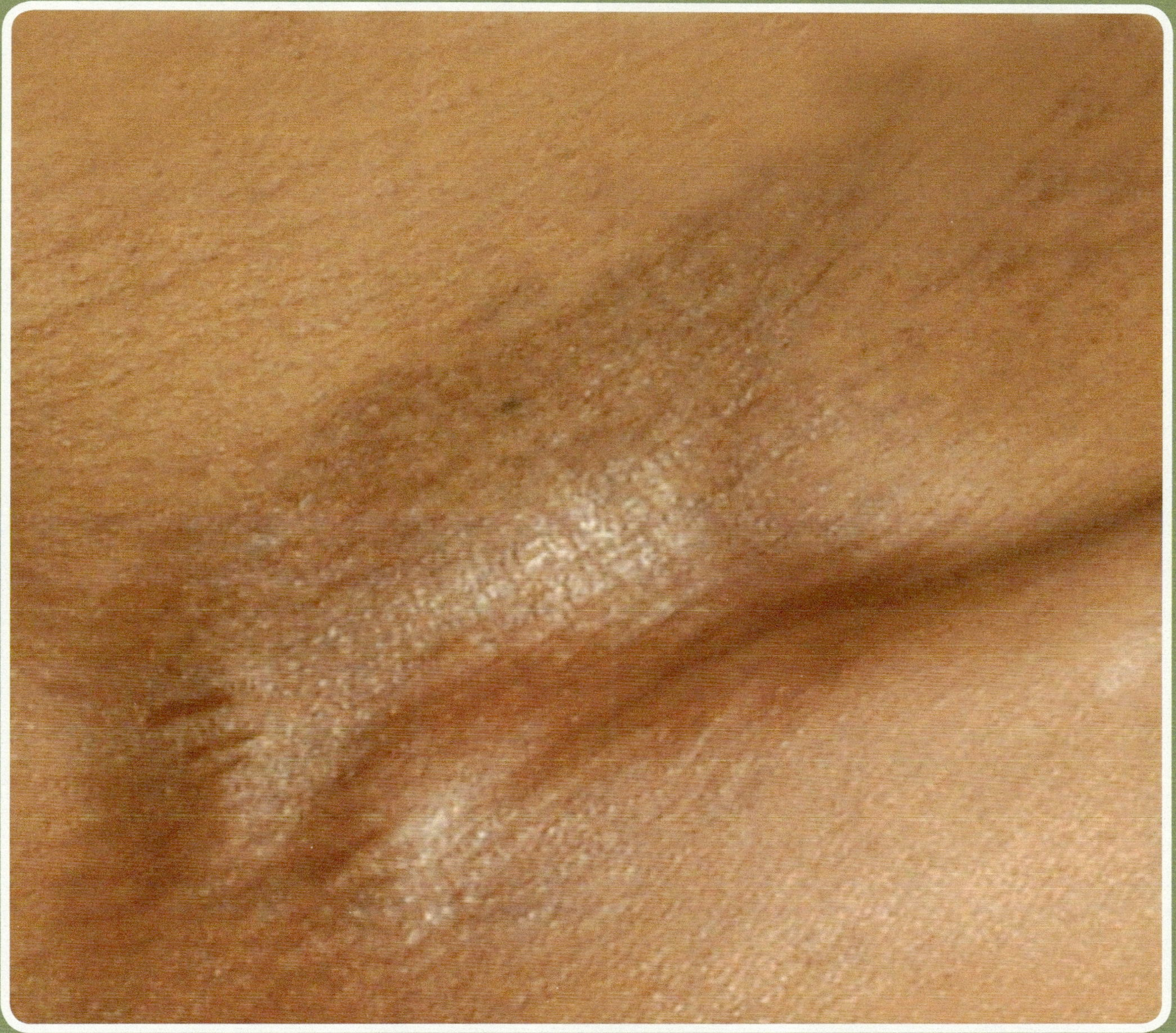

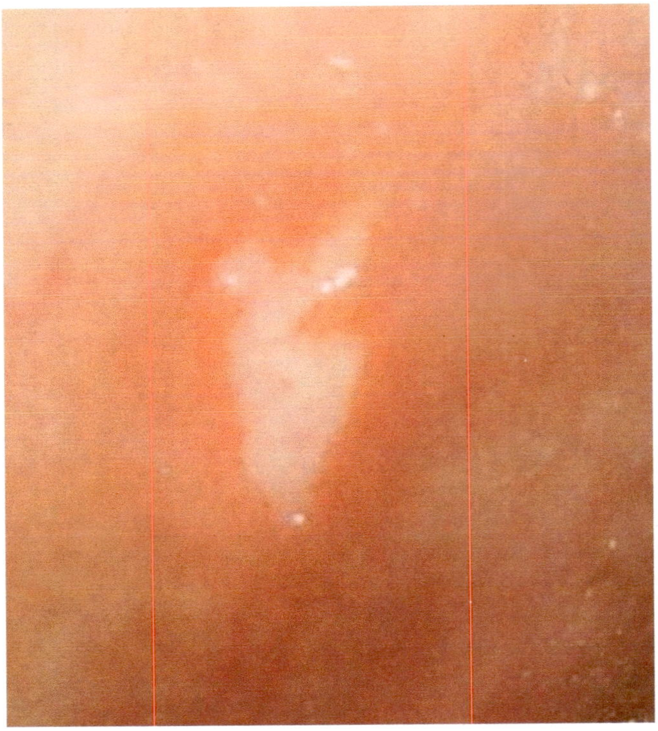

Lymphogranuloma venereum: Primary stage. Superficial irregular herpetic erosion. Usually not seen.

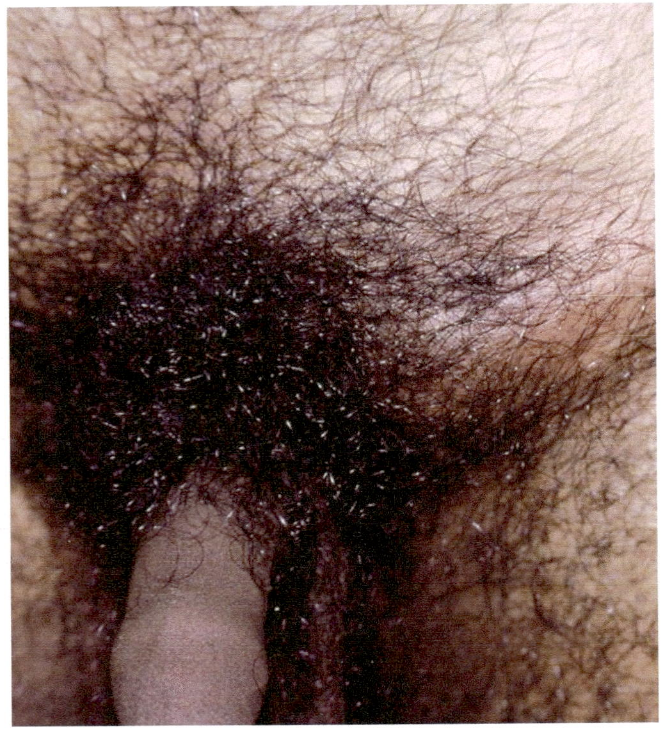

Lymphogranuloma venereum: Inguinal syndrome. Unilateral tender lymphadenopathy. Lymph nodes in LGV are matted and eventually adhere to skin.

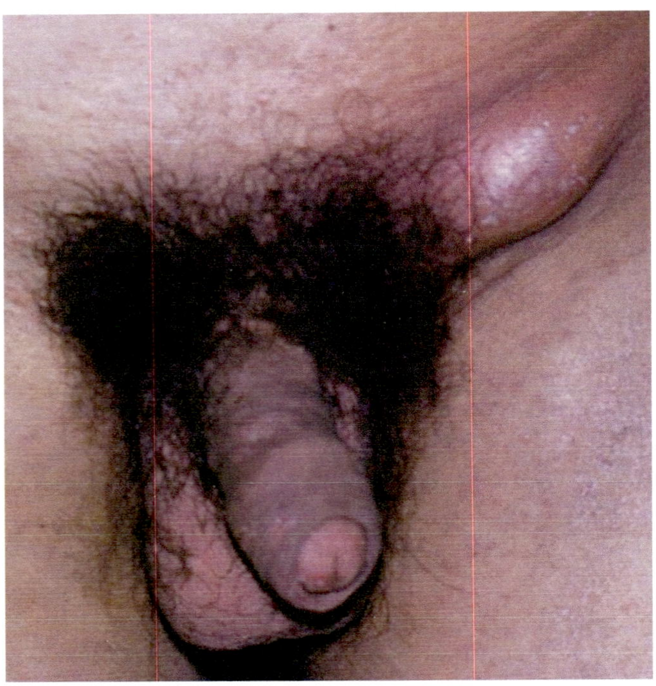

Lymphogranuloma venereum: Inguinal syndrome. Unilateral lymphadenopathy in the absence of concurrent genital ulcer. Lymphnodes have adhered to the skin, indicating impending rupture.

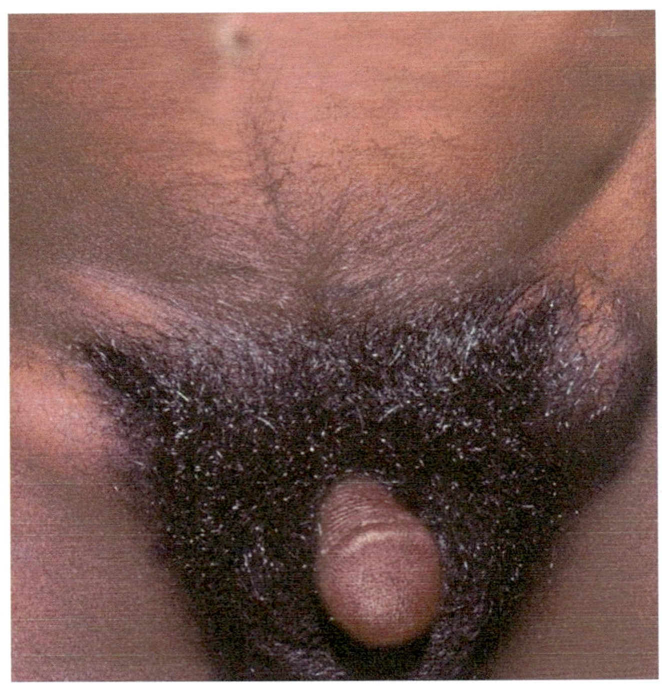

Lymphogranuloma venereum: Bilateral lymphadenopathy with sign of groove. In LGV, one-third of patients have bilateral lymphadenopathy. Other lymphnodes which may be involved include iliac lymph nodes and perirectal group.

Also known as climatic bubo, tropical bubo, lymphogranuloma inguinale.

ETIOLOGY

Etiological Agent

- *Chlamydia trachomatis,* biovar L 1-3 responsible for LGV. Biovar L2b (Amsterdam variant) responsible for lymphogranuloma (LGV) in MSM.
- Lymphotropic, obligate intracellular organisms. Obligate anaerobe.
- Produce intracellular iodine-staining inclusions known as elementary bodies.

Transmission

- Sexually transmitted.
- Non venereal transmission in health care personnels from ruptured bubos or infected tissue reported.

EPIDEMIOLOGY

Geographic Distribution

- Worldwide distribution.
- Endemic in India, South East Asia.

Demographic Distribution

- Six times more frequent in men compared to women.
- Less common in women, probably because remains unrecognized in them for longer.

CLINICAL FEATURES

Incubation Period

- Variable, 7–12 days. Can be longer (6 months).

Morphology

Three stages described in LGV—primary, secondary, tertiary.

Primary Stage

- Often not noticed by patient, especially women.
- ***Morphology:*** Small, transient, asymptomatic lesion (papule, pustule, vesicle or herpetic erosion); heals without residue. Edema of labia, phimosis may develop.
- ***Common sites:*** Coronal sulcus, frenulum, prepuce, glans penis, urethral meatus in males. Vagina, cervix in females. Anorectal area in MSM.
- Cord like lymphangitis of dorsal aspect of penis. May form a tender lymphoid nodule known as 'bubonolus'.

Secondary Stage (Inguinal Syndrome)

- After 2-6 weeks of primary lesion.
- Tender lymphadenopathy. Matted, fixed, to overlying skin which becomes dusky (in case of impending rupture). Upon rupture, sinuses with bluish undermined edge formed. Discharge: Thin, serous. Or thick, sticky, blood-stained. Or caseous.
- Unilateral in 2/3rd cases, bilateral in remaining. Inguinal, perirectal and deep iliac lymph nodes in women.
- ***Groove-sign of Greenblatt:*** Enlargement of lymph nodes both above (inguinal) and below (femoral) the inguinal ligament leading to groove formation.
- Persists for months and heals with thick, contracted scars.
- ***Variable constitutional symptoms:*** Fever, malaise, nausea, vomiting, abdominal pain, arthralgia, photosensitive skin lesions. Also leucocytosis and hyperglobulinemia.

Tertiary Stage (Genito-Ano-Rectal Syndrome)

- Frequent in females, homosexual males.
- Secondary to perirectal and pelvic lymphatic involvement.
- ***Manifestations:***
  - *Genital syndrome:* lymphedema leads to elephantiasis and distortion. Vascular compromise leads to ulcers.
  - *Anorectal syndrome:* hyperplastic ulcers in lower anorectal mucosa. Later fibrosis leading to strictures.

Skin Findings Associated with LGV

- Hypersensitivity reaction (? id eruption).
- Transient generalized exanthem, erythema nodosum, erythema multiforme, erythema annulare centrifugum, urticaria and widespread papules and pustules.

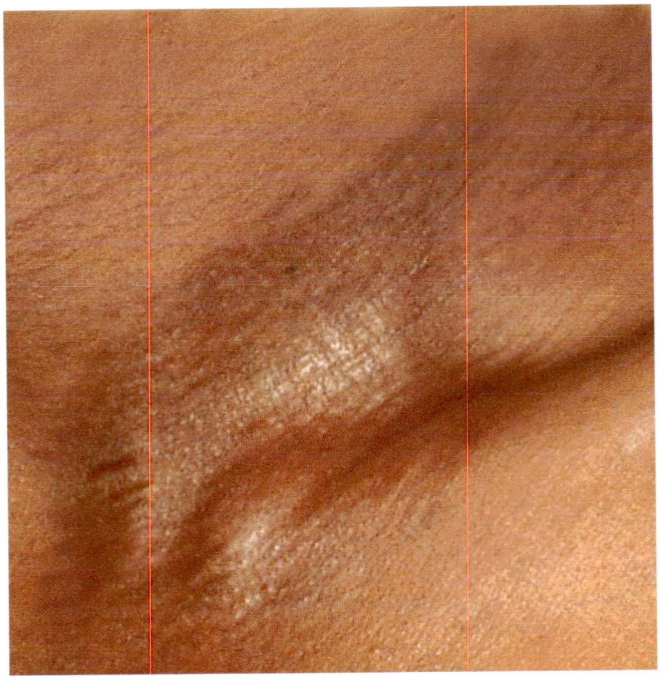

Lymphogranuloma venereum: Sign of groove. Lymph nodes enlarged both above (inguinal group) and below (femoral group) inguinal ligament result in a groove.

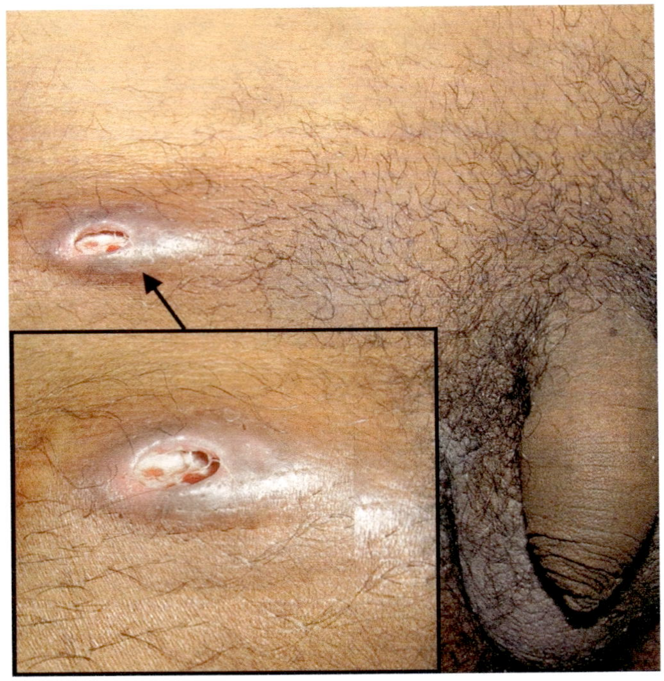

Lymphogranuloma venereum: Ruptured bubo forming a chronic non-healing sinus with elongated mouth and bluish undermined edge (inset).

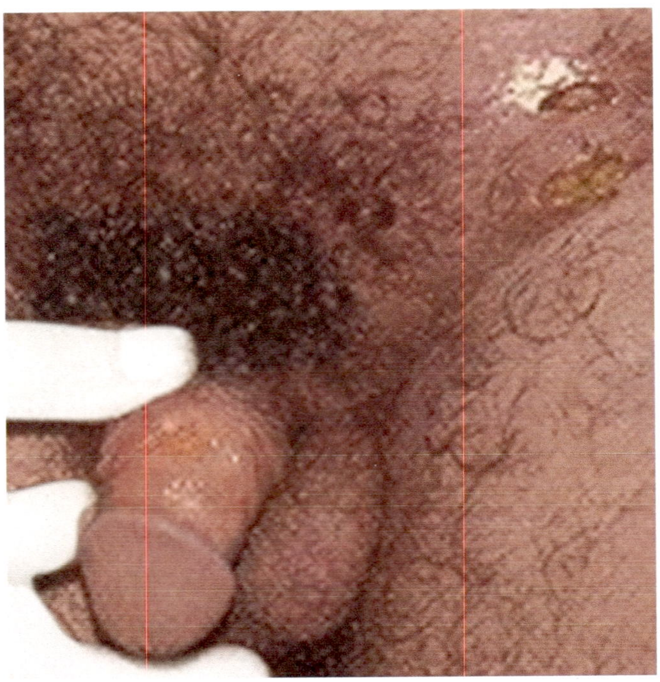

Lymphogranuloma venereum: Bilateral lymphadenopathy which has ruptured to form multiple sinuses. Lymphadenopathy of LGV is associated with multilocular abscesses.

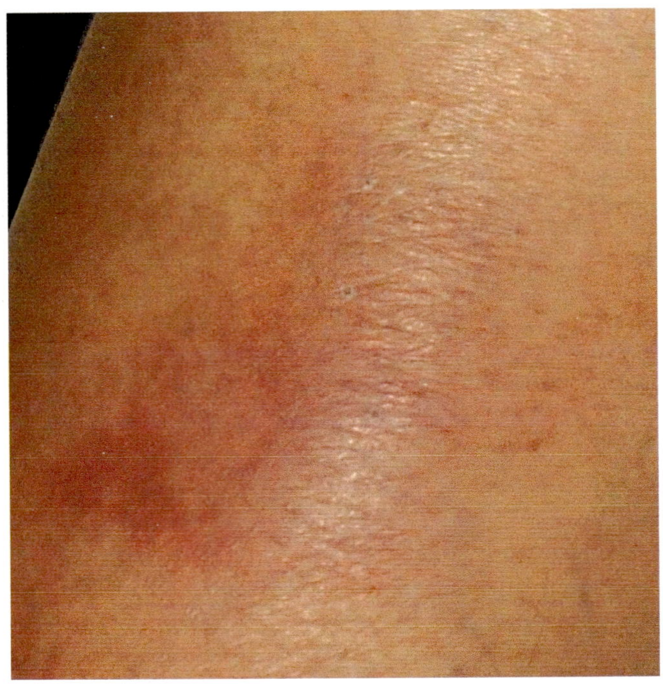

Lymphogranuloma venereum: Erythema nodosum may occur in secondary stage (and rarely in tertiary stages).

COMPLICATIONS

Of Secondary Stage

- Rupture of inguinal bubo. Can lead to chronic non-healing sinuses, rapidly spreading phagedenic infection, slowly spreading cutaneous lymphogranuloma.

Of Tertiary Stage

- ***Esthiomene:*** Lymphedema of vulva associated with polypoid growths ulcers and fistulae.
- ***Distorted genitalia:*** 'Ramrod penis', 'saxophone penis'.
- ***Rectal strictures:*** Annular, tubular or funnel shaped. Located about 5 cm from anal orifice.
- ***Stenosis:*** Of vagina, urethra, rectum.
- ***Fistulae:*** Between rectum and vagina; and urethra and vagina.
- ***Perianal area:*** Lymphedema with ulcers and sinuses. In MSM.

HIV AND LGV

- ***Effect of LGV on HIV:*** Increased transmission of HIV, in presence of primary.
- ***Effect of HIV on LGV:*** No effect generally noted.

DIAGNOSIS

Based on Clinical Features

- Small asymptomatic, non-indurated ulcer, occurring after few days of sexual intercourse suggestive of primary stage often not noticed.
- Tender, matted, fluctuant inguinal lymphadenopathy. May rupture later to form sinuses with elongated mouth and undermined bluish margins characteristic of secondary stage.
- Lymphedema, fistulae, strictures and stenosis occur in tertiary stage.

Laboratory Investigations

Isolation and Identification of Organism

- ***Direct staining:***
  - Specimens taken from pus from bubo.
  - Giemsa or iodine staining shows intracellular inclusion bodies. Low sensitivity.
- ***Microimmunoflourescence identification:*** And typing helpful but not universally available.
- ***Antigen detection:*** Using ELISA, rapid assays (as point of care tests) and polymerase chain reaction. From ulcer scrapings, bubo aspirates, cervix, rectum, urethra.
- ***Tissue culture:*** On HeLa 229, McCoy cells and baby hamster kidney cell lines.

Serological Tests

- ***Complement fixation test:*** Four-fold rise in antibodies. Or titer > 1:64 to *C. trachomatis* L1, 2, 3 indicative of LGV.
- ***Microimmunofluorescence test:*** Most specific but limited availability as laborious.

Others

- ***Frei's skin test:*** Unreliable and outdated.

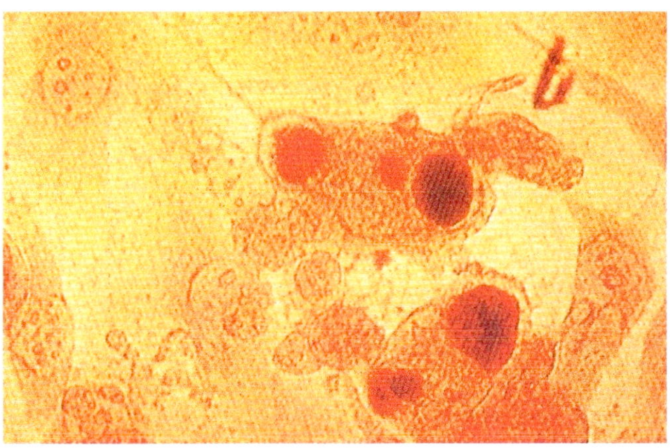

Lymphogranuloma venereum: Iodine staining showing iodine stained intracytoplasmic elementary bodies.

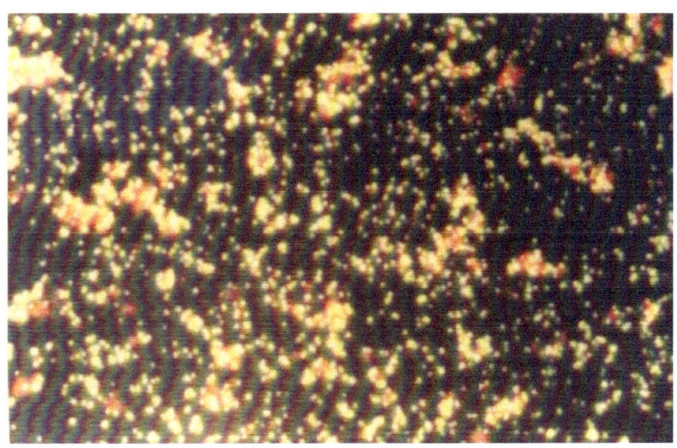

Lymphogranuloma venereum: Microimmunofluorescence test to detect chlamydial antigen (seen as greenish refractile particles 100x).

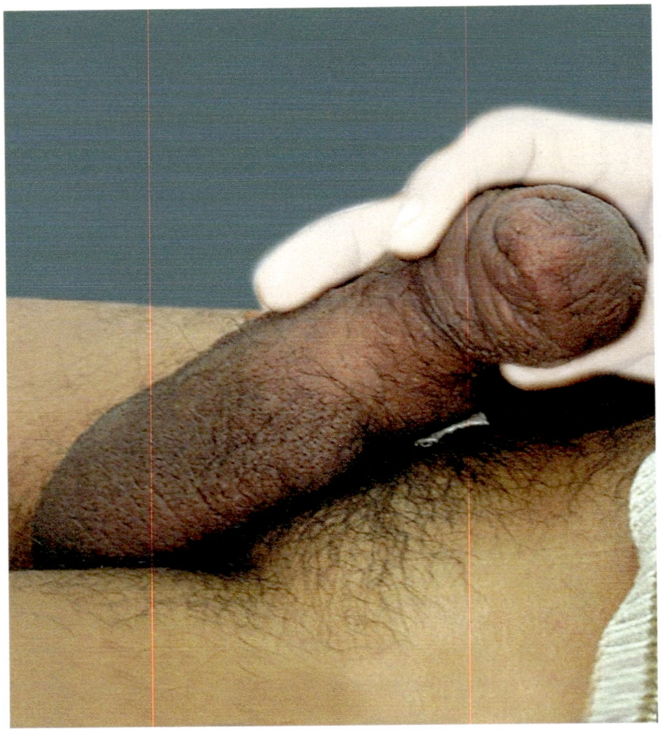

Lymphogranuloma venereum: Ramrod penis. Solidification of penis follows lymphedema.

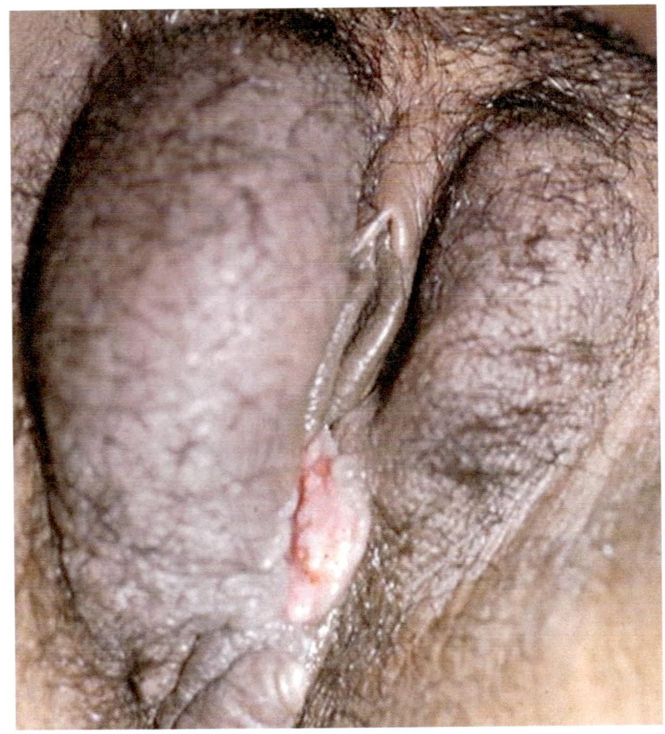

Lymphogranuloma venereum: Esthiomene. A serious complication due to lymphedema of the female genitalia resulting in enlargement of female external genitalia.

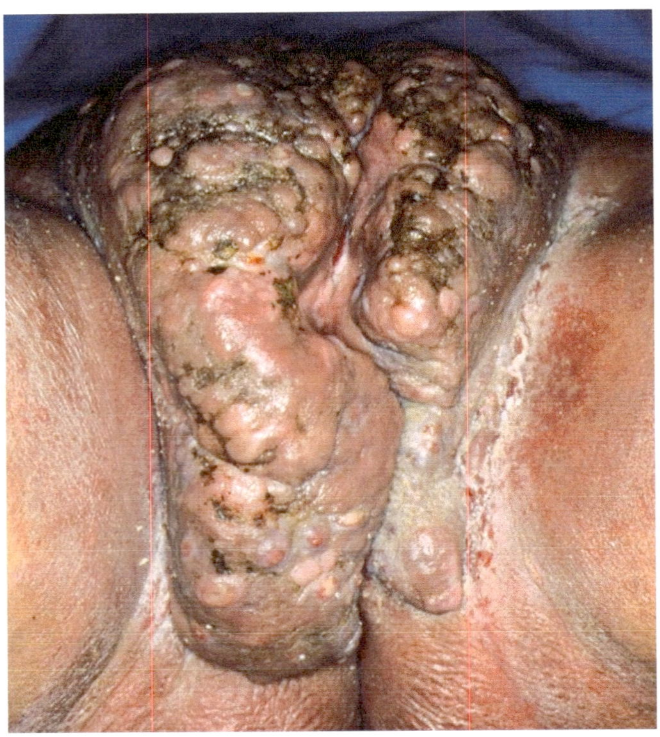

Lymphogranuloma venereum: Esthiomene. Enlargement, formation of fistulae, polyploidal growths and gross distortion of female external genitalia.

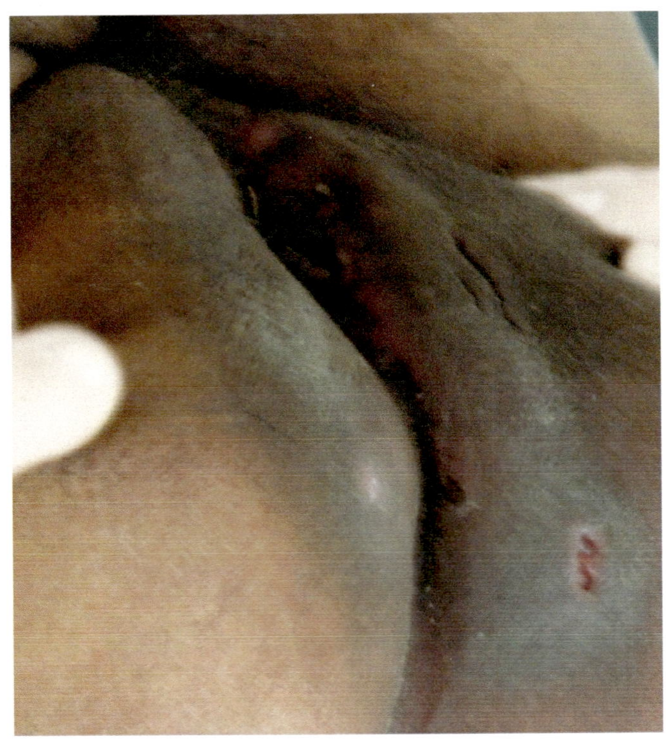

Lymphogranuloma venereum: Lymphedema of perianal region with sinus tracts and ulcers.

TREATMENT

Specific Treatment

- Doxycycline mainstay of treatment (Table 4.1).
- Longer regimens needed in advanced disease.
- Sequelae such as strictures and/or fistulae require surgery.

General Measures

- Fluctuant lymph nodes aspirated through healthy skin from non-dependent area. Incision and drainage or excision of nodes avoided.

Partner Management

Treat partner (symptomatic and asymptomatic) who have had sexual contact with patient in preceding 60 days.

Pregnant Woman

Erythromycin base 2 g daily (in 4 divided doses) for 3 weeks. Doxycycline and ciprofloxacin avoided.

In HIV Infected

- Same as in non-HIV individuals.

Follow-up

- Re-examine till all lesions have completely healed.

Other Considerations

- Rule out HIV, HBV and syphilis at first visit.
- If negative, retest for syphilis and HIV 3 months after initial visit.

Table 4.1: Various treatment regimens for lymphogranuloma venereum

	CDC 2010	WHO 2003	NACO 2007
Recommended regimens	• Doxycycline 100 mg bid × 21 days	• Doxycycline 100 mg bid × 14 days OR • Erythromycin 500 mg qid × 14 days	• Doxycycline 100 mg bid × 21 days
Alternative regimens	• Erythromycin 500 mg qid × 21 days	• Tetracycline 500 mg qid × 14 days	

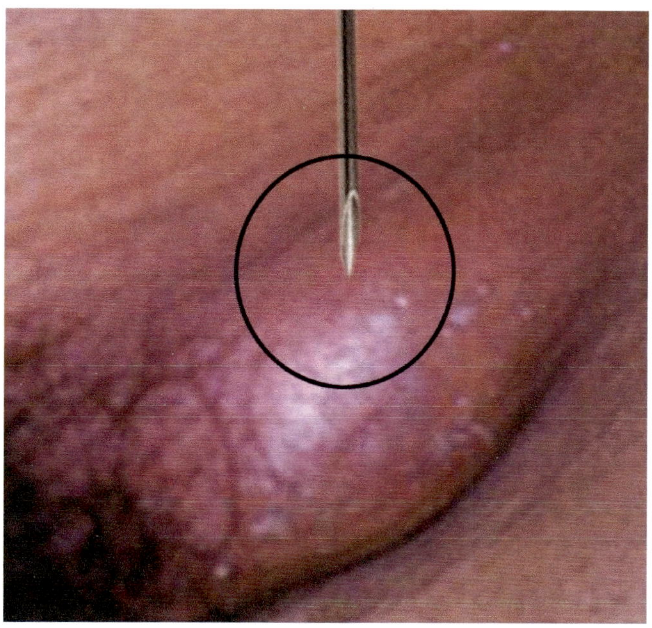

Lymphogranuloma venereum with bubo: Aspirated through healthy skin from nondependent area.

CHAPTER 5

Donovanosis

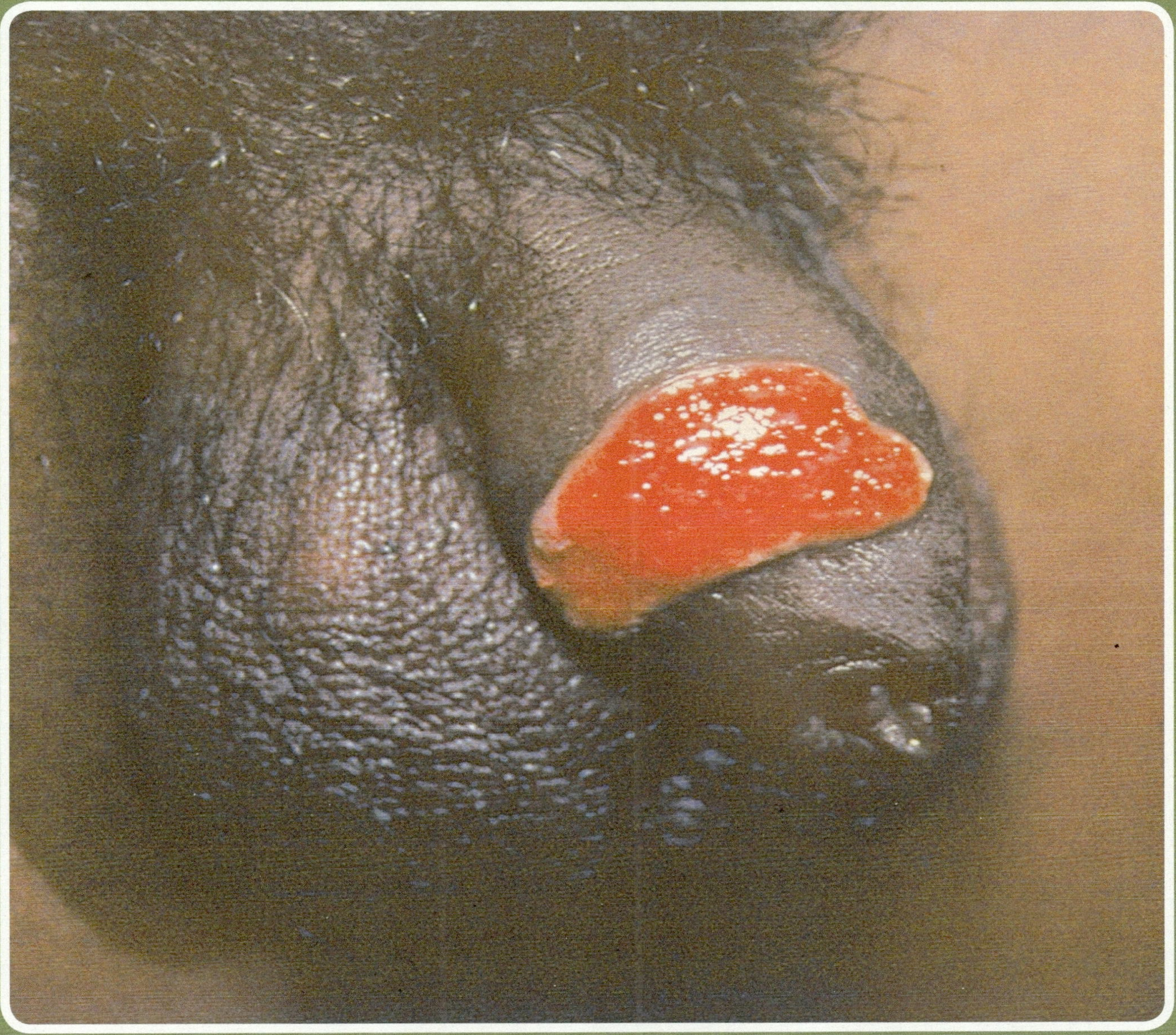

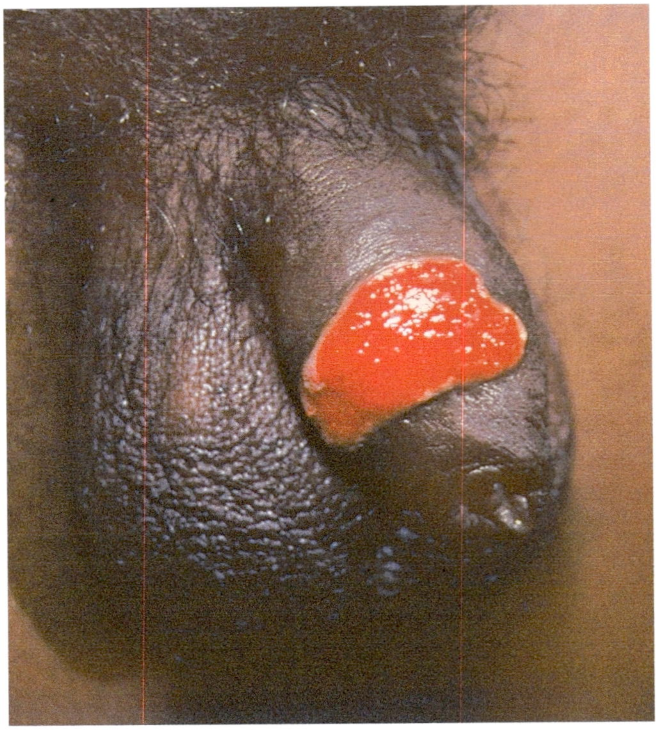

Donovanosis: Classical type. Well-defined ulcer on penile shaft with beefy red granulation tissue and irregular margin.

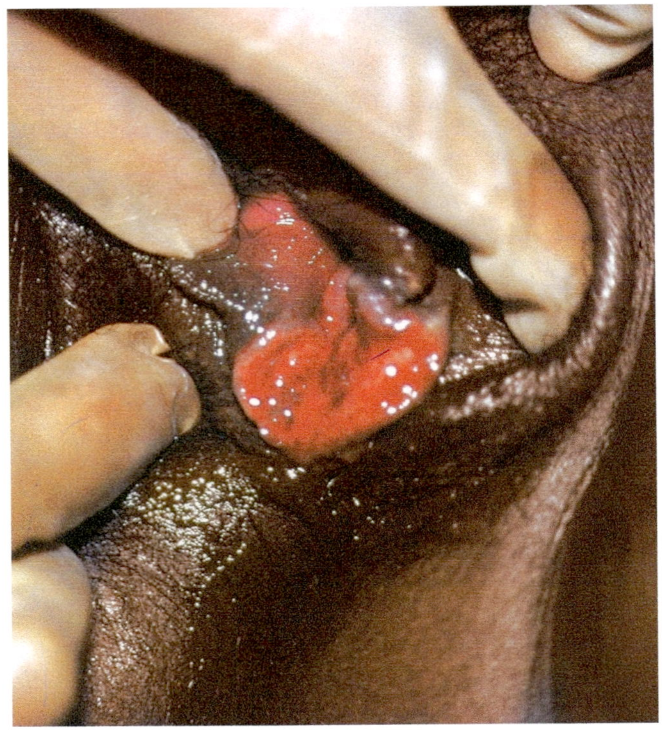

Donovanosis: Classical type. Well-defined ulcer with beefy granulation tissue.

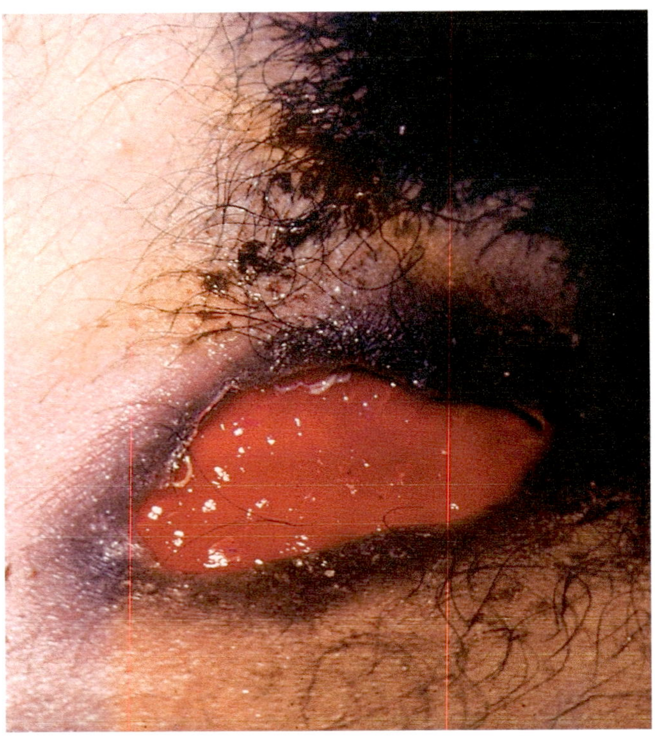

Donovanosis: Classical type. Well-defined ulcer with beefy granulation tissue on floor.

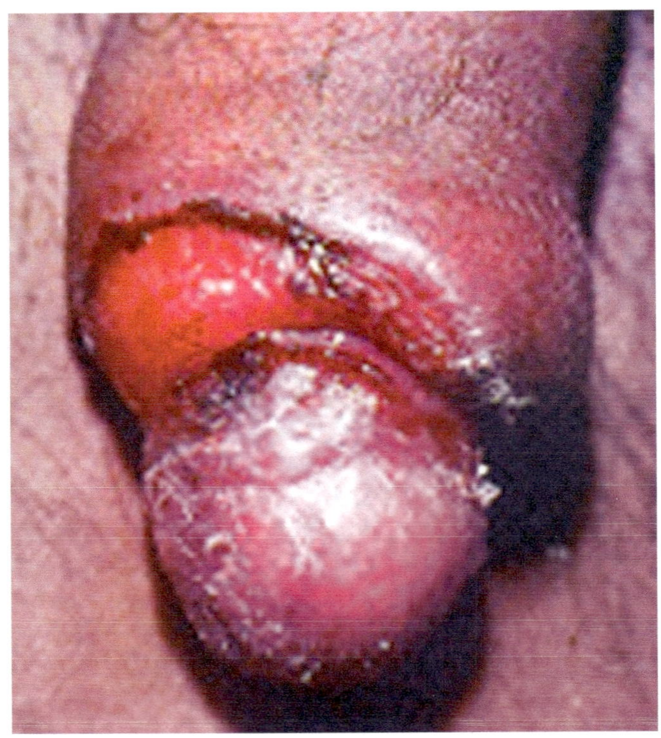

Donovanosis: Classical type. Well-defined ulcer with undermined edges and clean granulaton tissue on floor.

Also known as granuloma venereum, granuloma inguinale, granuloma inguinale tropicum, granuloma contagiosa, genito-inguinale.

ETIOLOGY

Etiological Agent

- *Klebsiella granulomatis* (previously known as *Donovania granulomatis*, *Calymmatobacterium granulomatis)*.
- Gram-negative bacteria, 1.5 × 0.7 μ.
- Intracellular parasite of histiocytes. Organism surrounded by a dense capsule. Shows bipolar staining—'safety-pin' appearance.
- Fastidious bacteria, difficult to culture consistently.

Transmission

Transmitted by unprotected sexual contact.

EPIDEMIOLOGY

Geographic Distribution

- Endemic in southern China, northern Australia, Africa, West Indies.
- In India, endemic along East coast.

Demographic Distribution

- Common in males (male:female ratio is 4:1).
- Frequent in lower socio-economic strata with poor personal hygiene. And people engaged in indiscriminate sex.

CLINICAL FEATURES

Incubation Period

- Variable, 3 days to 3 months.

Morphology

- Starts as single or multiple papules which ulcerate.
- ***Classical ulcer:*** Painless ulcers; beefy red, friable, floor which bleeds easily on touch. Elevated, irregular (serpiginous) edge. Firmly indurated base. Size variable, few to many cms.
- ***No lymphadenopathy:*** Lesions in inguinal area mimic lymphadenopathy (but not). So known as pseudo-buboes.

Sites of Lesions

- Genitals, perianal area, inguinal region.
- ***Extragenital lesions:*** Lips, gums, cheeks, palate, pharynx, larynx, neck.

Variants

- ***Granulomatous type:*** Exuberant granulation tissue, undermined edge, foul smelling discharge. Inguinal area.
- ***Hypertrophic type:*** Raised ulcer with thick everted edges without any exudate.
- ***Sclerotic or cicatricial type:*** Common in women. Fibrotic scars leading to deformity of genitalia.
- ***Destructive necrotic type:*** Superadded anaerobic infection. Rapid spread with necrotic inflammation and foul smelling exudate.

COMPLICATIONS

- Phimosis, distortion of genitalia, partial or complete amputation of penis.
- Genital lymphedema and elephantiasis.
- Vaginal stenosis. And rectovaginal fistula.

HIV AND DONOVANOSIS

- ***Effect of Donovanosis on HIV:*** Amplified transmission of HIV (like any other genital ulcer disease).
- ***Effect of HIV on Donovanosis:***
  - Treatment failure and slower response.
  - Regimens same as in non-HIV individual. Consider adding parenteral aminoglycosides (vide infra).

DIAGNOSIS

Based on Clinical Features

- Painless, fleshy, exuberant, ulcerated plaque ulcer with irregular serpiginous margin.
- No inguinal lymphadenopathy. Inguinal lesions, if present, pseudobuboes.

Laboratory Investigations

Isolation and Identification of Organism

- ***Crush smear from lesion:*** Stained with Giemsa stain. Donovan bodies appear as pinkish bipolar intracellular bodies (safety pin appearance) under oil immersion.

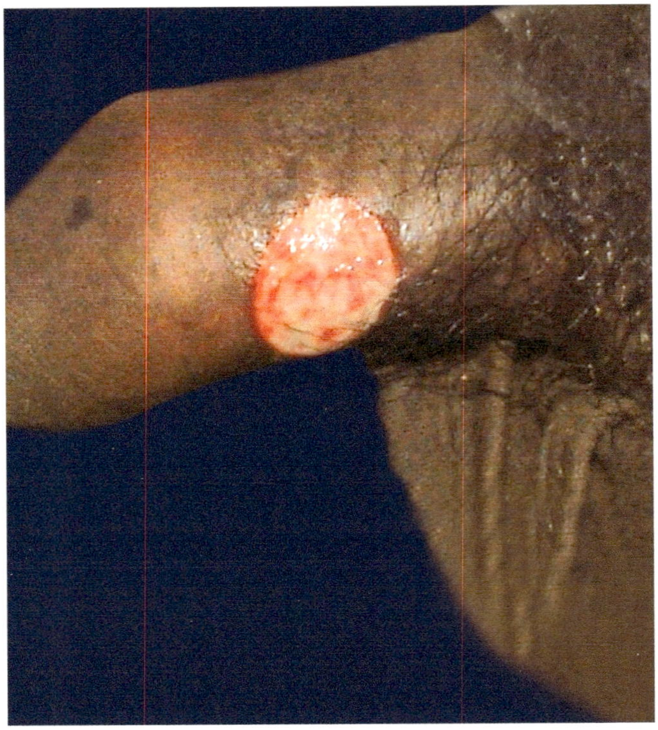

Donovanosis: Granulomatous type. Well-defined ulcer with exuberant granulation tissue on floor.

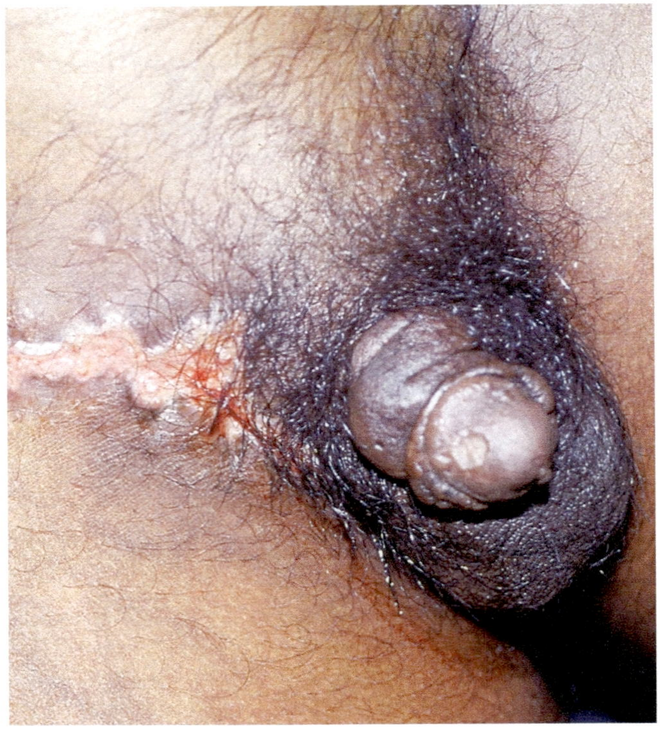

Donovanosis: Cicatricial type. On healing, ulcers form linear scars.

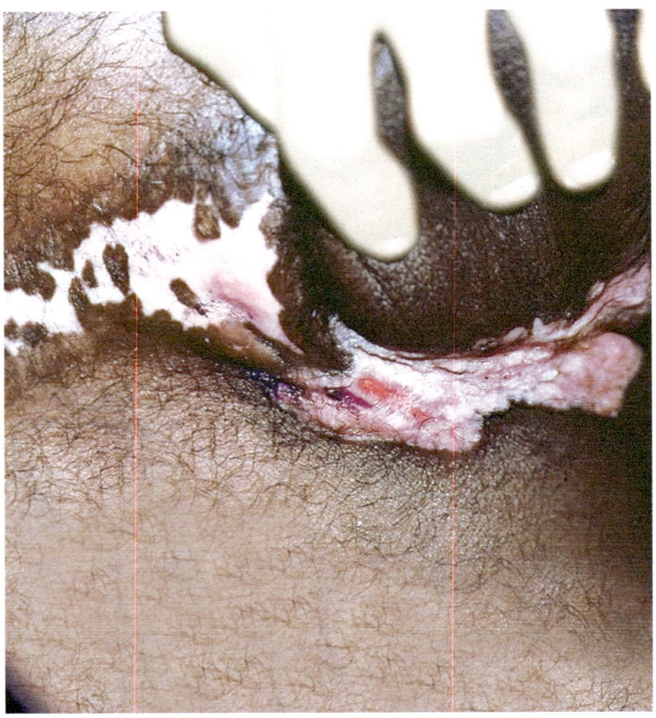

Donovanosis: Cicatricial type. Elongated scars formed on healing of ulcers distorting the genitalia.

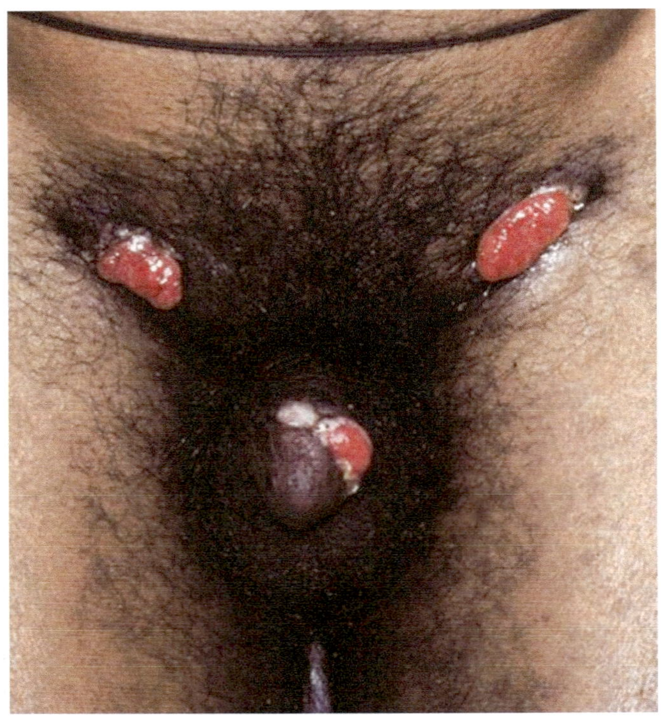

Donovanosis: Genital lesion with pseudo buboes. Subcutaneous nodules in inguinal area rupture to form donovanosis-like ulcers.

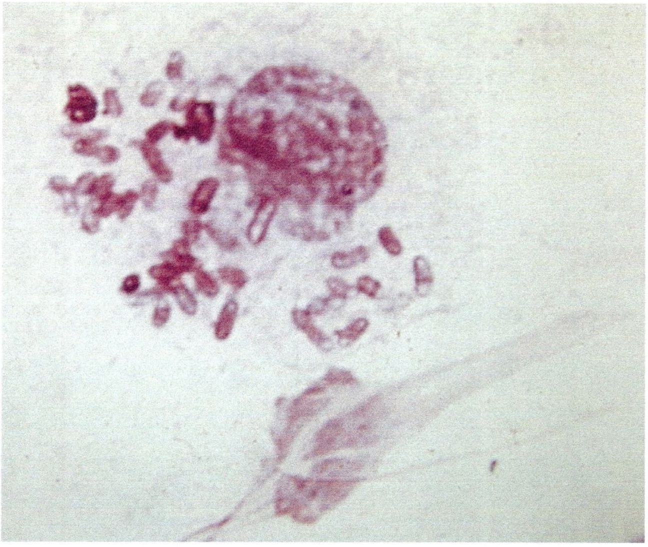

Donovanosis: Crush smear of material from ulcer stained with Giemsa stain. Visualized under oil immersion for multiple intracellular pink, bipolar stained organisms.

- ***Culture:*** Difficult and controversial. In yolk sac of chick embryo, Hep-2 cell lines. Not available routinely.
- ***PCR:*** In research settings only.

Others

- ***Skin biopsy:*** Important in 2 situations:
  - Confirm diagnosis of donovanosis.
  - Rule out malignancy.
- ***Serological tests:*** None available.

TREATMENT

Specific Treatment

- All treatment regimens continued for 3 weeks. Or till lesions heal completely (Table 5.1).
- Addition of aminoglycosides (e.g. gentamicin 1 mg/kg IV every 8 hours) considered in:
  - Patients responding poorly during 1st few days of conventional therapy.
  - HIV positive individuals.

Partner Management

Treat partner (symptomatic and asymptomatic) who have had sexual contact with patient in preceding 60 days.

Pregnant Woman

Erythromycin base 500 mg orally qid (for at least 3 weeks) until all lesions have completely healed. Doxycycline and ciprofloxacin avoided.

Follow-up

- Re-examine till all lesions have completely healed.

Other Considerations

- Rule out HIV, HBV and syphilis at first visit.
- If negative, retest for syphilis and HIV 3 months after initial visit.

Table 5.1: Recommended treatment regimens for donovanosis

	CDC 2010*	WHO 2003**	NACO 2007
Recommended regimens	• Doxycycline 100 mg bid	• Azithromycin 1 g on first day, then 500 mg od OR • Doxycycline 100 mg bid	No specific mention
Alternative regimens	• Azithromycin 1 g weekly OR • Ciprofloxacin 750 mg bid OR • Erythromycin 500 mg qid OR • Trimethoprim-sulfamethoxazole one double-strength (160 mg/800 mg) tablet bid	• Erythromycin 500 mg qid OR • Trimethoprim-sulfamethoxazole one double-strength (160 mg/800 mg) tablet bid OR • Tetracycline 500 mg qid	

*Treatment continued for 3 weeks or till all lesions heal. **Treatment continued till all lesions heal.

CHAPTER 6

Gonorrhoea

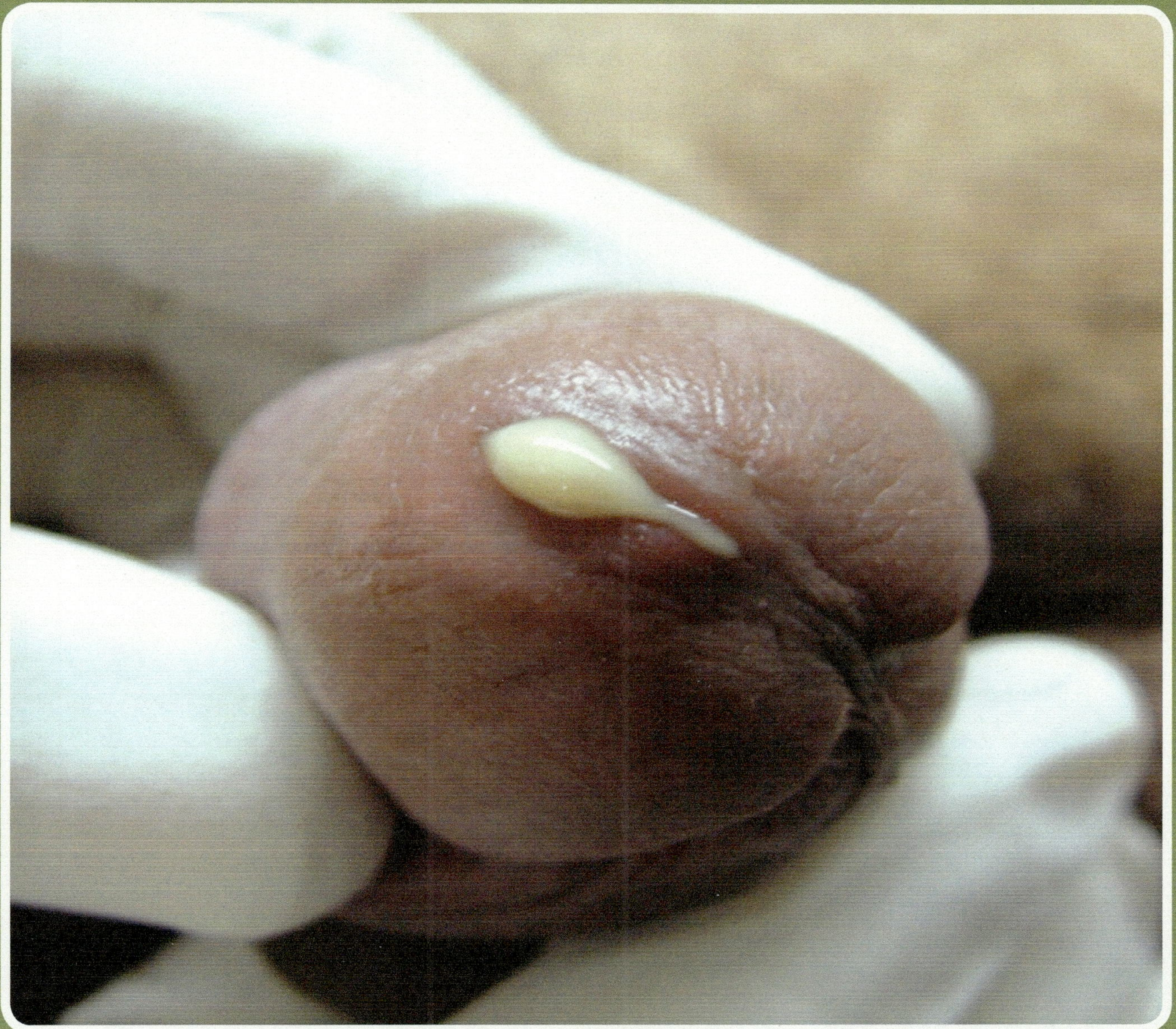

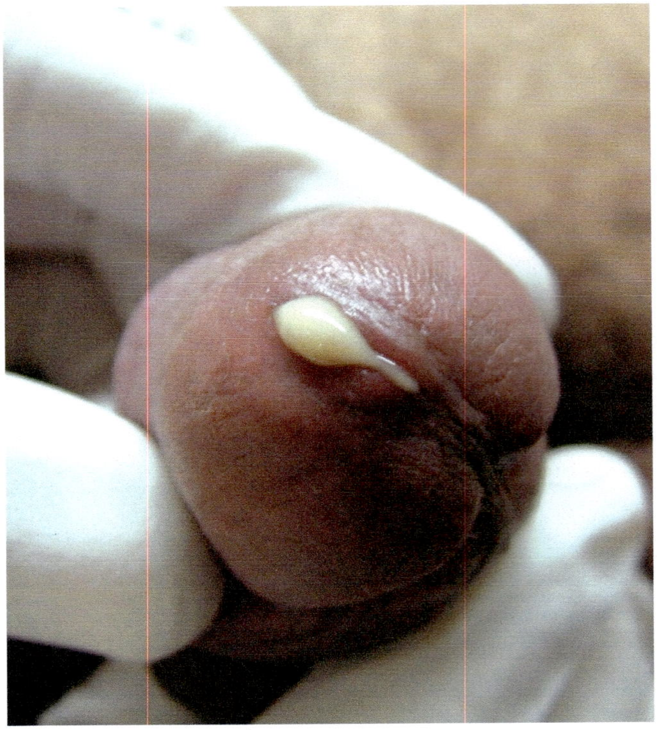

Gonorrhoea: Profuse purulent discharge at urethral meatus.

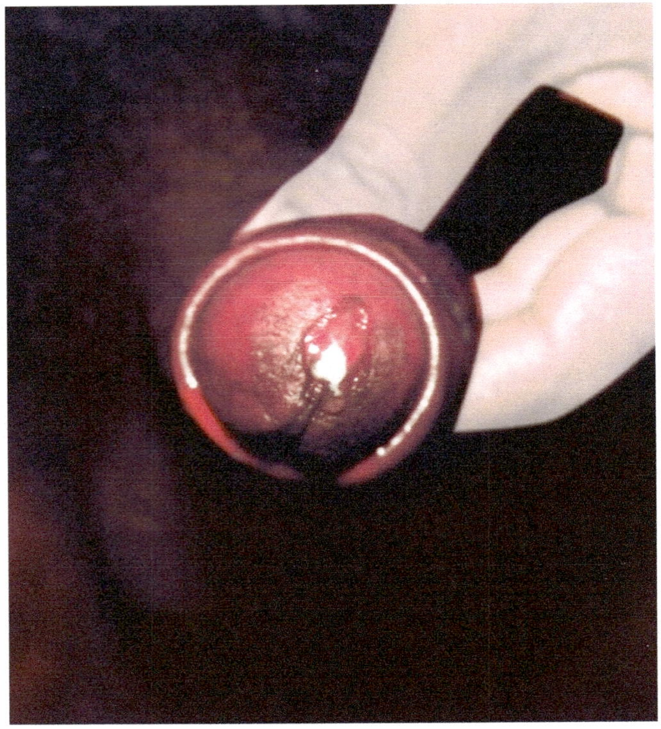

Gonorrhoea: Mild mucopurulent discharge at urethral meatus. Made obvious by milking urethra. If discharge absent, ask patient to hold urine.

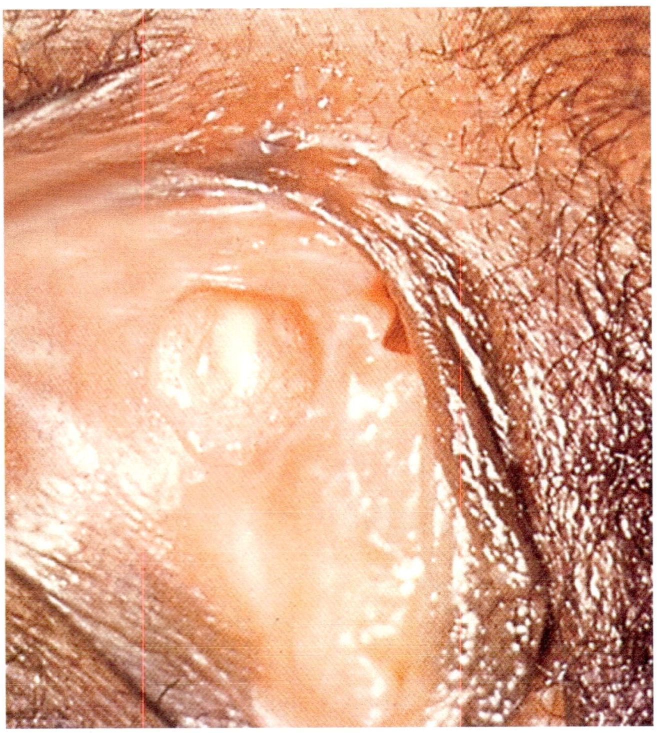

Gonorrhoea: Profuse creamy discharge from urethra, presenting as vaginal discharge.

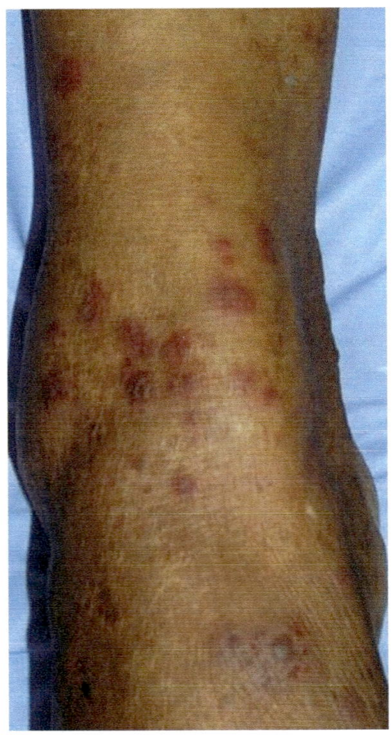

Gonorrhoea: Disseminated gonococcal infection. Tender necrotic vesicles and pustules with irregular purpuric margin on acral parts (feet in this case).

ETIOLOGY

Etiological Agent

- Gram-negative diplococci, *Neisseria gonorrhoeae*. Aerobic, oxidase positive, intracellular organism.
- Bear pili (hair-like projections) that facilitate adherence to epithelial surfaces; invade columnar or cuboidal epithelium.
- Penicillinase (β lactamase) producing gonococcal infections pose serious therapeutic problems.

Transmission

- ***Sexual:***
  - Predominant mode—hetero- or homosexual; genital, anogenital and orogenital contact.
  - Often transmitted from asymptomatic partner particularly women. Male to female transmission better-several reasons, including prolonged contact with infected secretions retained in vagina.
- ***Non-sexual transmission:*** Uncommon. Includes mother (infected) to child transmission during birth, resulting in ophthalmic infection (ophthalmia neonatorum).

EPIDEMIOLOGY

- Worldwide prevalence declining.
- Commoner in young girls in the developed world.

CLINICAL FEATURES

Incubation Period

1-10 (generally 2-5) days.

Signs and Symptoms in Males

- ***Urethritis:***
  - *Anterior urethritis:* yellowish or greenish yellow purulent discharge, accompanied by burning or painful micturition. Meatal lips everted, erythematous and edematous. Sometimes balanitis or balanoposthitis. Occasionally (10-15%) males asymptomatic.
  - *Posterior urethritis:* urgency and frequency of micturition. And painful erections (priapism).
- ***Anorectal infection:*** Homosexual contact in males. Anal pruritus; pain on defecation and tenesmus. Mucoid or mucopurulent discharge; bleeding. Anal mucosa unaffected but rectal mucosa reveals erythema (mild to severe) with mucopus in lumen.

Signs and Symptoms in Females

- ***Endocervical infection:*** Often asymptomatic (in 75%). Symptoms, when present, mild and non-specific. Vaginal discharge, dysuria and postcoital bleeding.
- ***Vulvovaginitis:*** In prepubertal girls. Due to sexual abuse.
- ***Anorectal infection:*** Anogenital contact. Or contamination with vaginal discharge. Symptoms milder in women.

Oropharyngeal Infection

- More frequent in MSMs and women than heterosexual males.
- Due to oro-genital contact (fellatio or cunnilingus).
- Asymptomatic. Or mildly symptomatic-sore-throat, mucopurulent discharge.

Gonococcal Conjunctivitis

- ***Neonates:*** Transmitted to neonate during birth through infected maternal passage. Acute purulent conjunctivitis. May end up with keratitis or panophthalmitis.
- ***Adults:*** Rare; occurs by inoculation with infected fingers.

COMPLICATIONS

- ***Males:***
  - *Acute:* tysonitis, littritis, infection of median raphe, funiculitis, epididymo-orchitis, watering can perineum periurethral abscesses, fistulae, prostatitis.
  - *Chronic:* urethral strictures.
- ***Females:***
  - *Acute:* bartholinitis or Bartholin's abscess, salpingitis, pelvic inflammatory disease.
  - *Chronic:* infertility, ectopic pregnancy.
- ***Disseminated gonococcal infection:*** Uncommon. Due to penicillin sensitive strains (AHU auxotype). Commoner in females and homosexual males.
  - *Primary site:* asymptomatic but acts as source of hematogenous dissemination.
  - *Arthritis-dermatitis syndrome:* fever. Asymmetrical, septic polyarthritis (gonococci demonstrable). Tender necrotic pustules with irregular hemorrhagic border. And discrete petechial lesions over the digits of the hands and feet. Blood cultures positive only in initial 'bacteraemic' phase.

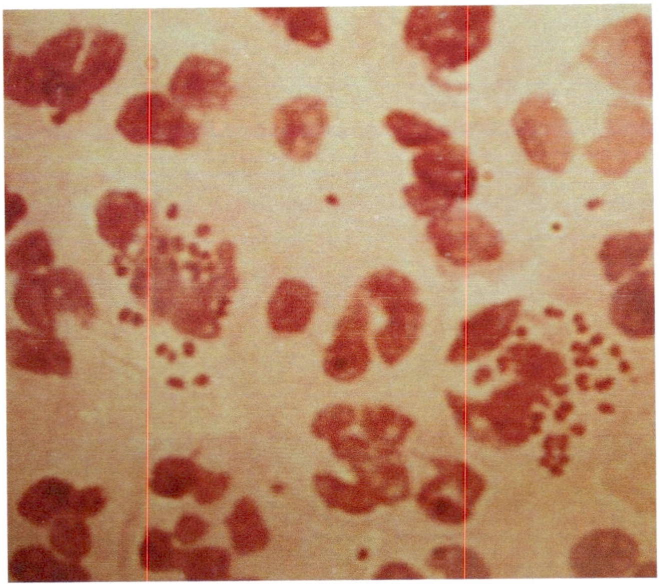

Gonorrhoea: Gram stain of urethral discharge showing several polymorphonuclear cells with intracellular Gram negative diplococci (100x). Gram stain very sensitive in males, not in females.

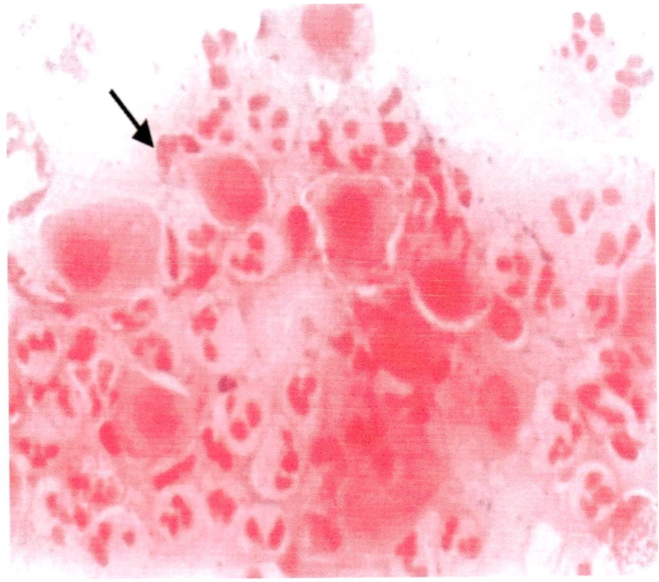

Gonorrhoea: Gram stain of cervical smear showing several polymorphonuclear cells with few intracellular Gram negative diplococci. Note several epithelial cells due to contamination with vaginal secretion (100x). Gram stain not sensitive in females.

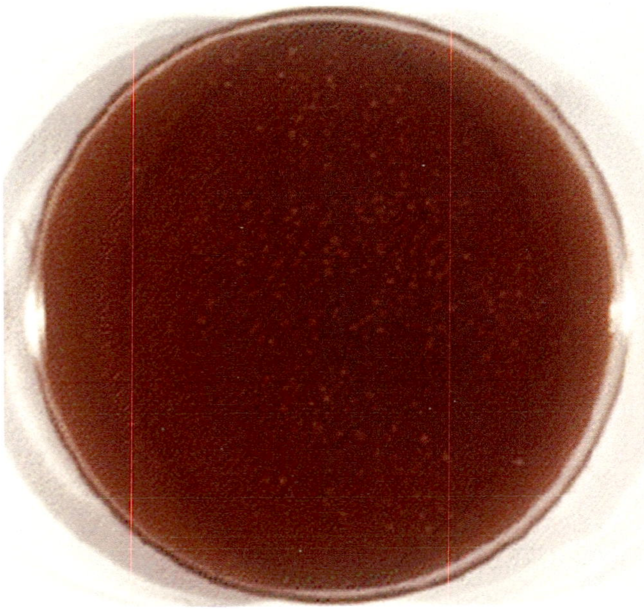

Gonorrhoea: Culture of *N. gonorrhoeae* on Thayer-Martin media showing small pin point colonies.
Courtesy: Dr Seema Sood, Department of Microbiology, AIIMS.

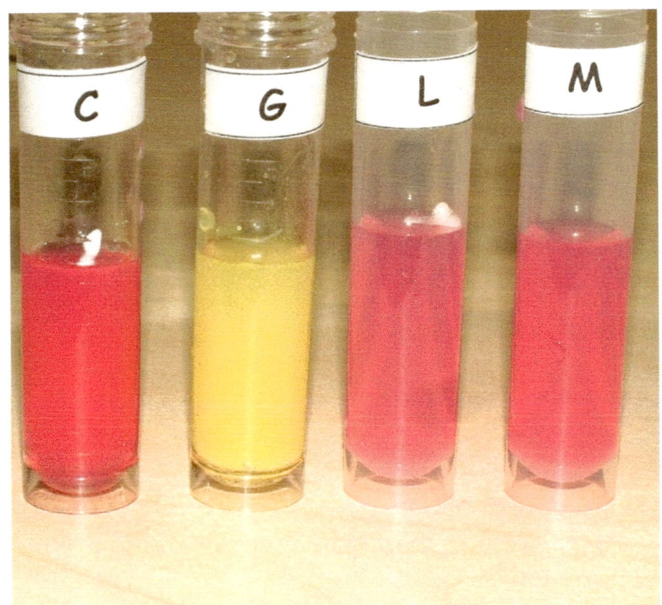

Gonorrhoea: Colonies of *N. gonorrhoeae* are confirmed by sugar fermentation tests. *N. gonorrhoeae* ferments glucose but not lactose, maltose and sucrose.

DIAGNOSIS

Based on Clinical Features

Diagnosis of gonorrhoea based on clinical features difficult.

- In males, profuse urethral discharge suggestive.
- In females, poor predictive value.

Lab Investigations

Demonstration of organism

- ***Sample:*** Urethral discharge (and if absent, swab from within urethra) after holding urine × 4 hours and massaging urethra. First void urine (FVU) for nucleic acid based tests. Endocervix (in women), rectum (in case of anal intercourse and in MSMs) and oropharynx (in case of orogenital sex and in MSMs).
- ***Gram stain:*** Shows many polymorphs and intracellular and extracellular Gram negative diplococci. Test sensitive in males but not in females.
- ***Culture:*** Essential in cervical, pharyngeal and rectal infections. Testing for antibiotic sensitivity (and penicillinase production) of great help in planning treatment.
    - Grow in selective media (Thayer-Martin medium; chocolate-agar with antibiotics), in presence of carbon dioxide.
    - Colonies small, rounded, glistening-gray.
    - Confirmed by sugar fermentation tests. Ferment glucose but not maltose, sucrose or lactose.
- ***Nucleic acid hybridization tests and nucleic acid amplification tests:*** Highly sensitive. Useful for FVU. Multiplex PCR with *C. trachomatis* available for patients with urethral discharge.

Serology

- Not useful.

TREATMENT

Specific Treatment

- Treatment regimens recommended based on geographic area (Table 6.1). Maintain high blood levels of appropriate antibiotics/chemotherapeutic agents with a single large dose (for uncomplicated gonorrhoea). Or repeated doses (for complicated cases). Treat sexual partners simultaneously.
- Simultaneous treatment for *C. trachomatis* recommended as coinfection common (syndromic treatment).

Special Situations

- ***Gonococcal conjunctivitis:*** Ceftriaxone 1 gm intramuscular, single dose.
- ***Gonococcal meningitis and endocarditis:*** Ceftriaxone 1-2 gm intravenous every 12 hours for 2 weeks.
- ***Disseminated gonococcal infection:*** Ceftriaxone 1 gm intramuscular or intravenous every 24 hours for 7 days.

Partner Management

Treat partner (symptomatic and asymptomatic) who have had sexual contact with patient in preceding 60 days.

Pregnant Woman

Ceftriaxone 250 mg intramuscular single dose. Or cefixime 400 mg single oral dose. Both with azithromycin 1 gm single oral dose (to cover *C. trachomatis*). Doxycycline and ciprofloxacin avoided.

In HIV Infected

Same as in HIV negative individuals.

Follow-up

- Re-examine after 3-5 days.

Other considerations

- Rule out HIV, HBV and syphilis at 1st visit.
- If negative, retest for syphilis and HIV 3 months after initial visit.

Table 6.1: Recommended treatment regimens for uncomplicated infection of urethra, cervix and rectum

CDC 2010	WHO 2003	NACO 2007
• Ceftriaxone 250 mg IM stat	• Ciprofloxacin 500 mg SOD*	• Cefixime 400 mg SOD*
OR	OR	PLUS
• Cefixime 400 mg SOD*	• Ceftriaxone 125 mg IM stat	• Azithromycin 1 gm SOD*
PLUS	OR	
• Azithromycin 1 gm SOD*	• Cefixime 400 mg SOD*	
OR	OR	
• Doxycycline 100 mg bid × 7 days	• Spectinomycin 2 gm IM stat	
Alternative regimens:		
• Cefpodoxime 400 mg oral SOD*		
• Cefuroxime 1 gm oral SOD*		
• Azithromycin 2 gm SOD*		

*SOD: Single oral dose. Azithromycin and doxycycline given to cover concomitant *C. trachomatis* infection.

CHAPTER 7

Non-Gonococcal Urethritis and Genital Tract Infections

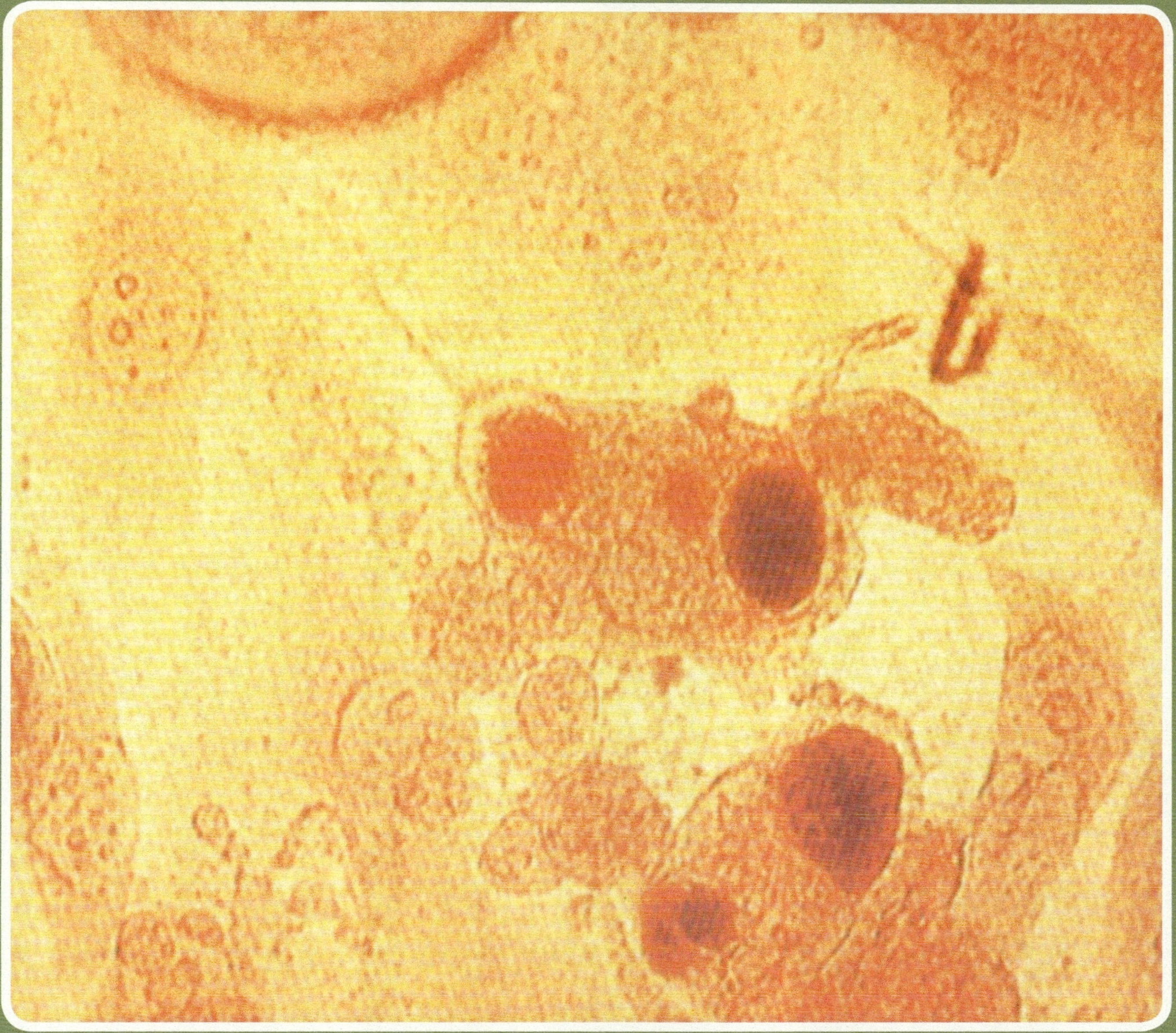

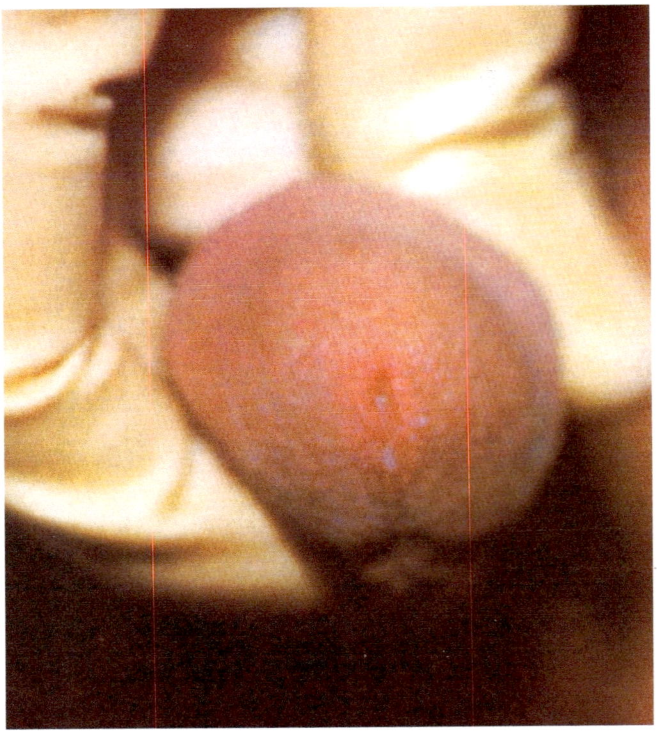

Chlamydial urethritis: Scant mucoid discharge present at urethral meatus in males.

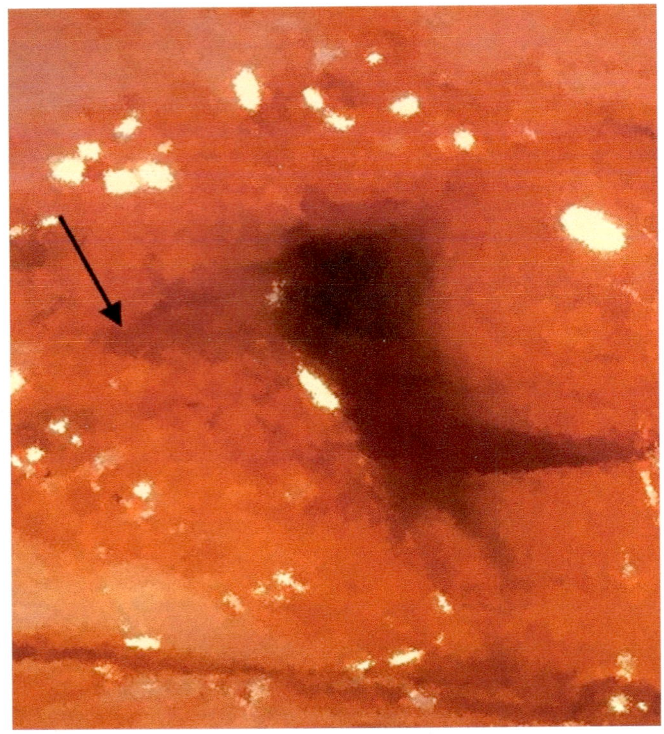

Chlamydial cervicitis: Minimal mucopurulent cervical discharge. Such a patient is asymptomatic. Or may have dysuria or postcoital bleeding. Note ectopy.

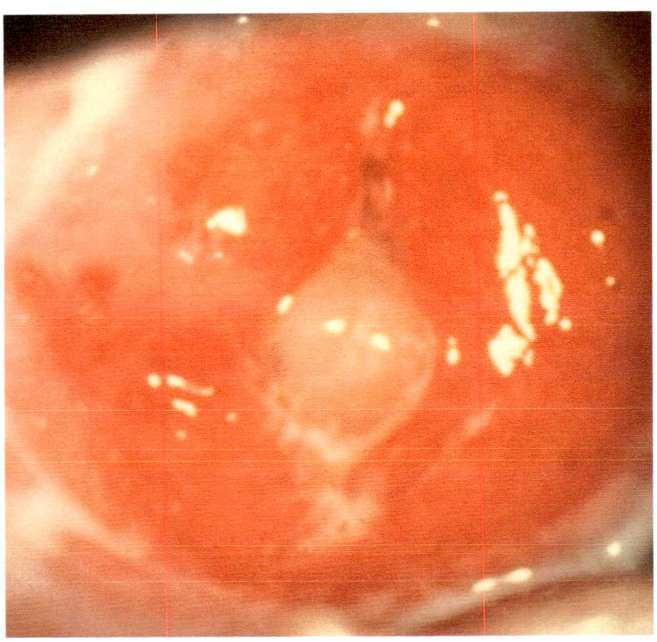

Chlamydial cervicitis: Sometimes discharge is profuse and patient presents with vaginal discharge.

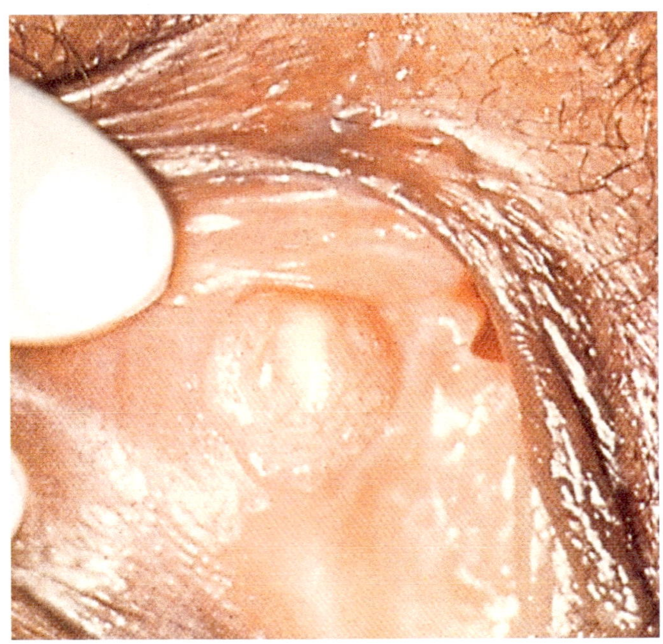

Chlamydial urethritis: Discharge present at urethral meatus in female. Urethritis occurs in more than half the patients with cervicitis and presents as dysuria.

DEFINITIONS

- ***Urethritis:*** Is presence of dysuria and urethral discharge. And on Gram stain of urethral smear, presence of ≥ 5 polymorphs/oil immersion field (OIF). Or persistent pyuria on first void urine (FVU). Includes infectious (gonococcal and nongonococcal) and noninfectious causes.
- ***Non-gonococcal urethritis (NGU):*** Is urethritis due to causes other than *Neisseria gonorrhoeae*. Gram stain of urethral discharge/swab shows ≥ 5 polymorphs/OIF and no Gram negative diplococci. Includes infectious and non-infectious causes (Table 7.1).
- ***Non-gonococcal non-chlamydial urethritis (NGNCU):*** Is urethritis due to causes other than *N.gonorrhoeae* and *Chlamydia trachomatis*. Is mainly caused by *Mycoplamsa genitalium, Ureaplasma urealyticum* and *Trichomonas vaginalis*.
- ***Recurrent urethritis:*** Is recurrence of urethritis within 90 days after response to treatment. And urethral smear showing ≥ 5 polymorphs/OIF. Recurrence of only symptoms without lab confirmation not considered recurrent urethritis. Due to reinfection because partner not treated. Or is not compliant. Or new infected partner.
- ***Persistent urethritis:*** Initial symptoms of urethral discharge persist despite compliant treatment by both partners. And urethral smear shows ≥ 5 polymorphs/OIF. Persistent symptoms without lab confirmation not considered persistent urethritis. Due to doxycycline or azithromycin resistant *Mycoplasma/Ureaplasma.* Or due to *T. vaginalis*.
- ***Cervicitis:*** Unlike urethritis, definition not standardised. Defined as > 30 polymorphs/HPF on Gram stain of endocervical smear. Or > 10 polymorphs/HPF of vaginal smear.

ETIOLOGY

Etiological Agents

Several organisms incriminated in causing non gonococcal genital infections (Table 7.1). Mixed infections due to more than one organism in 10-30%.

Transmission

Sexually transmitted, during unprotected intercourse.

EPIDEMIOLOGY

Geographic Distribution

- Worldwide distribution, no specific endemic areas.
- Now more frequent than gonococcal infection– increased prevalence partly because of better methods of detection of chlamydia, mycoplasma and ureaplasma.

Demographic Distribution

- More common in younger males.
- NGU in adolescents, mostly due to *M. genitalium* and *U. urealyticum*.
- NGU in young adults, mostly due to *C. trachomatis*.

CLINICAL FEATURES

Incubation Period

4 days to 2 months.

Signs and Symptoms in Males

- ***Urethritis:*** Generally mucoid discharge; less frequently, profuse creamy discharge. And dysuria. But often asymptomatic.
- ***Anorectal infections:*** Symptomatic proctitis rare. MSM may present with anorectal pain, discharge, tenesmus.

Table 7.1: Etiology of nongonococcal urethritis and genital tract infections

Commonly detected organisms	Less common organisms	Noninfective causes
Chlamydia trachomatis	*Herpes simplex*	*Trauma*
Ureaplasma urealyticum	*Adenovirus*	*Chemicals*
Mycoplasma genitalium	*Candida spp*	*Foreign bodies*
Trichomonas vaginalis	*Escherichia coli*	*Stricture*
	Staphylococcus saprophyticus	*Carcinoma*
	Hemophilus spp	*Urolithiasis*
	Neisseria meningitides	
	Streptococcus pneumonia	

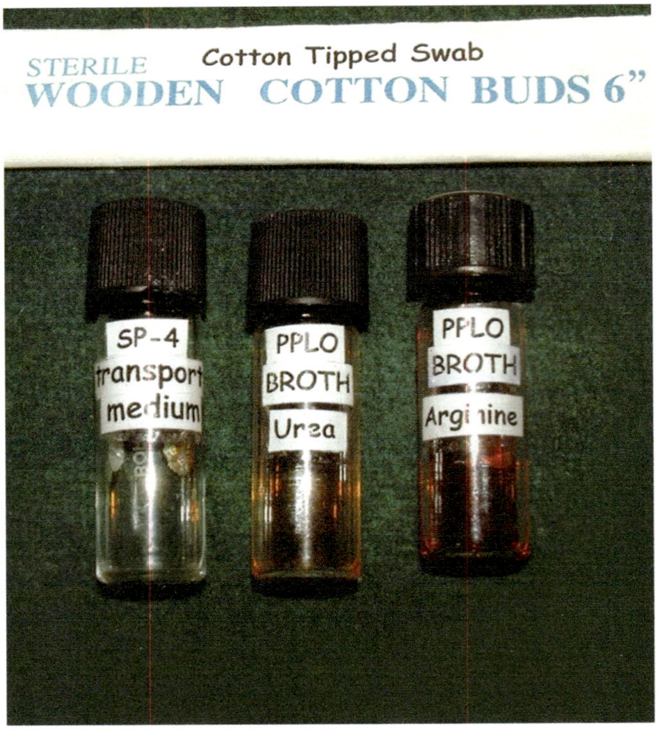

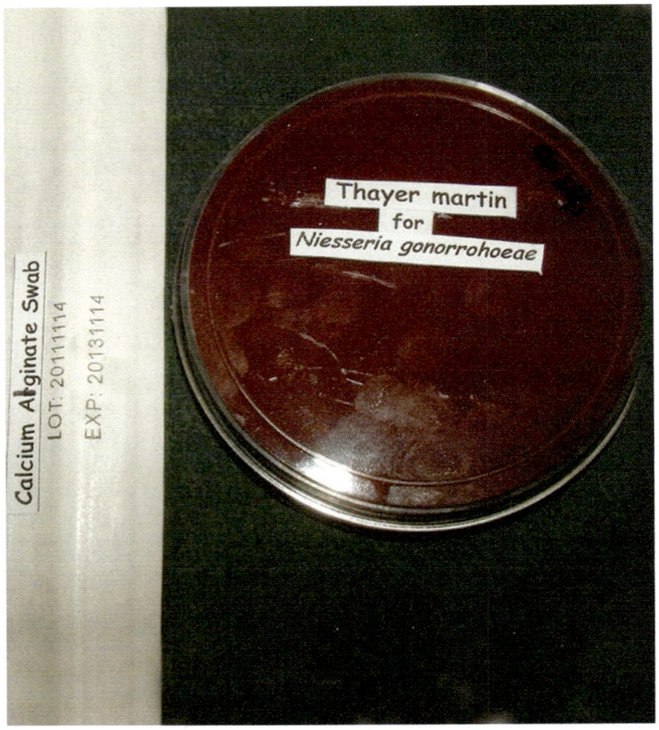

Non-gonococcal urethritis: Sample collection in urethral/cervical discharge. Samples collected for chlamydial culture (on cell lines) in transport medium, for ureaplasma culture in PPLO broth with urea, for mycoplasma culture in PPLO broth with arginine using wooden cotton tipped swabs. Always important to screen for *N.gonorrhoeae,* as coinfections common. Specimens for gonococcus collected using calcium alginate swabs and cultured on modified Thayer Martin medium.

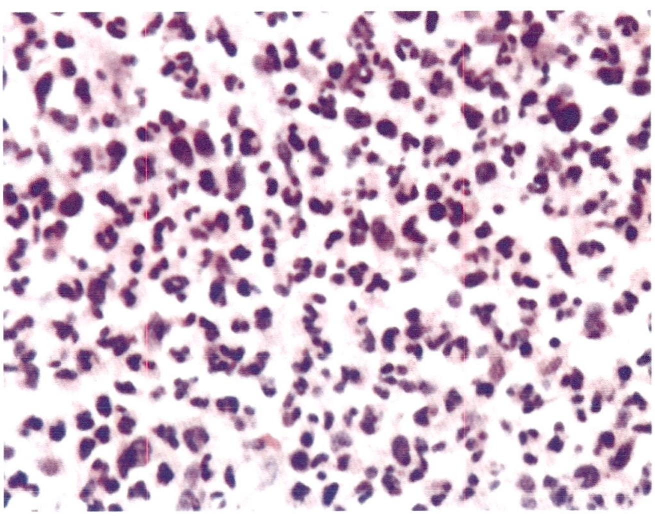

Non-gonococcal urethritis: Gram stain from urethral discharge showing ≥ 5 polymorphonuclear leucocytes in the absence of Gram-negative diplococci.

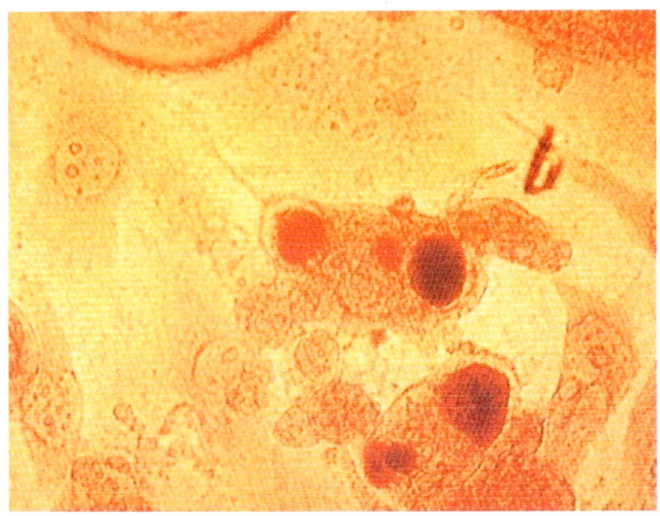

Chlamydial urethritis: Iodine staining of smear showing intracytoplasmic iodine stained chlamydia bodies.

Signs and Symptoms in Females

- ***Cervicitis:*** Most often asymptomatic. Or mild mucoid vaginal discharge. Other symptoms include post coital/intermenstrual bleeding. And lower abdominal pain. Per- speculum evaluation: cervical friability.
- ***Urethritis:*** Frequency, dysuria. Also suprapubic pain.
- ***Anorectal infections:*** Symptomatic proctitis rare.

Nongonococcal Conjunctivitis

- ***Neonates:*** Transmitted during birth through infected maternal passages.
- ***Adults:*** May be associated with concomitant genitourinary infection.

COMPLICATIONS

- ***Men:*** Epididymorchitis. Doubtful role in infertility. Reactive arthritis (Reiter's syndrome).
- ***Women:*** Pelvic inflammatory disease (10-40%), leading to tubal factor infertility, ectopic pregnancy and chronic pelvic pain. Rarely perihepatitis (Fitz-Hugh- Curtis syndrome).

HIV AND NONGONOCOCCAL GENITAL TRACT INFECTIONS (NGGTI)

- ***Effect of NGGTI on HIV:*** Increased transmission (4 fold).
- ***Effect of HIV on NGGTI:*** No definite alterations described.

DIAGNOSIS

Based on Clinical Features

Not sensitive not specific.

- ***In males:*** Dysuria with or without discharge. Discharge scant, mucoid in contrast to profuse purulent discharge of gonorrhoea. May be asymptomatic.
- ***In females:*** Asymptomatic mostly. Vaginal discharge minimal. Post coital/intermenstrual bleeding. Often lower abdominal pain.

Laboratory Investigations

For chlamydial infection

- ***Samples collected:***
  - *In males:* Intraurethral swab. Preferably after holding urine. First Void Urine (FVU) may be used for sensitive tests (PCR).
  - *In females:* Endocervical swab. Self obtained vaginal samples (SOVS). Or FVU in PCR.
- ***Direct microscopy[1]:***
  - *Giemsa staining:* Not sensitive. Shows basophilic intracytoplasmic bodies in epithelial cells.
  - *Iodine staining:* Not sensitive. Shows brown intracytoplasmic bodies.
  - *Direct fluorescent test:* Sensitive, specific but expensive and laborious.
  - *EIA:* Sensitive and specific. And simple.
  - *Point of care (rapid) tests:* Several available like chlamydia rapid test.
- ***Nucleic acid- based tests:***
  - *PCR:* Very sensitive and specific. Multiplex PCR for *C.trachomatis* and *N. gonorrhoeae* also available.
  - *Others:* Like ligase chain reaction.
- ***Culture:*** Earlier considered gold standard. On radiated McCoy cells, Hela-229 and BHK-2. Confirmed by Giemsa/iodine staining or fluorescence labeled antibodies.
- ***Serology:*** Not reliable for lower genital infection. May help for upper genital infection in women where isolation not possible.

For mycoplasma and ureaplasma infections

- ***Samples collected:*** As for *C.trachomatis*.
- ***Culture:*** Using PPLO broth and agar. Mycoplasma colonies have classical fried egg appearance. Ureaplasma colonies pinpoint (difficult to see without magnification). Stain blue with Dienes stain. Colonies further serotyped to determine serovars.
- ***PCR:*** Used both for identification of direct samples. And for identification of colonies on culture.
- ***Serological tests:*** Not standardised.

For T.vaginalis

- ***Samples collected:*** In females, sample from posterior fornix. In males, from urethra. For nucleic acid based tests, urine and SOVS also useful.
- ***Wet mount:*** Under 40x. Visible as pear shaped flagellate motile (jerky movements) organisms.
- ***Culture:*** On modified Diamond's media.

---

[1]Urethritis in males defined as ≥ 5 OIF on Gram stain of urethral secretions. Or persistent pyuria in FVU. Cervicitis defined as (though definition varies) > 30 polymorphs/HPF on Gram stain of endocervical smear. Or > 10 polymorphs/HPF field of vaginal smear.

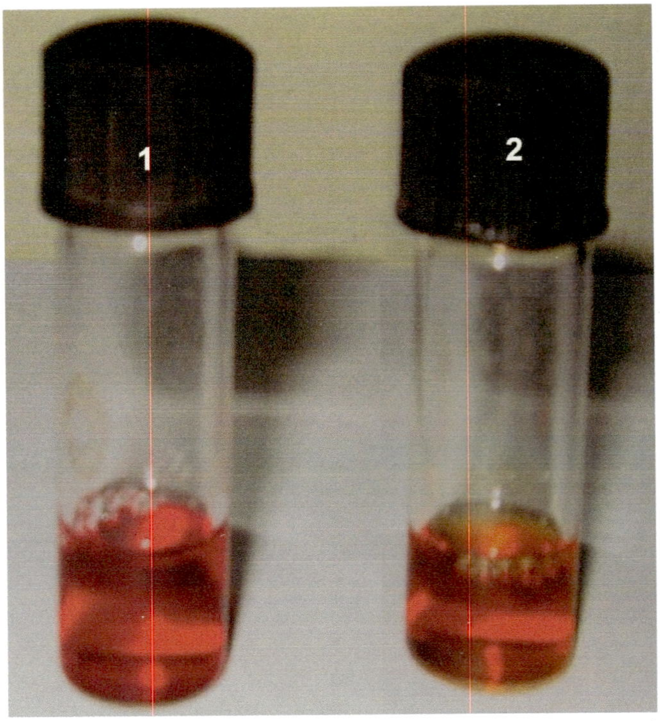

Culture of Mycoplasma spp: Sample taken using cotton tipped swab stick and inoculated in PPLO broth containing arginine. Tube 1: Culture positive. Tube 2: Culture negative. Positive broth tubes: subcultured on PPLO agar for further identification.
Courtesy: Dr B. Dhawan, Ms J. Rawere, Dept of Microbiology, AIIMS, New Delhi.

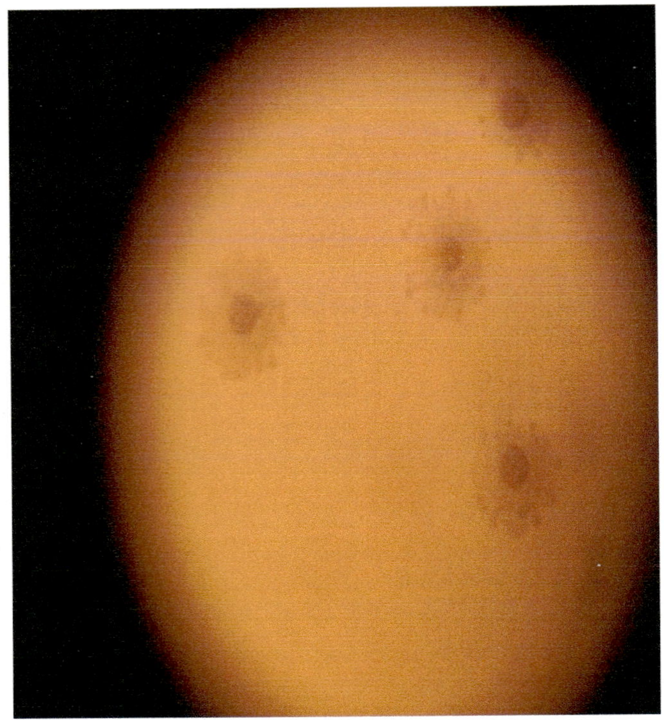

Colonies of M.hominis: Characteristic colonies on PPLO agar showing fried egg appearance.
Courtesy: Dr B. Dhawan, Ms J. Rawere, Dept of Microbiology, AIIMS, New Delhi.

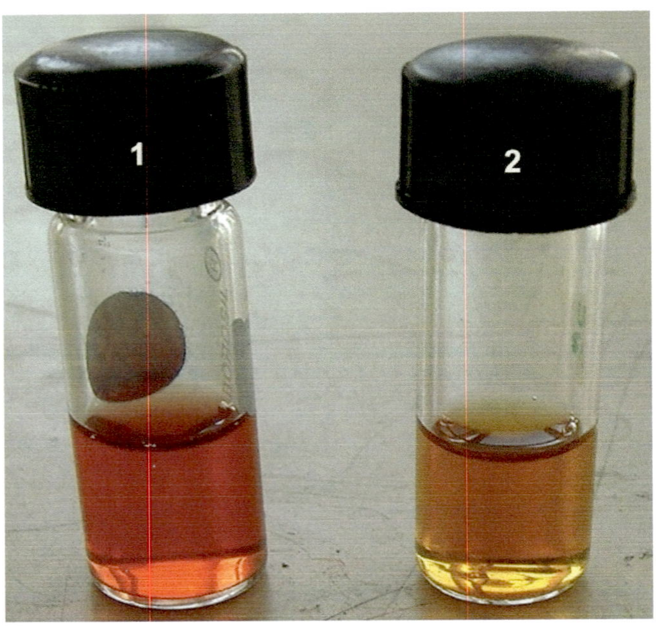

Culture of Ureaplasma spp: Sample taken using cotton tipped swab stick and inoculated in PPLO broth containing urea. Tube 1: Culture positive. Tube 2: Culture negative. Positive broth tubes: subcultured on PPLO agar for further identification.
Courtesy: Dr B. Dhawan, Ms J. Rawere, Dept of Microbiology, AIIMS, New Delhi.

Colonies of U. urealyticum: Diene's stained colonies of *U.urealyticum* on PPLO agar.
Courtesy: Dr B. Dhawan, Ms J. Rawere, Dept of Microbiology, AIIMS, New Delhi.

Table 7.2: Treatment guidelines for non gonococcal urethritis

CDC 2010	WHO 2003	NACO 2007
• Azithromycin, 1 gm SOD* **OR** • Doxycycline, 100 mg bid	• Doxycycline, 100 mg bid × 7 days **OR** • Azithromycin, 1 g SOD*	• Azithromycin, 1 gm SOD*
Alternative regimens • Erythromycin base, 500 mg qid × 7 days • Levofloxacin 500 mg od • Ofloxacin 300 mg bid × 7 days	Alternative regimens • Amoxycillin, 500 mg tid × 7 days **OR** • Erythromycin, 500 mg qid × 7 days **OR** • Ofloxacin, 300 mg bid × 7 days **OR** • Tetracycline, 500 mg qid × 7 days	

*SOD: Single oral dose

Table 7.3: Treatment guidelines for recurrent and persistent urethritis

CDC 2010	WHO 2003	NACO 2007
If patient non-compliant or re-exposure • Azithromycin 1 gm SOD* **OR** • Doxycycline 100 mg bid If patient compliant and no history of re-exposure: • Metronidazole or tinidazole, 2 gm SOD* **PLUS** • Azithromycin, 1 gm SOD*	• Metronidazole, 400 mg or 500 mg bid × 7 days **OR** • Tinidazole, 500 mg bid × 5 days	• Secnidazole, 2 gm SOD*

*SOD: Single oral dose

- ***Others:*** Latex agglutination: Sensitive and rapid, point of care test. Nucleic acid based tests (sensitive; also used on urine and SOVS).

TREATMENT

- Treatment for *C.trachomatis* often combined with that of *N.gonorrhoeae* (Table 7.2) because of frequent co-infection (syndromic approach).
- If symptoms persist, to treat *T. vaginalis* (Table 7.2).

SEXUALLY ACQUIRED REACTIVE ARTHRITIS

- Previously known as Reiter's syndrome (triad of urethritis, arthritis and conjunctivitis). New term, reactive arthritis.
- Aseptic arthritis following non-gonococcal urethritis in a genetically predisposed individual termed sexually acquired reactive arthritis (SARA).
- May also follow other infections as a trigger (dysentery or respiratory tract infection).

Epidemiology

Geographic distribution

- Prevalence correlates with prevalence of HLA B27 seropositivity in population.
- Common in parts of Western Europe, South East Asia.

Demographic distribution

- SARA occurs mainly (only!) in males.
- Common in young adults (of 20-40 years age group).
- Occurs in 1-3% of patients after NGU.

Etiology

- Occurs following NGU, *C.trachomatis* the commonest pathogen.
- HLA-B27 most commonly correlated with SARA.

CLINICAL FEATURES

Incubation Period

Varies from less than a month to 3 months.

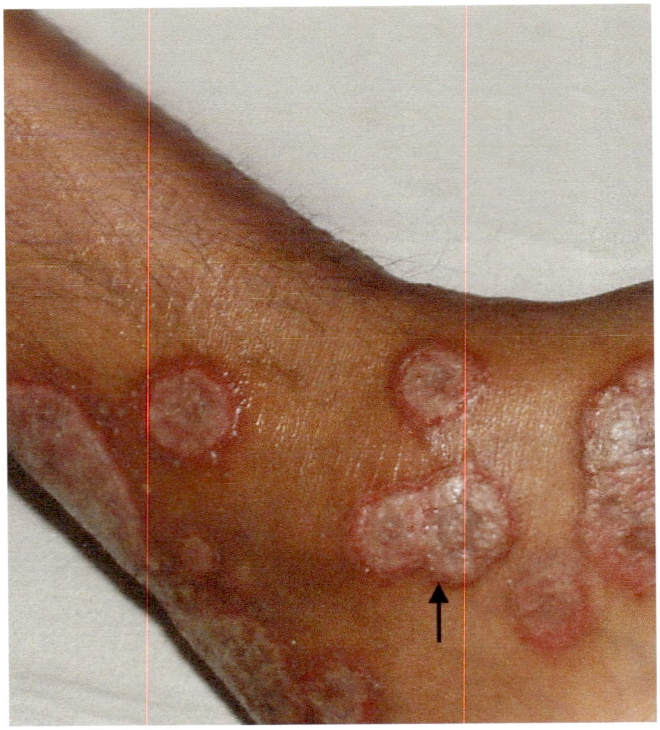

Skin lesions of Reiter's syndrome: Well defined annular plaques with heaped up scales at the periphery, which is often studded with pustules.

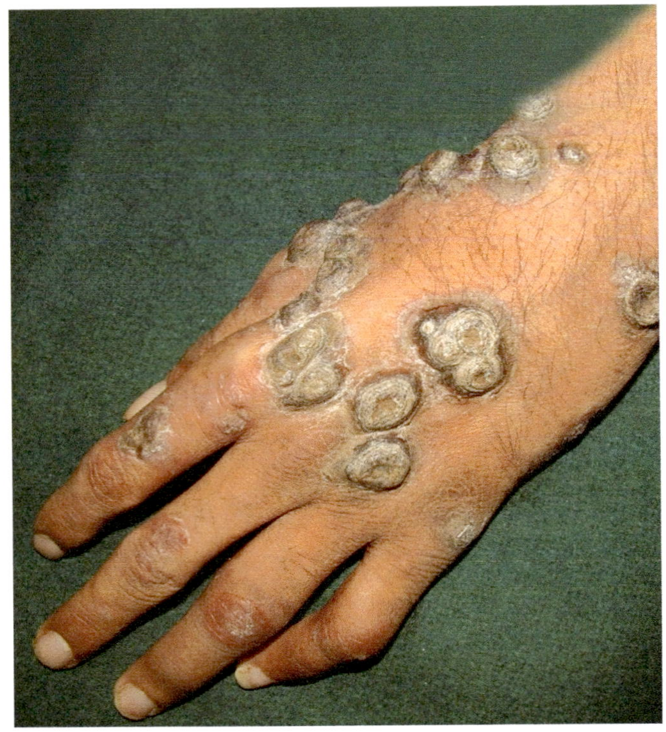

Skin lesions of Reiter's syndrome: Hyperkeratotic lesions some conical resembling a limpet-the so called rupioid lesions. Many of have a central cupping, similar to an oyster shell.

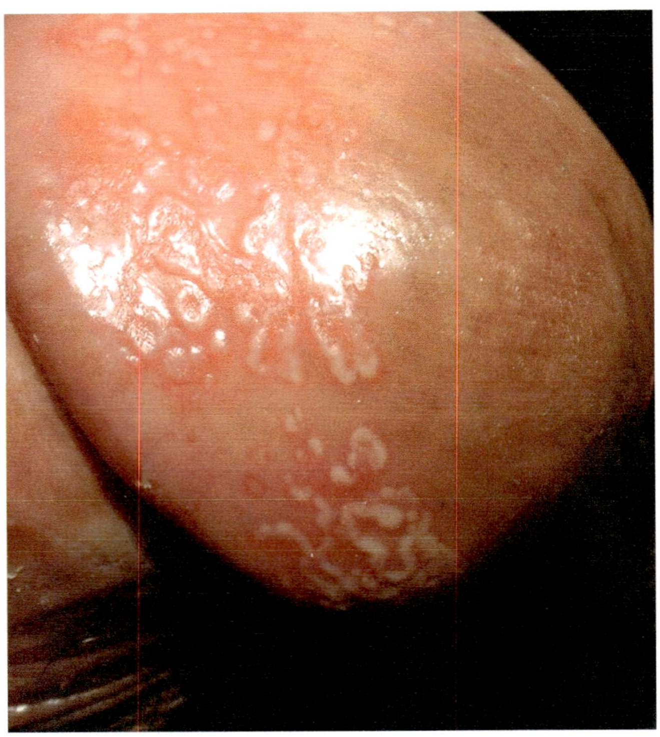

Circinate balanitis: Moist annular plaques with serpiginous margin.

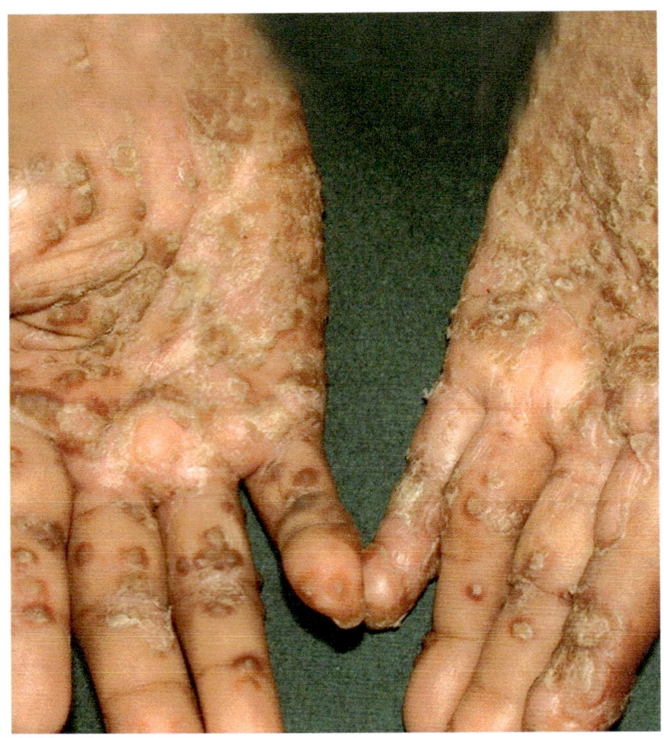

Keratoderma blenorrhagicum: Erythematous hyperkeratotic plaques on palms (and soles).

Manifestations

- ***Spondyloarthropathy:*** Involves single or multiple joints asymmetrically (at least initially):
  - Relapses and remissions frequent.
  - Lower limb (knee, ankle) joints most often affected. Also sacroiliitis.
  - Destructive arthritis.
- ***Conjunctivitis:***
  - Bilateral or unilateral.
  - Variable severity with spontaneous clearance.
  - Occasionally uveitis.
- ***Mucocutaneous lesions:***
  - *Skin lesions:* Well-defined erythematous scaly plaques, usually annular with heaped up scales and frequently pustules, crusts and sometimes vesicles at periphery. Sometimes lesions conical (limpet-like)-the so called rupioid lesions.
  - *Circinate balanitis:* Moist, superficial, erythematous plaques with serpiginous margins occurring on glans penis.
  - *Keratoderma blenorrhagicum:* Erythematous well defined plaques with heaped up keratotic crusts, occurring on palms and soles. Removal of crusts reveals underlying erosions.
  - *Oral mucosa:* Geographic tongue. And painless, superficial mucosal ulcers.
  - *Nail changes:* Subungual hyperkeratosis, pitting, yellowish discolouration of nail plate, onycholysis.

COMPLICATIONS

- Mutilating arthritis.
- Contractures leading to immobility.
- Anemia of chronic disease.

DIAGNOSIS

No definite diagnostic test. Diagnosis based on a combination of clinical features, histopathology, negative rheumatoid factor and HLA-B27 positivity.

Based on Clinical Features

- Several criteria for diagnosis of reactive arthritis. Many include molecular tests.
- Commonly used clinical criteria include:
- Seronegative asymmetrical arthropathy affecting predominantly lower limbs and lasting more than 1 month.
- **Plus** at least 2 (some use 1) of following:
  - History of genital discharge/dysuria/diarrhoea for at least 1 day antecedating arthritis by 3-42 days.
  - Inflammatory eye disease.
  - Mucocutaneous disease including circinate balanitis, keratoderma blennorrhagicum, pustular or rupioid lesions.

Laboratory Investigations

- ***Skin biopsy:*** Massive hyperkeratosis, parakeratosis, acanthosis. Plenty of neutrophils within epidermis forming microabscesses; dilated capillaries in superficial dermis, neutrophils in perivascular location.
- ***Rheumatoid factor:*** Negative.
- ***HLA-B27:*** Positive. Expensive and not freely available.
- ***Urethral swab:***
  - *Gram's stain:* ≥ 5 polymorphs/HPF.
  - Detection of chlamydia, mycoplasma and ureaplasma by various techniques.
- ***Radiology:*** Of affected joints to look for enthesitis and arthritis. X-ray of heel to look for calcaneal spur.
- ***Serological tests for other STIs:*** HIV, syphilis, HBV.

TREATMENT

- ***Skin and mucosal lesions:***
  - *Mild to moderate disease:* Topical steroids with or without salicylic acid.
  - *Severe involvement:* Oral methotrexate, retinoids, cyclosporine.
- ***Joints:***
  - *Oligoarthritis:* NSAIDS, intra-articular corticosteroids.
  - *Polyarthritis. Or disabling arthritis:* Systemic steroids, methotrexate, cyclosporine.
- ***Role of antibiotics:***
  - *If chlamydial antigen positive:* Doxycycline for two weeks.
  - *If chlamydial antigen negative:* No proven advantage (in changing course of disease. Or prognosis) of giving short or long course of antibiotics.

3 SECTION

VIRAL SEXUALLY TRANSMITTED INFECTIONS

Chapter 8

Genital Herpes

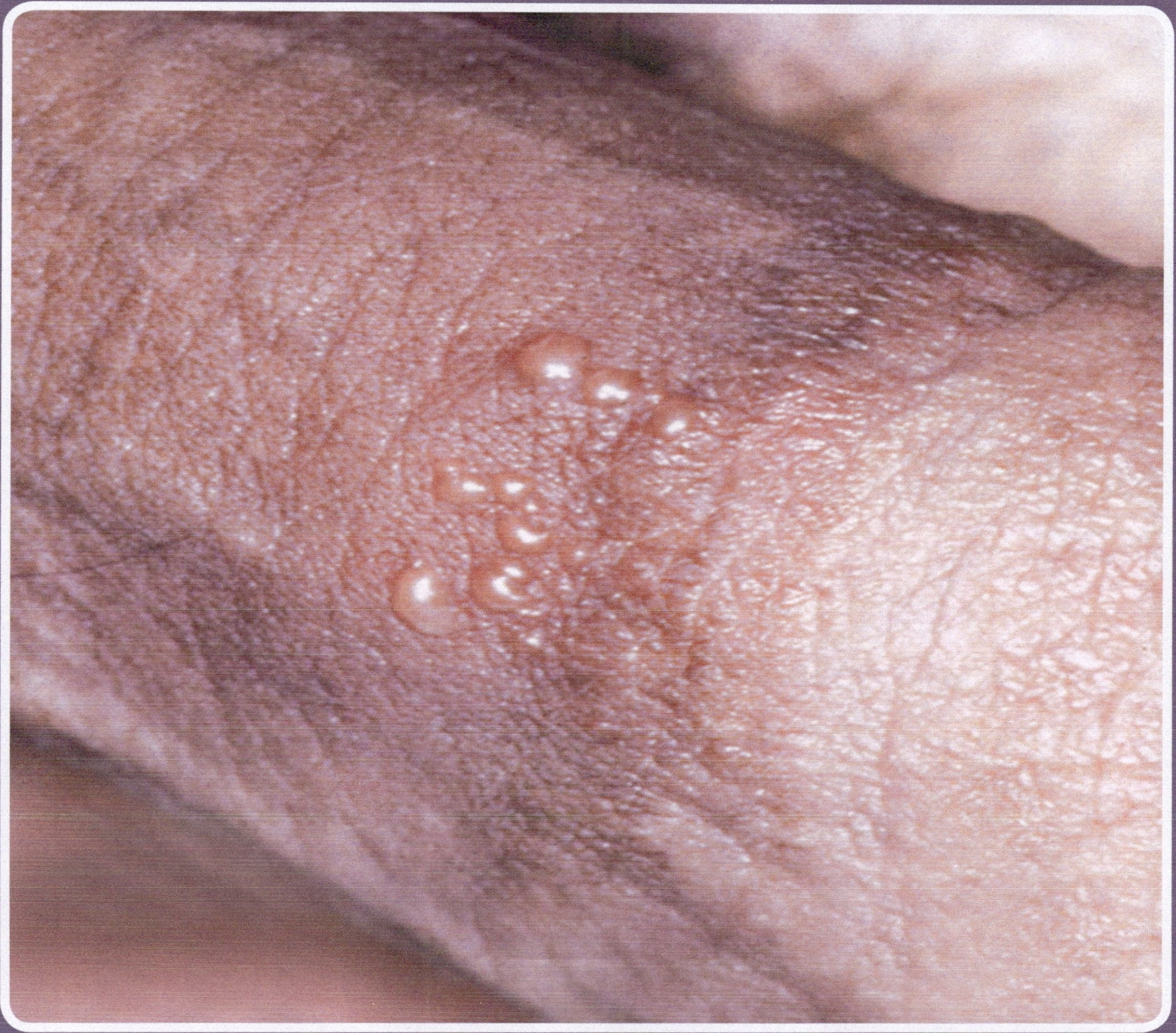

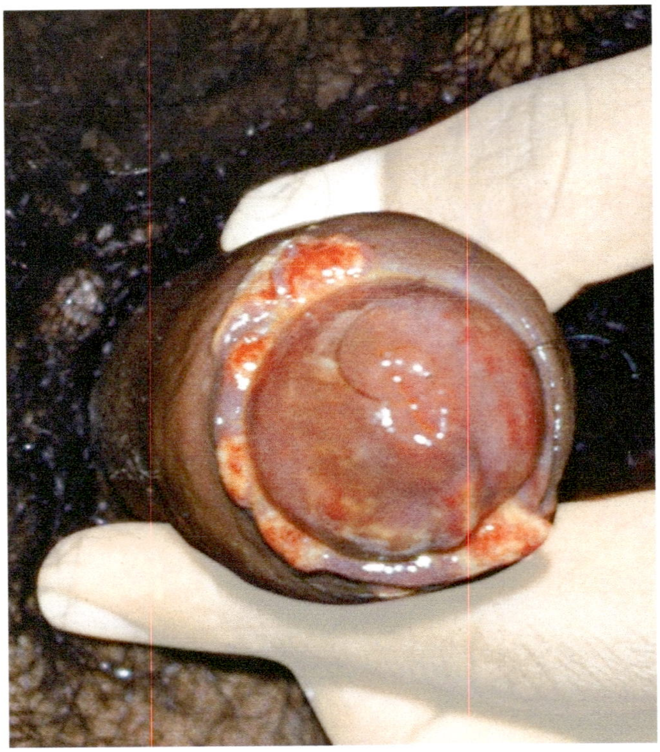

Primary genital herpes: Multiple, erythematous superficial erosions, present circumferentially on prepuce and on glans. Difficult to retract the prepuce. Patient had bilateral tender lymphadenopathy and constitutional symptoms.

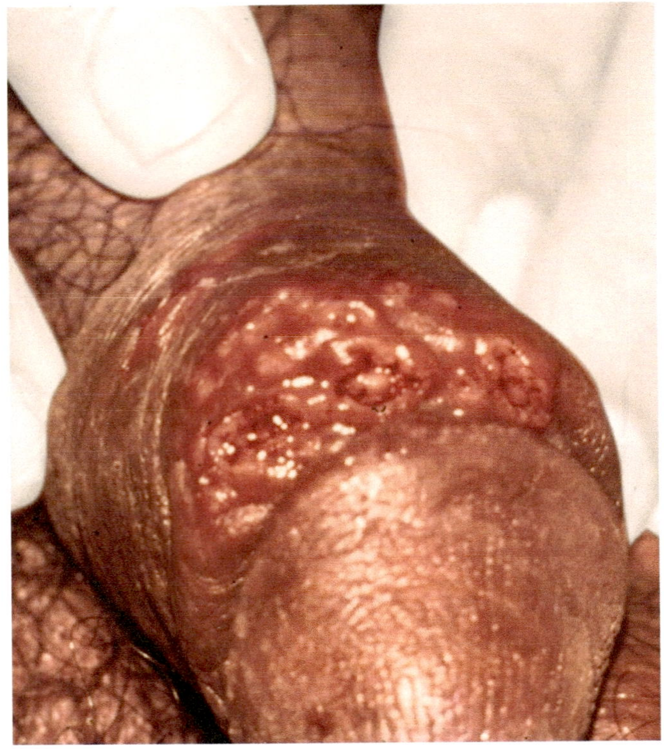

Primary genital herpes: Large erosion with polycyclic margins involving under surface of prepuce. Patient had bilateral tender inguinal lymphadenopathy and constitutional symptoms.

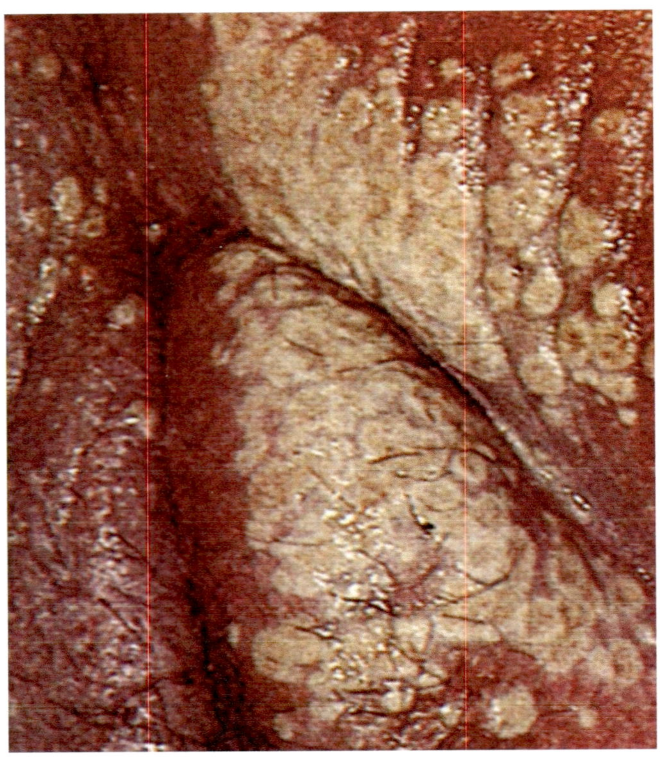

Primary genital herpes: Closely grouped vesicles (some umbilicated) on the vulva, almost appearing as a white plaque. This patient is pregnant.

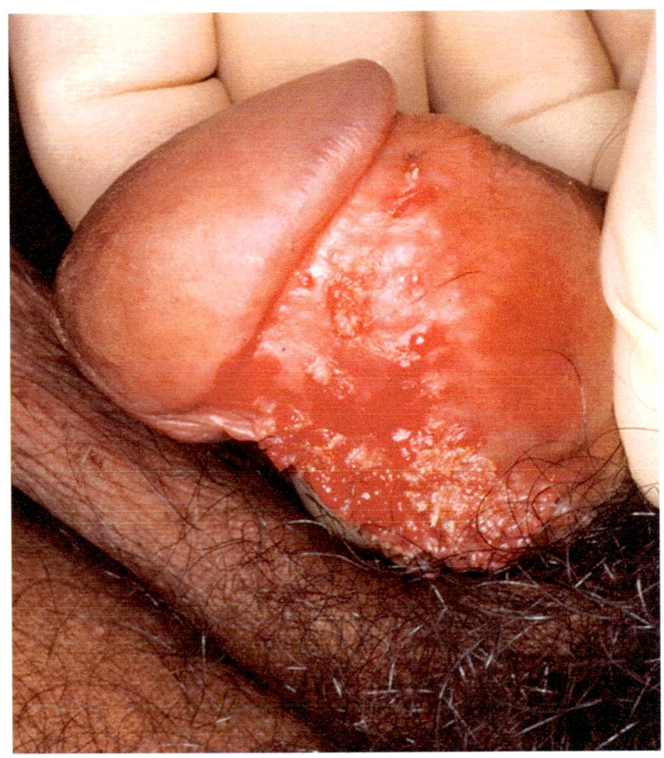

First episode genital herpes: Grouped vesicles and superficial erythematous erosions on prepuce, seen on retraction of prepuce. Patient did not have previous history of lesions-so labelled 1st episode GH.

Genital herpes (GH), a recurrent viral infection.

ETIOLOGY

Etiological Agent

- Herpes simplex virus (HSV).
- Has a double-stranded, linear DNA genome (core) encased within icosahedral protein cage (capsid). Which is wrapped by proteinaceous cover (tegument) which is surrounded by outer lipid membrane (envelope) with spikes.
- Two main subtypes: HSV-1, HSV-2.
  - Prevalence of HSV-1 as a cause of anogenital herpes, specially 1st episode, increasing (50%).
  - Majority cases of recurrent GH due to HSV-2.
- Clinical features of HSV-1 and HSV-2 GH almost similar but with some differences (Table 8.1).

Transmission

- ***Sexual contact:*** Genital, anogenital and oro-genital intercourse.Contact during asymptomatic shedding[1], commonest mode of transmission. Shedding of HSV-2 >> HSV-1.
- ***Non-sexual:*** Direct skin to skin contact.

Table 8.1: Differences between HSV-1 and HSV-2 infection

	HSV-1	HSV-2
Prevalence	Lower	Higher
Subclinical shedding of virus	Less	More
Risk of transmission	Less	More
Recurrences	Fewer	More
Mother to child transmission	More	Less

- ***Vertical transmission:*** Transmission to infant before, during or after delivery. Mothers mostly asymptomatic. Vertical transmission of HSV1 > HSV2.

EPIDEMIOLOGY

Geographic Distribution

Worldwide distribution. Now commonest cause of genital ulcer disease globally.

Demographic Distribution

- Acquired in adolescence. Or young adulthood.
- More males clinically symptomatic. More women serologically affected.

CLINICAL FEATURES

Incubation Period

3-14 days.

Classification

Clinically classified as:

- Primary GH.
- First episode GH.
- Recurrent GH.

Morphology

Primary GH

- Often silent. Sometimes clinically overt. Local prodrome (pain, itching) followed by vesicles (small,

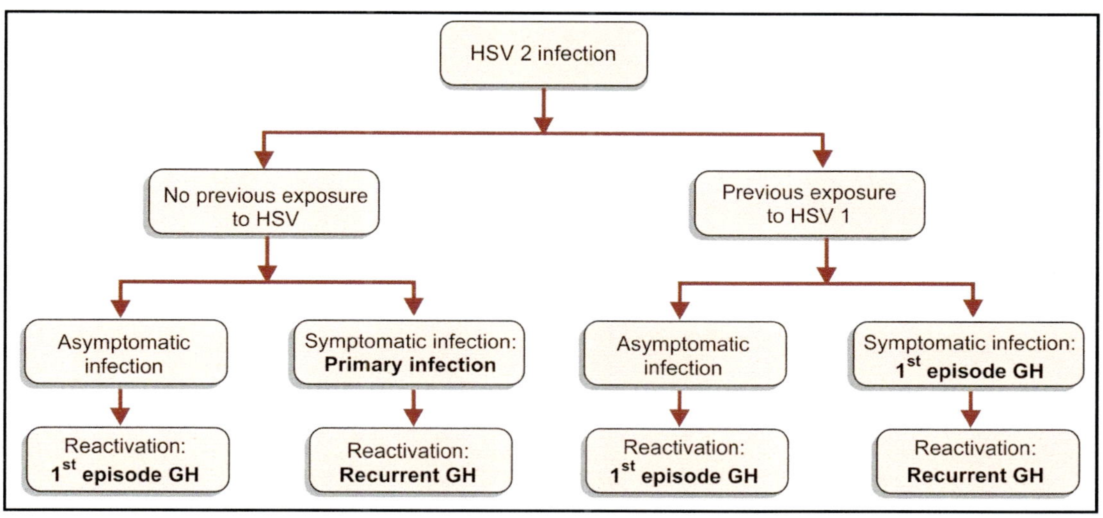

Classification of genital herpes

[1]**Asymptomatic shedding:** Shedding of virus in absence of lesions.

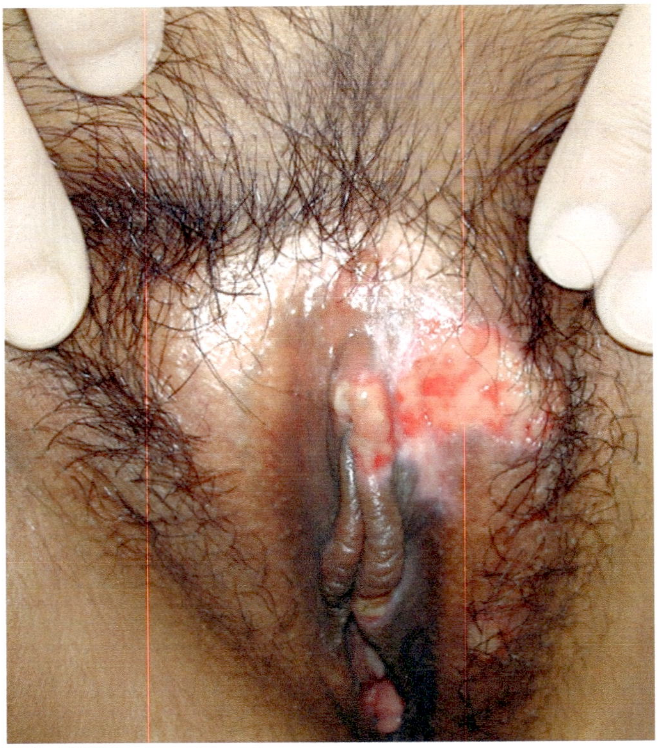

First episode genital herpes: Well-defined erosions with circinate margins present on inner aspect of labia majora and labia minora.

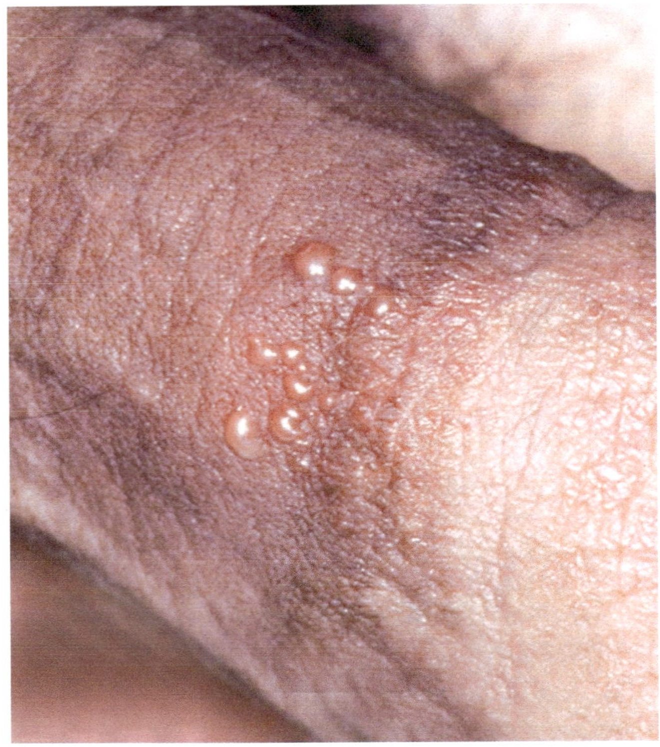

Recurrent genital herpes: Grouped tiny vesicles on shaft of penis. No lymphadenopathy or constitutional symptoms.

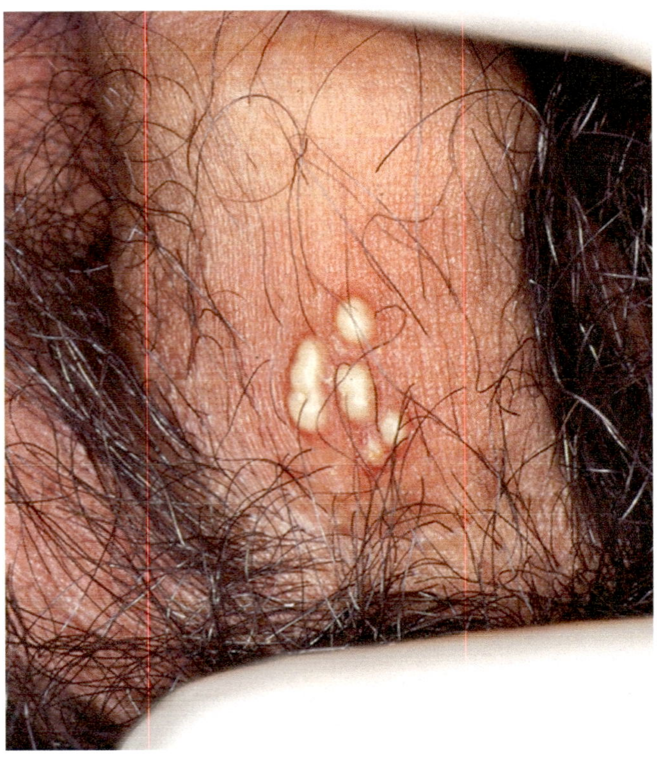

Recurrent genital herpes: Grouped pustules appearing at site of previous lesions.

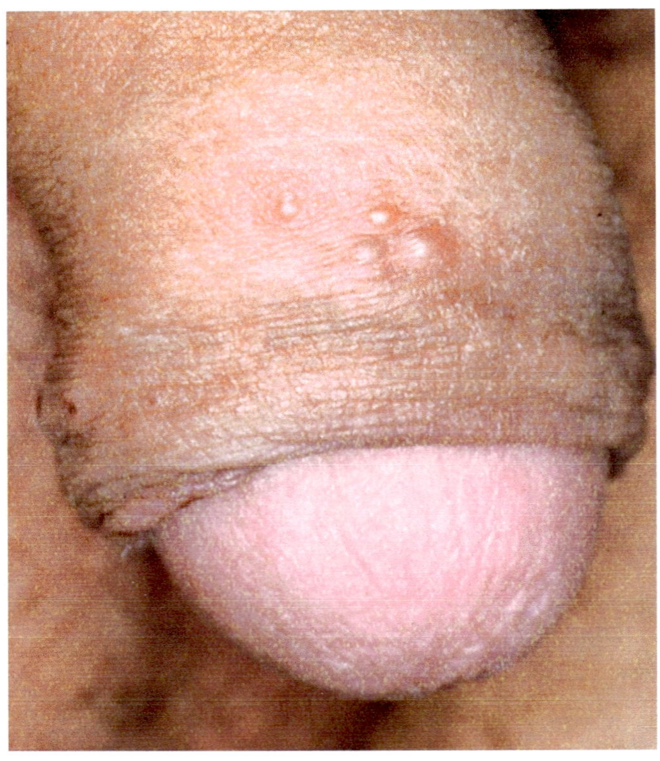

Recurrent genital herpes: Few tiny grouped vesicles on prepuce.

grouped, painful) or pustules on erythematous base. Rupture in 2-4 days to form erosions or ulcers (polycyclic). Often large areas (including adjoining extragenital) involved. Heal without scarring in 2-3 weeks. May present as balanoposthitis or vulvovaginitis. Or as urethral (if intraurethral)/vaginal (if on cervix) discharge.

- Tender, non-suppurative inguinal (often bilateral) lymphadenopathy.
- Constitutional symptoms frequent.

First episode GH

- First clinical manifestation of GH in a patient with serological evidence of previous HSV-1/HSV-2 infection.
- Smaller lesions, shorter course, less viral shedding.
- Lymphadenopathy less conspicuous.
- Constitutional symptoms less frequent and less severe.

Recurrent GH

- Common.
- Duration of remissions unpredictable. Recurrences more common with HSV-2, more frequent in men, in patients with prolonged primary infection and probably decrease with time.
- ***Precipitating factors:*** Emotional stress, physical fatigue, menstruation, febrile episodes.
- Prodrome of itching or burning. Few, small grouped vesicles on normal or erythematous base. Vesicles rupture easily to form tiny, shallow, painful erosions with polycyclic margins.
- Heal in about a week leaving normal skin. Or depigmentation.
- Recurrences occur at or around the same site.
- Lymphadenopathy and constitutional symptoms uncommon.

Sites of Lesions

- Labia majora and minora, cervix in females. Glans, prepuce in males. Also penile skin and urethral meatus.
- Bilateral and extensive in primary episode; localized in recurrent episodes.

Variants

Atypical features often immunocompromised states (HIV-infection):

- Hyperkeratotic, verrucous plaques.
- Chronic non-healing ulcers.
- Pseudogranuloma herpeticum: vegetative plaque resembling donovanosis.

COMPLICATIONS

- ***Extragenital lesions:*** Over thighs, lower abdomen.
- ***Pelvic inflammatory disease.***
- ***Erythema multiforme:*** Often recurrent.
- ***Hematogenous dissemination:*** To internal organs aseptic meningitis, encephalitis, radiculomyopathy.
- ***Neonatal herpes:***
  - Most neonatal infections acquired from asymptomatic mothers.
  - *Factors affecting acquisition of neonatal infection:*
    - Higher with primary 1st episode infection acquired in 3rd tremester (30-50%) than recurrent GH (<1%).
    - Higher with HSV-1 than HSV-2.
  - *Manifestations:* 3 types recognised:
    - Localized form: Vesicles, bullae occurring around eyes, mouth or localized area of skin.
    - Disseminated form: Dissemination to internal organs. Serious condition.
    - Central nervous system: Encephalitis. Serious condition, with poor prognosis.

GENITAL HERPES AND HIV

- ***Effect of GH on HIV:*** Amplified (7-10 fold) sexual transmission of HIV in presence of genital lesions of herpes.
- ***Effect of HIV on GH:***
  - Prolonged and severe episodes of genital, perianal or oral herpes. Chronic nonhealing ulcers, lasting more than a month and with herpetiform margins in perianal area characteristic of GH in HIV infected.
  - Increased asymptomatic shedding.
  - Lesions atypical—verrucous plaques, chronic non healing ulcers, pseudogranulomatous herpes.

DIAGNOSIS

Based on Clinical Features

Diagnosis of GH based on clinical features both insensitive and nonspecific. So requires lab confirmation. Clinical clues to diagnosis include:

- Recurrences.

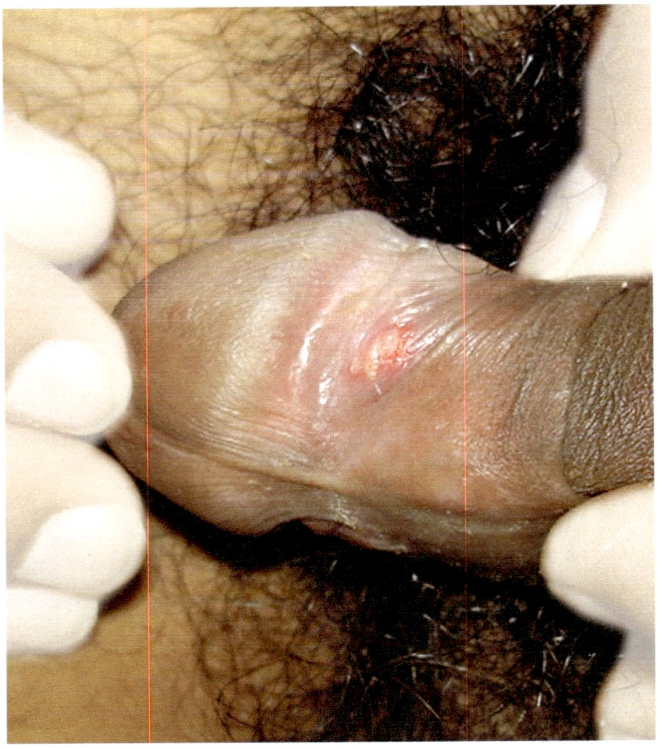

Recurrent genital herpes: Small grouped erosions on undersurface of prepuce.

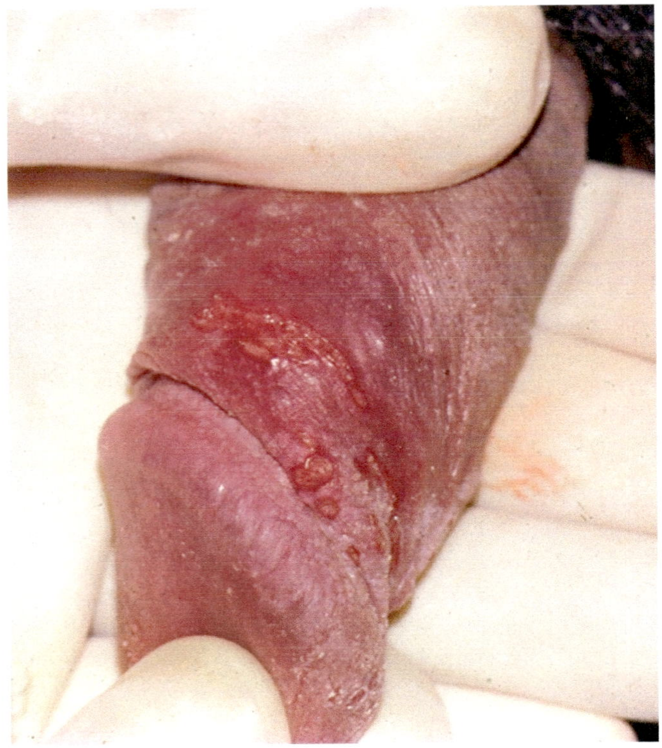

Recurrent genital herpes: Multiple erosions with polycyclic margins, nonindurated base.

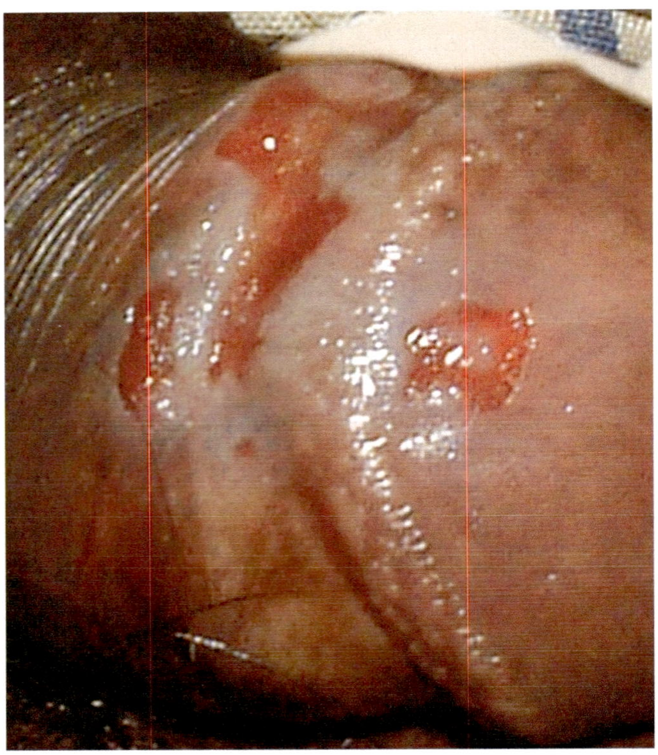

Recurrent genital herpes: Well-defined erosions with polycyclic margins.

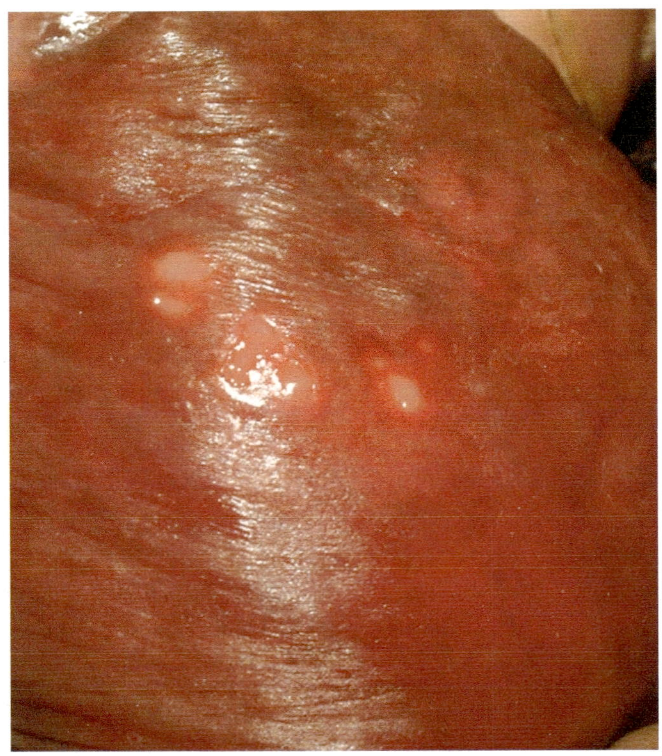

Recurrent genital herpes: Tiny well-defined erosions formed by rupturing of vesicles. Minimal involvement common in recurrent episodes.

- Grouped vesicles rupturing to form non-indurated painful erosions with polycyclic margins. Symptoms severe in primary *vis-a-vis* recurrent GH.

Laboratory Investigations

Demonstration of organism

- ***Samples:*** For Tzanck smear: floor of erosion. For culture: fluid from vesicle, larger the better. If crusted lesions, from floor after removing crust. Ectocervix better than endocervix.
- ***Tzanck smear:***
  - Easy to perform, inexpensive.
  - Multinucleated giant cells (MNGCs) with intranuclear eosinophilic inclusion bodies with a clear halo.
  - Does not differentiate between HSV-1 and HSV-2 infection.

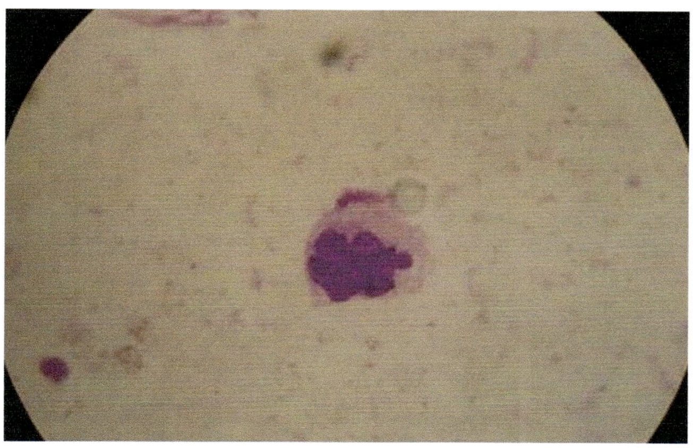

Tzanck smear in genital herpes: Multinucleated giant cell. Enlarged cell with multiple clustered nuclei containing eosinophilic bodies.

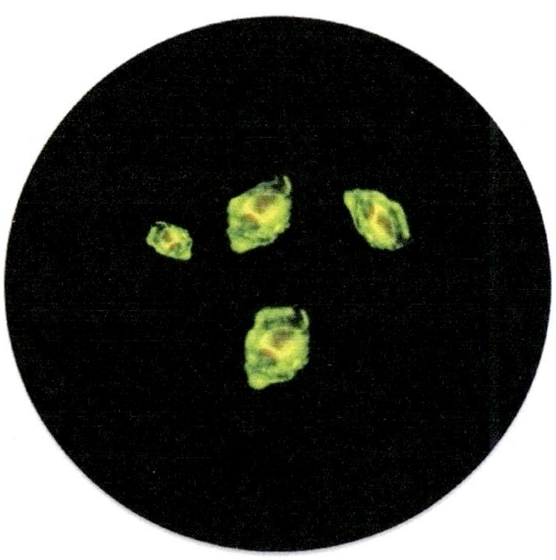

Direct immunofluresence test on Tzanck smear in genital herpes: Showing apple green intracellular fluorescence.

  - Good sensitivity in vesicular and early erosions; low in healing lesions.
- ***Direct immunofluorescence test:*** Rapid. More sensitive than culture. Shows apple green intracellular fluorescence.
- ***Polymerase chain reaction (PCR):*** Preferred test. Rapid, sensitive and specific especially in late lesions. Also multiplex PCR with *T. pallidum* and *H. ducreyi* (common pathogens for genital ulcer disease) available.
- ***Others:*** Immunoperoxidase tests and enzyme immunoassay.
- ***Culture:***
  - On human diploid fibroblast cell lines. Or vero cell line.
  - Cytopathic effect noted. Isolates further typed to determine whether HSV-1 or HSV-2.
  - Specific. But low sensitivity, especially in recurrent and late (healing) lesions.
  - Antiviral sensitivity can also be tested.

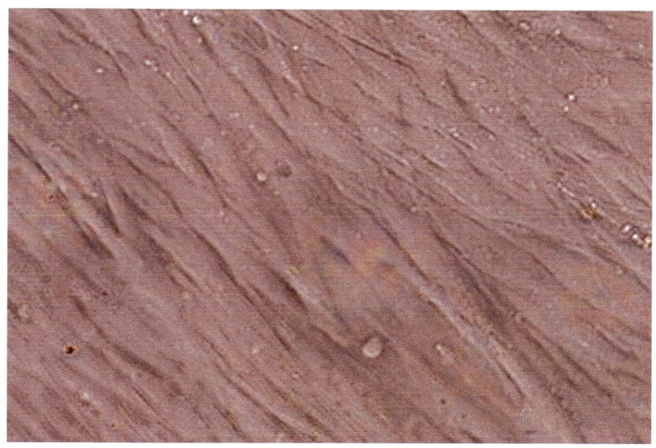

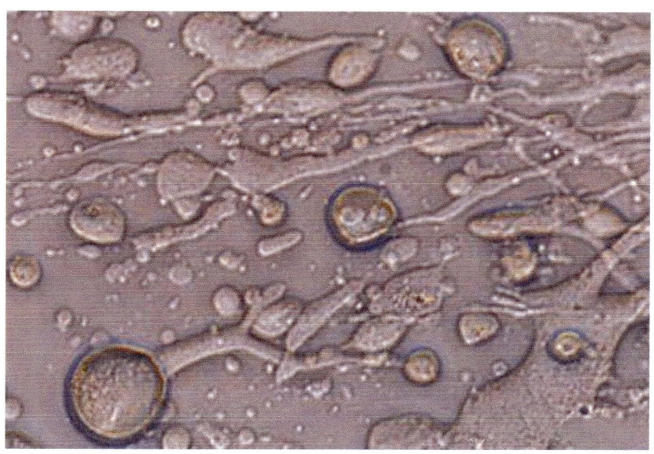

Herpes simplex virus on tissue culture causing a cytopathic effect usually within 48 hours. Further typed to determine whether HSV-1 and HSV-2.

Courtesy: Dr. Lalit Dhar, Department of Microbiology, AIIMS, New Delhi.

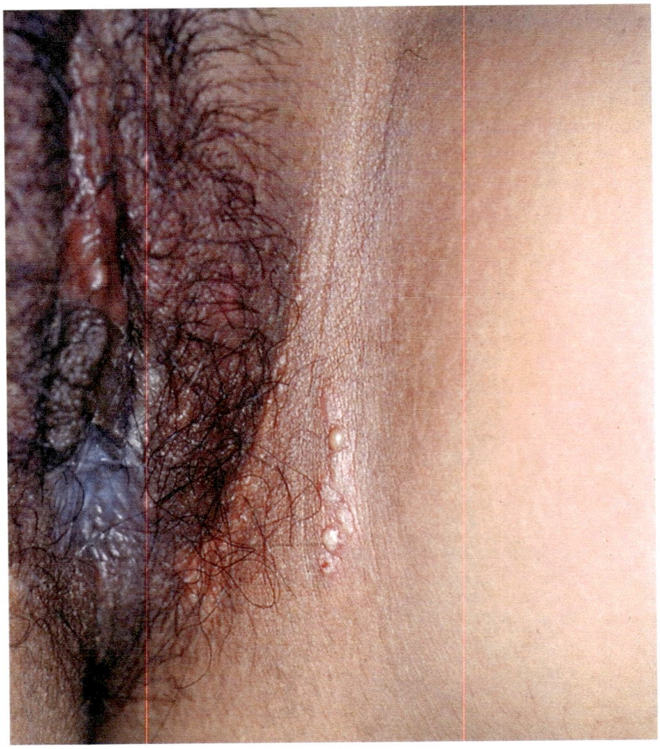

Recurrent genital herpes: Multiple grouped vesicles on inner aspect of thigh and erosions on labia minora.

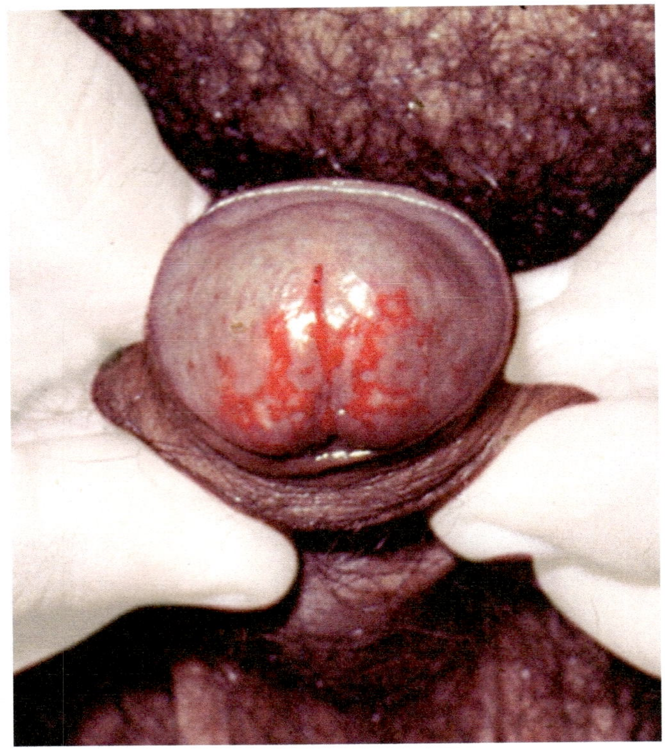

Meatal genital herpes: Erosions on tip on glans extending into urethral meatus. Such a patient presents with dysura.

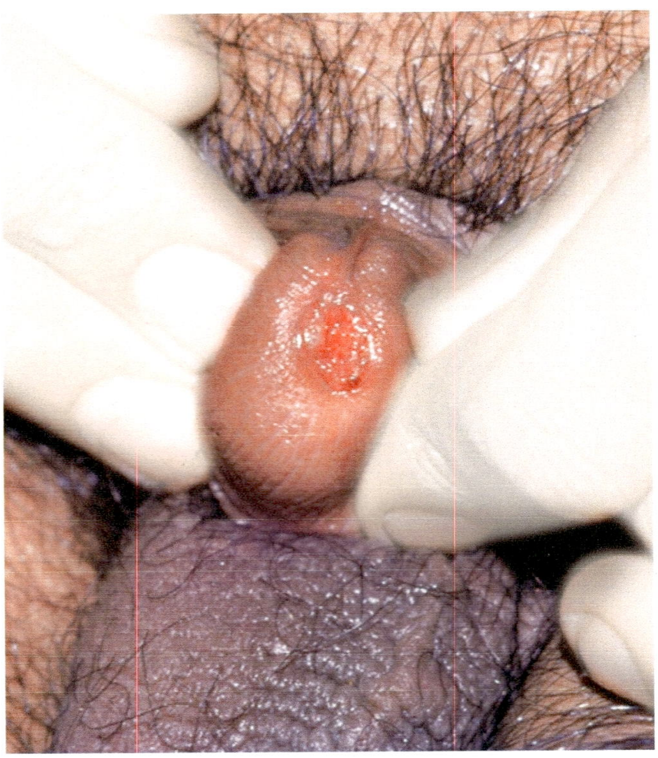

Meatal genital herpes: Small erosion on urethral meatus visible on careful examination. This patient presented with recurrent episodes of dysuria and minimal mucoid urethral discharge.

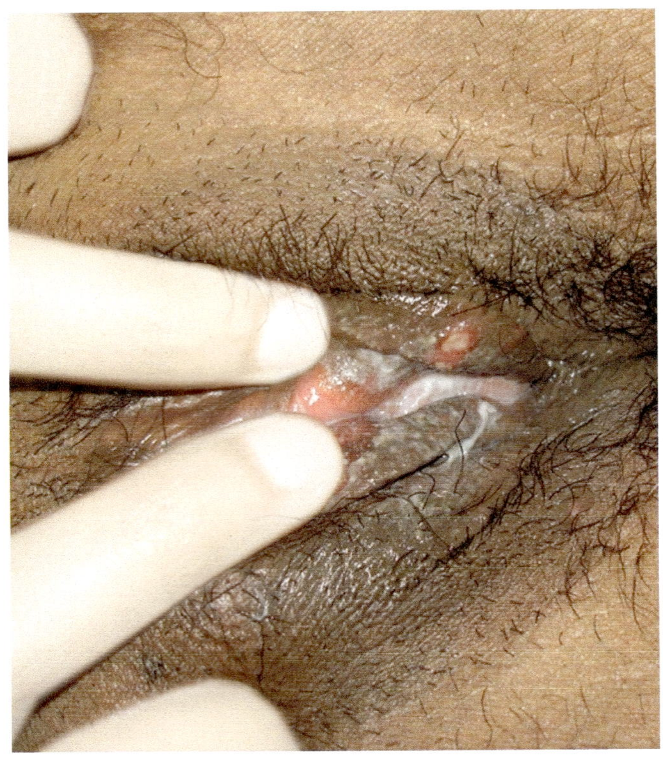

Meatal genital herpes: Recurrent GH. Well-defined erosions on inner aspect of labia minora and urethral meatus. Patient presented with recurrent episodes of dysuria and vaginal discharge.

Serology

- ***Serological response to HSV infection:*** Both IgM and IgG develop.
  - IgM detectable at week 1 and lasts 2 weeks. Also positive in 30% of recurrences. Often negative in 1st episode GH. Not reliable in differentiating HSV-1 and HSV-2.
  - IgG detectable at 6 weeks and lasts life long. So negative test after 6 weeks rules out HSV infection. Can differentiate between HSV-1 and HSV-2. Common commercially available kits detect IgG.
- ***Common tests available:***
  - *Lab-based test:* Western blot (expensive, not freely available), but gold standard for specificity and sensitivity. ELISA (for HSV-1, HSV-2) and immunoblot tests.
  - *Point of care-tests (POCT)*[2]*:* Provide rapid results with sensitivity and specificity comparable to ELISA.
- ***Indications for HSV serology:*** Type specific HSV serology indicated in:
  - Recurrent genital lesions with negative HSV cultures.
  - Strong clinical suspicion, but negative culture (IgM test preferred if primary episode).
  - In partner of patient with GH (to detect discordancy).

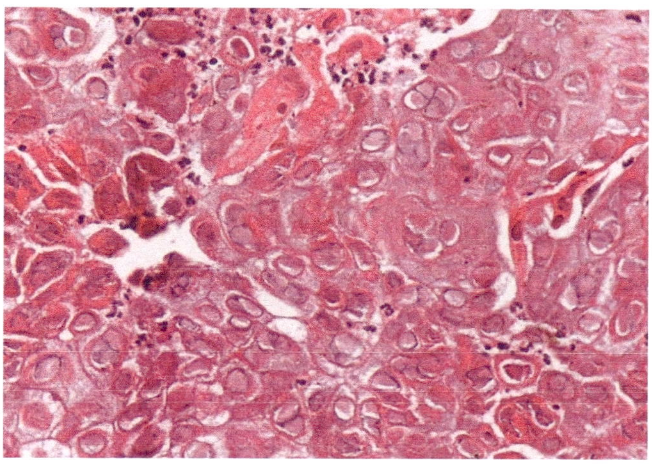

Biopsy of herpetic lesion: Showing ballooning degeneration of keratinocytes leading to vesicle formation. Other features include multinucleated giant cells and intranuclear eosinophilic inclusions (Cowdry bodies).
Courtesy: Prof. M. Ramam, Department of Dermatology, AIIMS, New Delhi.

[2]Tests done at clinic where patient presents. Results available immediately.

  - Evaluation of patients with STIs especially if multiple sex partners, HIV infection and if MSM.
- ***Interpretation of serological tests:***
  - In recurrences, IgM test negative in 70%.
  - In recurrent genital ulcers of > 6 weeks duration, a negative IgG rules out HSV infection.

Biopsy

- ***Indication:*** In doubtful cases where other laboratory tests like culture, PCR not available.
- ***Shows:*** Ballooning degenration of keratinocytes leading to vesicle formation. And multinucleated giant cells and intranuclear eosinophilic inclusions called Cowdry's bodies.

TREATMENT

Besides antiviral therapy, counselling patient paramount.

Counseling

- ***Goal of counseling:***
  - Help patients cope with GH infection.
  - Prevent sexual and perinatal transmission.
- ***Counsel about:***
  - *Natural course of GH:* About potential for recurrences, asymptomatic viral shedding, and sexual and perinatal transmission.
  - *Availability of therapy:* Episodic and suppressive, to reduce recurrences and transmission.
  - *Safe sexual practices: Viz* abstinence during prodrome and active lesions. And use of latex condoms consistently and correctly during asymptomatic periods.
  - *Informing partners:* Current and future. Type specific serological testing available for partners to ascertain risk of transmission. Never symptomatic persons with HSV-2 type-specific antibodies to receive same counseling as persons with symptomatic infection.
  - *Risk for neonatal HSV infection:*
    - Pregnant women to inform their antenatal care providers about HSV infection.
    - Pregnant women not infected with HSV-2 to avoid intercourse during 3rd trimester with men who have GH.

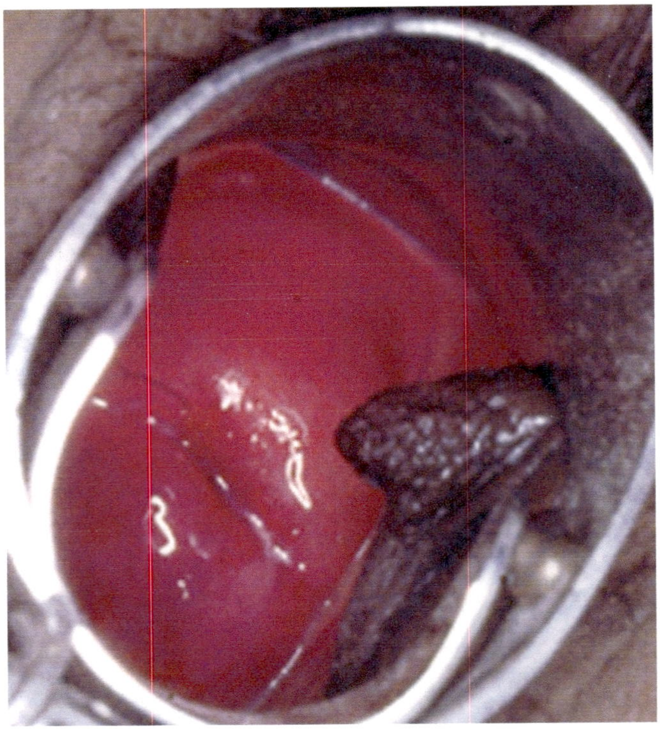

Cervical genital herpes: Polycyclic erosions on the cervical os. Such a patient is either asymptomatic or presents with vaginal discharge.

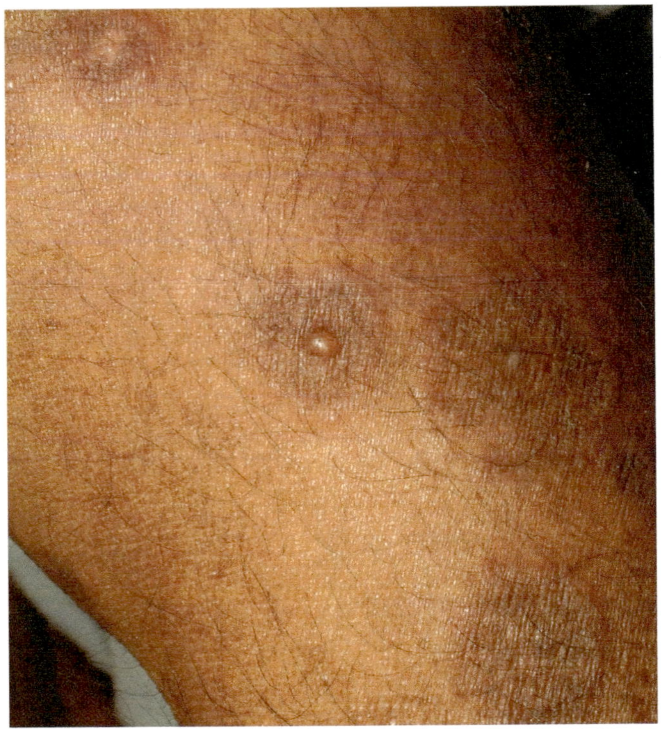

Complication of genital herpes: Recurrent erythema multiforme associated with recurrented GH.

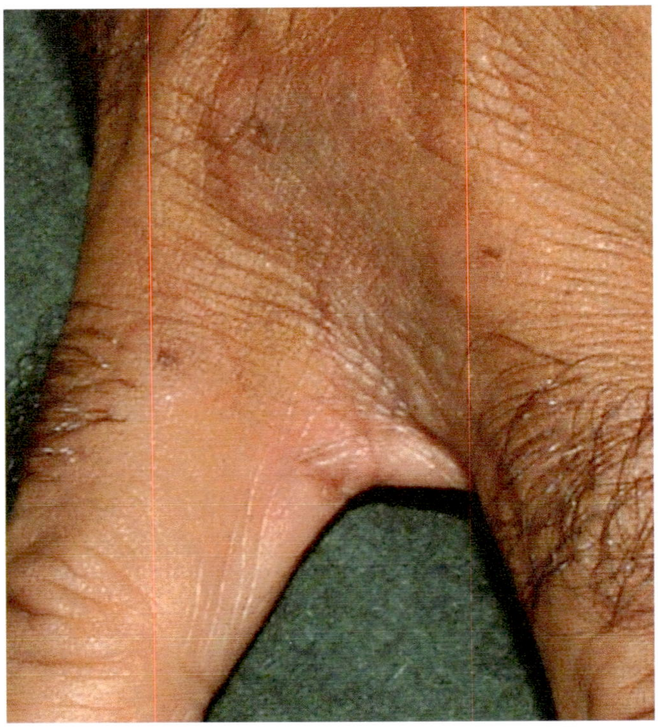

Complication of genital herpes: Erythema multiforme with central necrosis and surrounding erythema and edema (targetoid lesions). Patient had recurrent episodes.

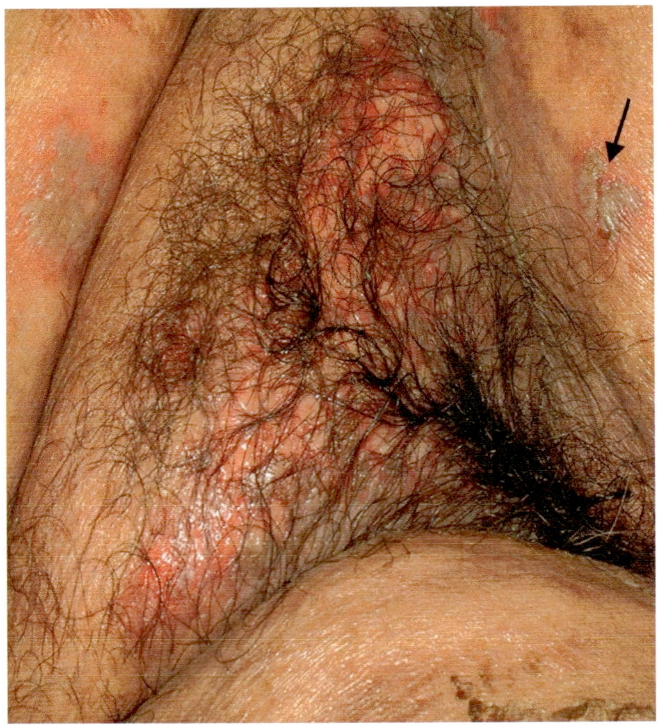

Genital herpes in HIV positive patient: Widespread polycyclic lesions on the vulva, mons and lower abdomen. Note grouped lesions on thighs.

- Pregnant women not infected with HSV-1 to avoid oro-genital exposure to HSV-1 during 3rd trimester (oral sex with partner with oral herpes and vaginal intercourse with partner with genital HSV-1 infection).

Specific Treatment

Systemic (not topical[3]) antiviral therapy (AVT) mainstay of therapy for symptomatic patients. Can be used episodically when lesions appear (or during prodrome). Or as daily suppressive therapy to prevent (almost) recurrences and reduce shedding. However, neither eradicate latent virus nor affect risk, frequency, or severity of recurrences after drug discontinued.

Three antivirals effective: acyclovir, valacyclovir, and famciclovir. Acyclovir has lower bioavailability and needs frequent dosing. Valacyclovir and famciclovir have high oral bioavailability. And all equally effective.

First episode of GH

- ***Indications:*** All patients with 1st episode GH; drugs preferably taken within 3 days of onset.
- ***Regimes:*** Tables 8.2 and 8.3.

Recurrent GH

AVT given episodically. Or continuously as suppressive therapy.

Table 8.2: Recommended regimens for treatment genital herpes (CDC 2010)

	1st episode*	Recurrent GH	
		*Episodic therapy**	*Suppressive therapy*
Acyclovir	• 400 mg tid × 7-10 days OR • 200 mg 5 times/days × 7-10 days	• 400 mg tid × 5 days OR • 800 mg bid × 5 days OR • 800 mg bid × 2 days	• 400 mg bid
Valacyclovir**	• 1,000 mg bid × 7-10 days	• 500 mg bid × 3 days OR • 1 g OD × days × 5 days	• 500 mg od OR • 1,000 mg od
Famciclovir	• 250 mg tid × 7-10 days	• 125 mg bid × 5 days OR • 1000 mg bid × 1 days	• 250 mg bid

*Treatment extended if healing incomplete after 10 days of therapy.
**If > 10 episodes/year

Table 8.3: Recommended regimens for treatment of genital herpes (WHO 2003)

	1st episode × 7-10 days	Recurrent GH	
		Episodic therapy × 5 days	*Suppressive therapy**
Acyclovir	• 400 mg tid OR • 200 mg 5 times/days	• 400 mg tid OR • 200 mg × 5 times/days OR • 800 mg × bid	• 400 mg bid
Valacyclovir	• 1,000 mg bid	• 1,000 mg × od OR • 500 mg × bid	• 500 mg od OR • 1,000 mg od
Famciclovir	• 250 mg tid	• 125 mg × bid	• 250 mg × bid

* If >6 episodes/year

[3]Topical antivirals offer no clinical benefit, so use discouraged.

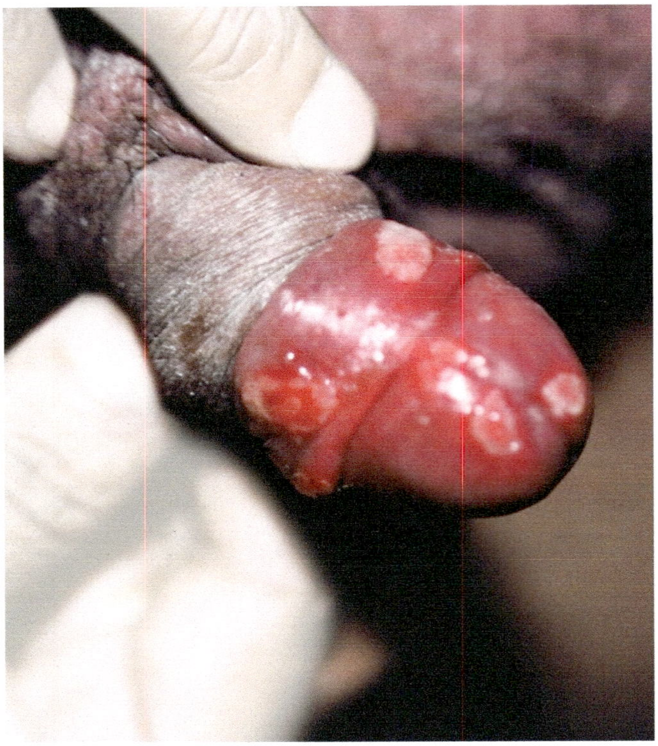

Genital herpes in HIV positive patient: Atypical lesions-multiple well-defined non-indurated deep ulcers with necrotic material on floor, suggestive of chancroid.

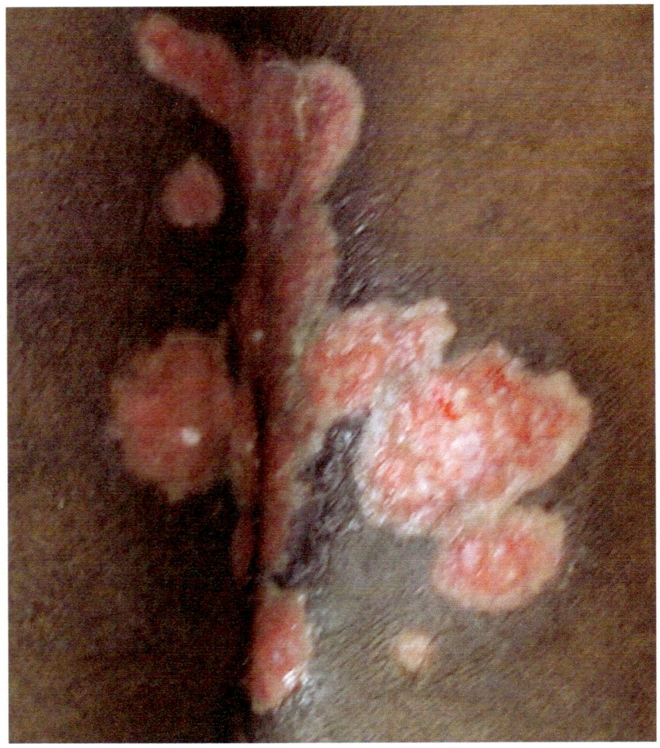

Genital herpes in HIV positive patient: Chronic non healing ulcer (lasting > 1 month) with polycyclic margins on perianal area warrants ruling out HIV infection.

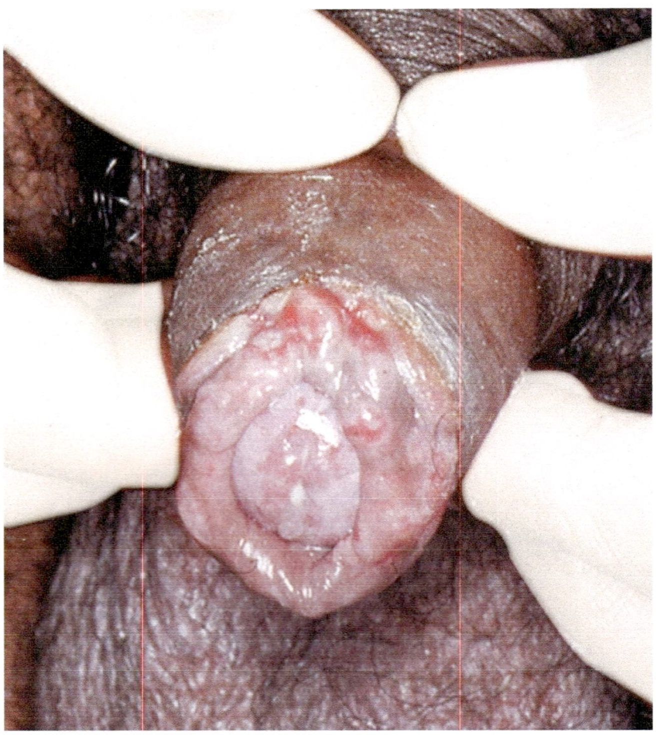

Genital herpes in HIV positive patient: Large polycyclic persistent erosions involving prepuce and glans. Persistent lesions not responding to adequate dose of acyclovir should arouse suspicion of acyclovir resistance.

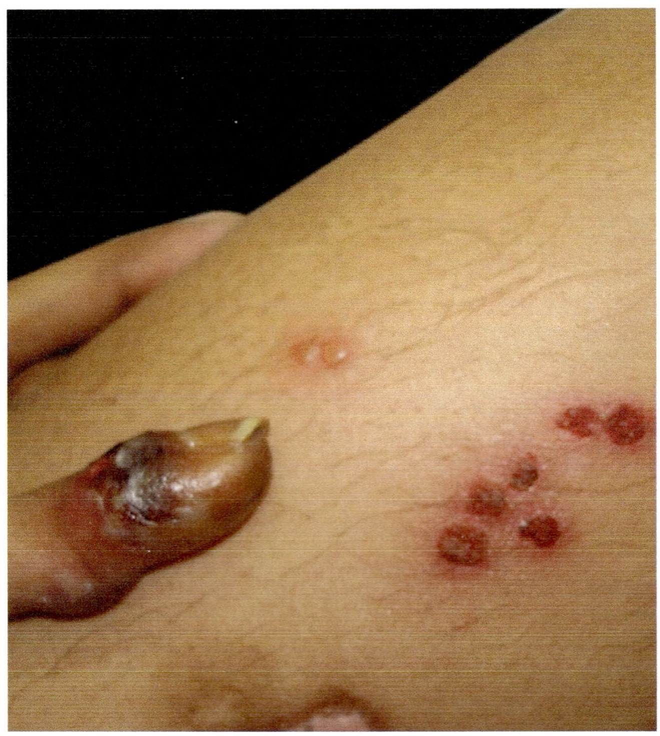

Genital herpes in HIV positive patient: Grouped crusted erosions on inner aspect of thigh. Finger affected with herpetic whitlow.

Episodic therapy for recurrent GH

- ***Indications:*** Less than 6 episodes/year.
- ***Effect:*** Reduces symptoms and shortens episode. Effective if initiated within a day of recurrence. Or during prodrome. So patient provided with a supply of drugs to self initiate therapy.
- ***Regimes:*** Tables 8.2 and 8.3.

Suppressive therapy for recurrent GH

- ***Indications:***
  - More than 6 episodes/per year.
  - Episodes associated with significant consitutional symptoms.
  - Episodes causing significant psychosocial distress.
- ***Effect of suppressive therapy:***
  - Reduces HSV shedding (both asymptomatic and during episodes).
  - Reduces frequency of GH recurrences (by 70–80%). And many patients report no recurrences.
  - Improves quality of life.
- ***Regimes:*** Tables 8.2, 8.3.

GH in HIV Infection

- Antiretroviral therapy reduces severity and frequency of symptomatic GH but subclinical shedding continues.
- Episodic or suppressive therapy decreases clinical manifestations of HG. Acyclovir, valacyclovir, and famciclovir safe in immunocompromised patients.
- Regimens:

Episodic therapy

- Acyclovir, 400 mg orally tid × 5–10 days.

OR

- Famiciclovir, 500 mg orally bid × 5–10 days.

OR

- Valacyclovir, 1 gm orally bid × 5–10 days.

Suppressive therapy

- Acyclovir, 400–800 mg orally bid/tid.

OR

- Famciclovir, 500 mg orally bid.

OR

- Valacyclovir, 500 mg orally bid.

Acyclovir Resistance

- Usually in HIV coinfected.
- Suspect if lesions persist. Or recur in patient receiving adequate acyclovir.
- Confirmed by HSV isolation and sensitivity testing.
- Cross-resistance to valacyclovir, and famciclovir noted.

GH in Pregnancy

Prevention of neonatal herpes

Depends on:

- Preventing acquisition of GH infection in late pregnancy. (see counselling)
- And avoiding exposure of infant to herpetic lesions during delivery, by ruling out GH at time of labour.
  - Women without symptoms or signs of GH delivered vaginally.
  - Women with GH at onset of labor delivered by Cesarean section[4] to prevent neonatal herpes.

Treatment in pregnancy

- ***1st episode GH:*** Acyclovir 400 mg tid × 7 days.
- ***Recurrent GH:*** Acyclovir 400 mg tid × 5 days.
- Treat with foscarnet, 40 mg/kg intravenous 8 hourly, until clinical resolution. Topical cidofovir gel 1% (prepared extemporaneously) od × 5 days also effective.

OTHER TREATMENT CONSIDERATIONS

Partner Management

- ***Symptomatic sex partners:*** Evaluation and treatment as in patients with genital lesions.
- ***Asymptomatic sex partners:*** Questioned about history of genital lesions. Offered type-specific serologic testing for HSV infection to detect discordancy.

Other Considerations

- Evaluate for presence of other STIs.
- Serologically rule out HIV, HBV and syphilis at 1st visit. If negative, retest for syphilis and HIV, 3 months after initial visit.

[4]Caesarian section: not completely foolproof.

CHAPTER 9

Anogenital Warts

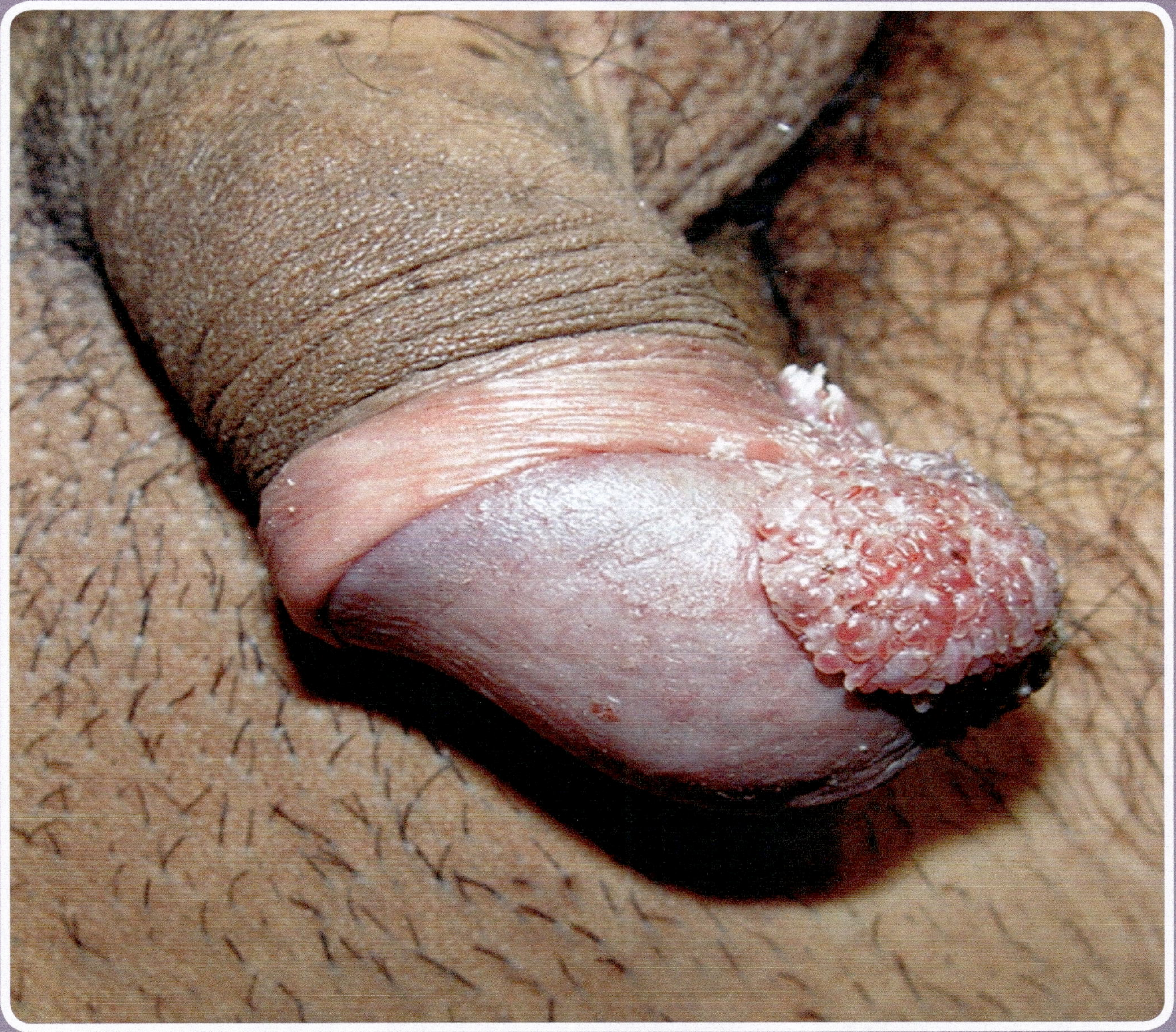

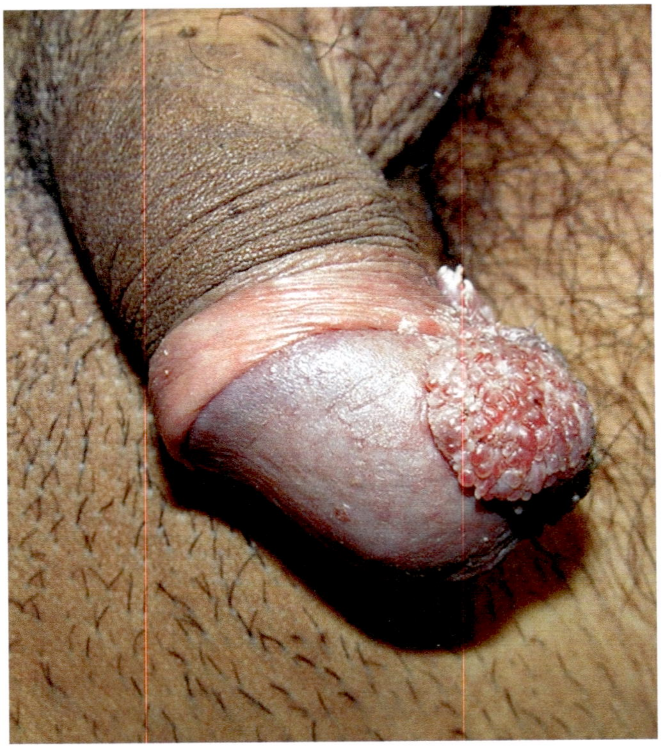

Condyloma acuminata: Verrucous, fleshy plaque on glans.

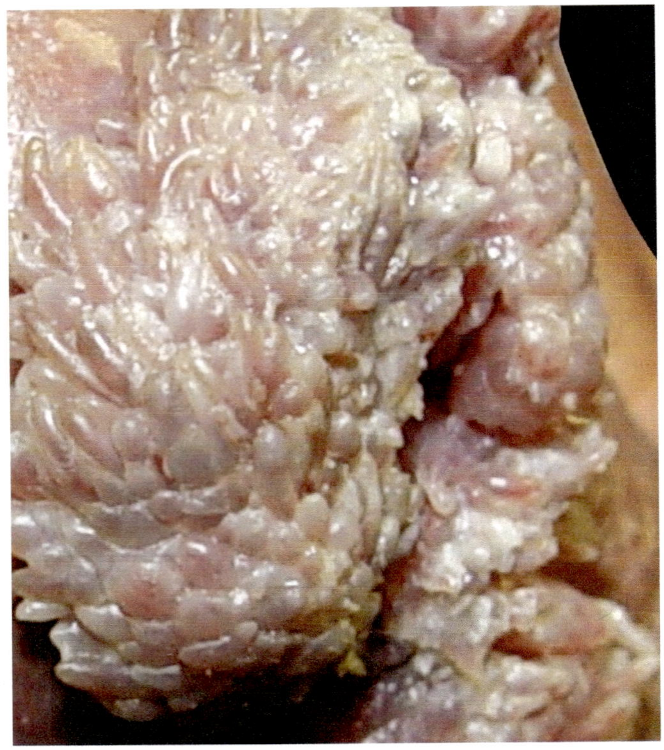

Condyloma acuminata: Close up showing filiform projections on a cauliflower like growth.

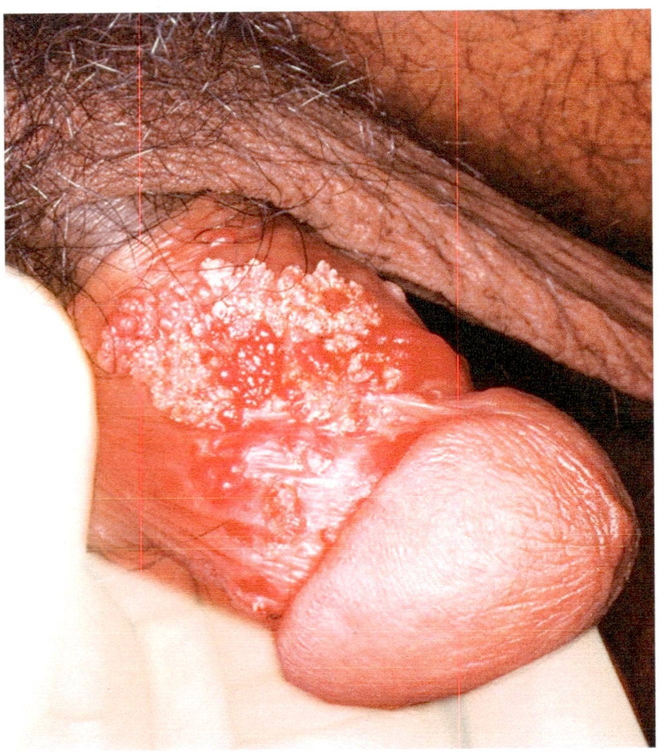

Condyloma acuminata: Verrucous plaque on inner aspect of prepuce, visible only on retracting the prepuce.

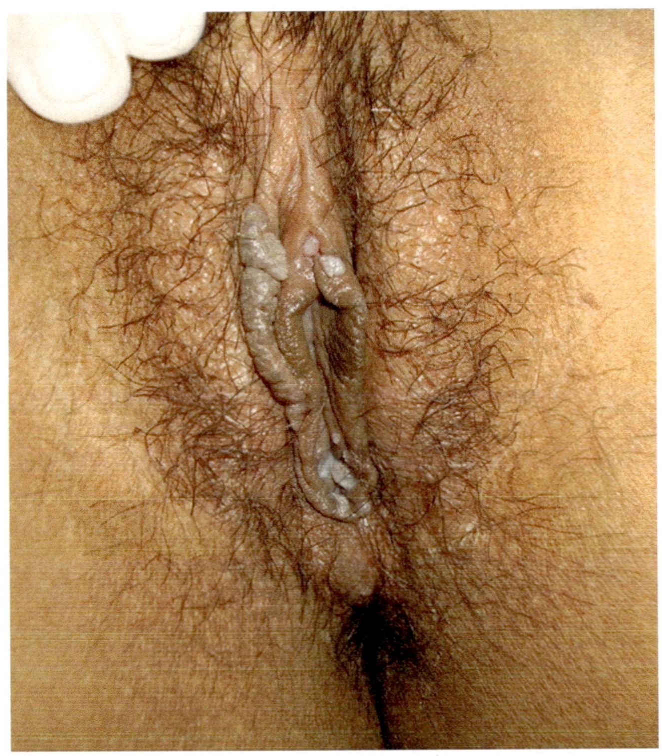

Condyloma acuminata: Small verrucous lesions on vulva.

Also known as venereal warts.

ETIOLOGY

Etiological Agent

- Human papilloma virus (HPV).
- Unenveloped DNA virus, of 55 nm diameter.
- HPV proteins of 2 types:
  - Early (E 1-7).
  - Late (L 1-2).
- HPV causing anogenital warts (AGW) classified (Table 9.1) into:
  - *High risk types:* High risk of malignant transformation; types 16, 18.
  - *Low risk types:* No or low risk for malignant transformation; types 6, 11.

Transmission

- ***Sexual transmission:***
  - Including vaginal, anal and oral.
  - Transmission common from asymptomatic partners.
  - Protection incomplete even with use of condoms.
- ***Vertical transmission:*** Mother (infected) to newborn, resulting in laryngeal papillomas in baby.
- ***Direct contact:*** Transmission from hand warts to genitalia. Very rare.

EPIDEMIOLOGY

Geographic Distribution

- Prevalent globally. Prevalence 1-13%.
- Probably the commonest STI.

Demographic Distribution

- Commoner in women.
- Young sexually active people (2nd-4th decade) at highest risk for acquiring AGW. But can affect any age.
- Infants of infected mothers born with laryngeal papillomas.

CLINICAL FEATURES

Incubation Period

Variable, 1-9 (average 2-3) months.

Symptoms

- Mostly asymptomatic.
- Sometimes bleeding on minor trauma in condyloma acuminata.

Morphology

Several morphological variants described:

- ***Condyloma acuminata:***
  - Erythematous fleshy, hyperplastic or papillomatous lesions (with finger-like projections).
  - Vascular, may bleed on minor trauma.
  - Can increase in size to form large fleshy cauliflower like masses.
  - On mucosal surface. Intrameatal lesions frequent.
- ***Papular:***
  - Flat surfaced, small papules, skin colored to brown.
  - On keratinized skin.

Table 9.1: Genital lesions associated with HPV type

Clinical manifestation	Common HPV types
Low risk HPV types	
Condyloma acuminata	6,11
Papular warts	6,11
Buschke Lowenstein tumor	6,11
High risk HPV types	
Condyloma acuminata	16, 18
Bowenoid papulosis	16, 34, 39, 45
Intraepithelial neoplasia (anal, vulval, cervical)	16, (most) 18, 31

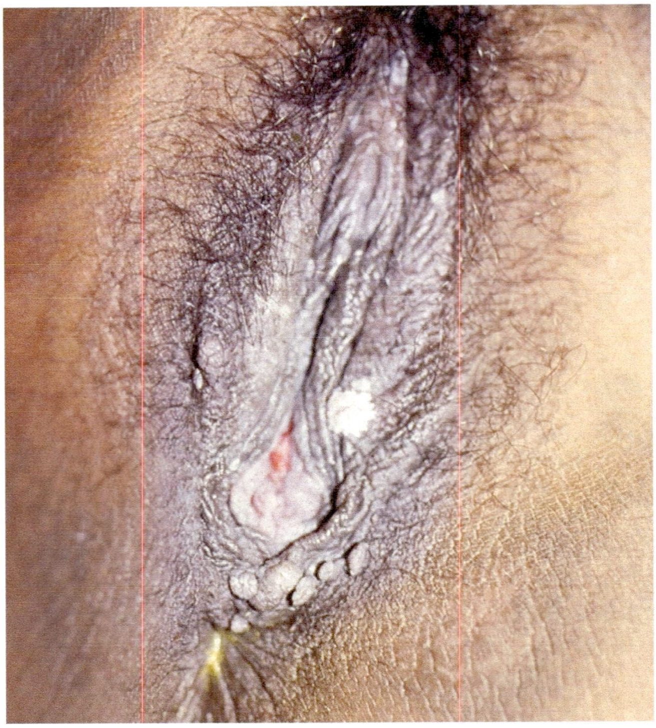

Condyloma acuminata: Small warts on perineum and in the introitus.

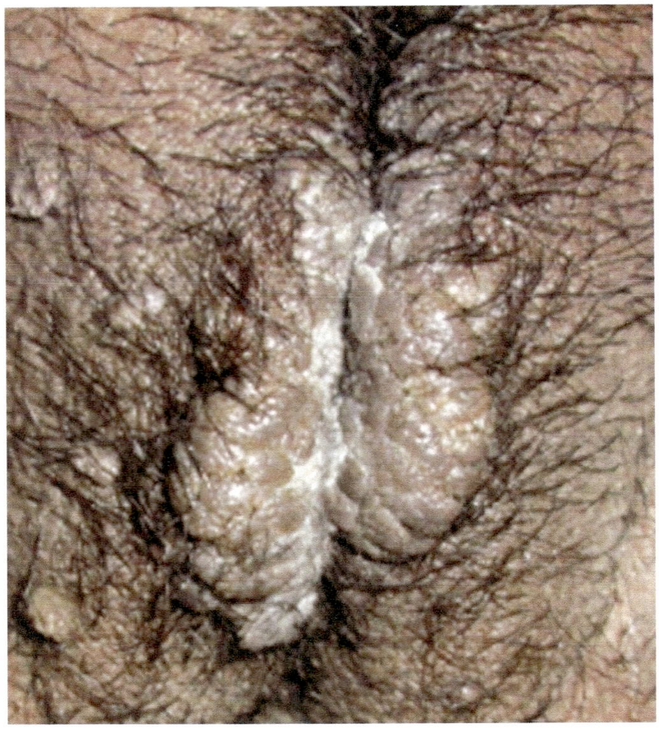

Condyloma acuminata: Large verrucous lesions on vulva of pregnant woman. AGW may become rapidly exuberant during pregnancy.

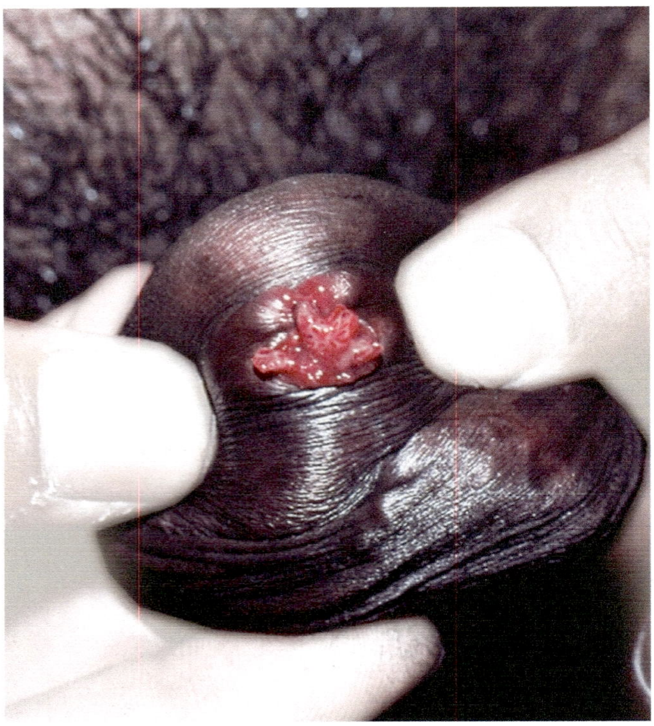

Intrameatal wart: Erythematous, fleshy, verrucous lesion growing within urethral meatus. True size of wart can only be judged by opening the meatus wide.

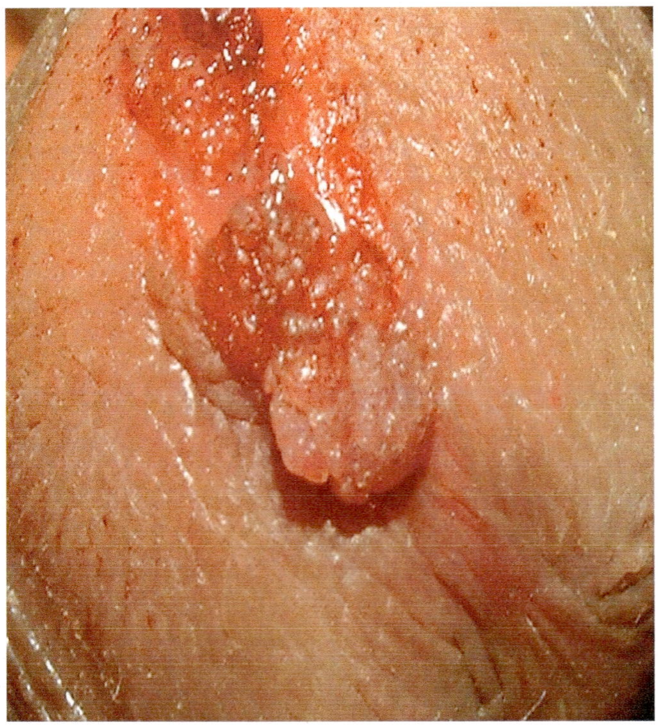

Intrameatal wart: Verrucous, erythematous lesion growing from within urethra. Surface shows bleeding spots.

- ***Variants of other warts:***
  - Like verruca vulgaris, filiform warts, etc.
  - Verrucous hyperkeratotic papules and plaques (verruca vulgaris-like) filiform lesions (filiform wart-like) and larger sessile lesions.
- ***Buschke Lowenstein tumors:***
  - Large verrucous plaques with exophytic as well as deeper growth (manifesting as induration).
  - Slow growing. Malignant potential (to locally invasive squamous cell carcinoma but not metastatic).
- ***Bowenoid papulosis:***
  - In younger patients.
  - Multiple, small, skin colored to reddish brown/ pigmented papules with velvety surface.
  - Premalignant condition (type of intraepithelial squamous cell carcinoma).

Sites of Lesions

- ***Condyloma acuminata:*** On non keratinised areas—corona, glans penis, prepuce and urinary meatus in men. And vaginal introitus, labia majora and minora in females.
- ***Other variants:*** On keratinised skin.
- ***Perianal area:*** Involved with or without genital involvement. Intra-anal warts in those who have had receptive anal intercourse.
- ***Internal warts:*** Cervical, anal and rectal warts. Hence, speculum examination in women with AGW. And proctoscopic examination in those indulging in receptive anal intercourse recommended. Often needs accentuation by acetowhitening.

COMPLICATIONS

- ***Psychological impact:*** Often huge!
- ***Secondary infection:*** Presenting as pus discharge, bleeding and foul smell.
- ***Obstetric complications:***
  - Increase in number and size during pregnancy. May become exuberant and obstruct vaginal delivery. Require episiotomy, sometimes even caesarian section.
  - Vertical transmission to newborn resulting in laryngeal papillomas.
- ***Malignancy:*** Malignant transformation in genital warts rare.
  - Some HPV types (16, 18) have higher association with intraepithelial neoplasia (vulval, anal ? penile) and cervical carcinomas.
  - Even in AGW caused by low risk type, possibility of concomitant transmission of high risk HPV types present.

ANOGENITAL WARTS AND HIV

- ***Effect of AGW on HIV:*** ? increased progression of HIV.
- ***Effect of HIV on AGW:***
  - AGW more frequent in HIV positive.
  - More numerous lesions, extensive involvement and larger nodules.
  - Higher prevalance of carcinoma *in situ* in cervix, vulva and anal canal. So regular monitoring of these areas.
  - More resistant to treatment. And more recurrences.

DIAGNOSIS

Based on Clinical Features

Diagnosis of AGW primarily clinical:

- Fleshy, erythematous or hyperpigmented verrucous papules and plaques.
- ***Acetowhitening test:*** Done to increase visibility of 'clinically invisible' lesions.

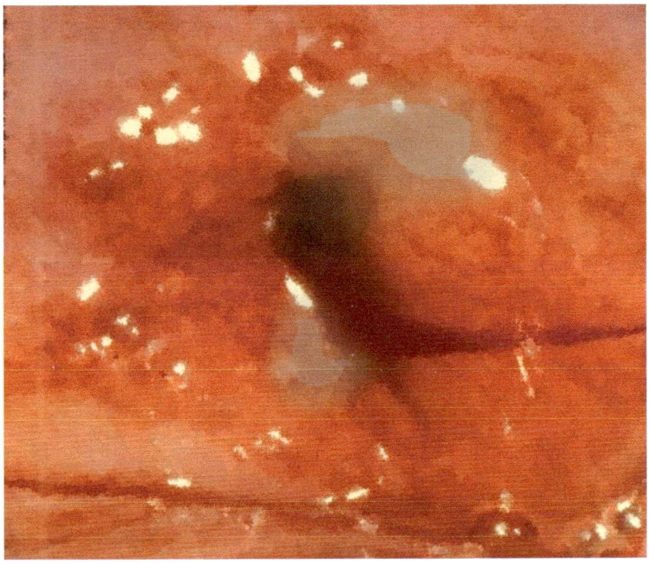

Acetowhitening test: Diluted acetic acid is applied to enhance visibility of clinically 'invisible' warts. In this case it is done on cervix.

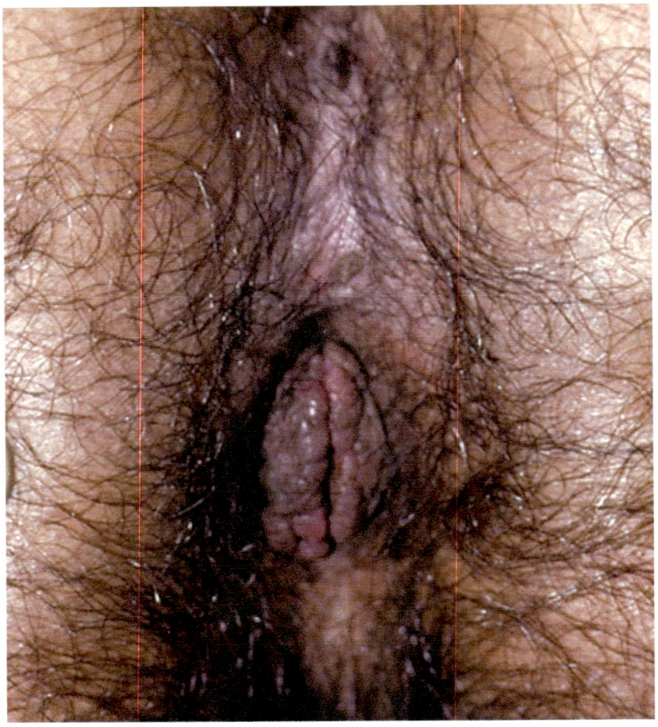

Perianal condyloma acuminata: Thorough perianal examination is mandatory in all patients with STI. This patient had penoanal sex. Such a patient would require proctoscopic evaluation.

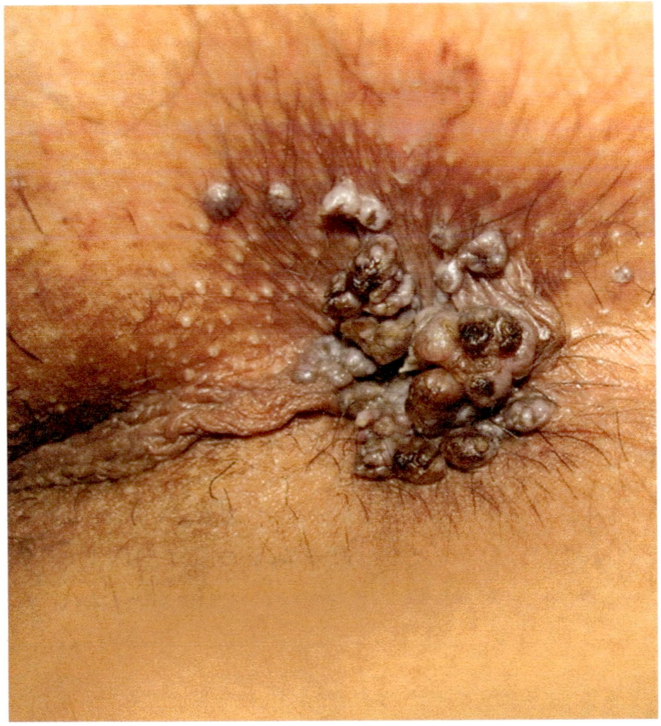

Perianal warts: Multiple discrete, grouped, hyperpigmented papules with verrucous surface surrounding the anal opening. Common in MSM.

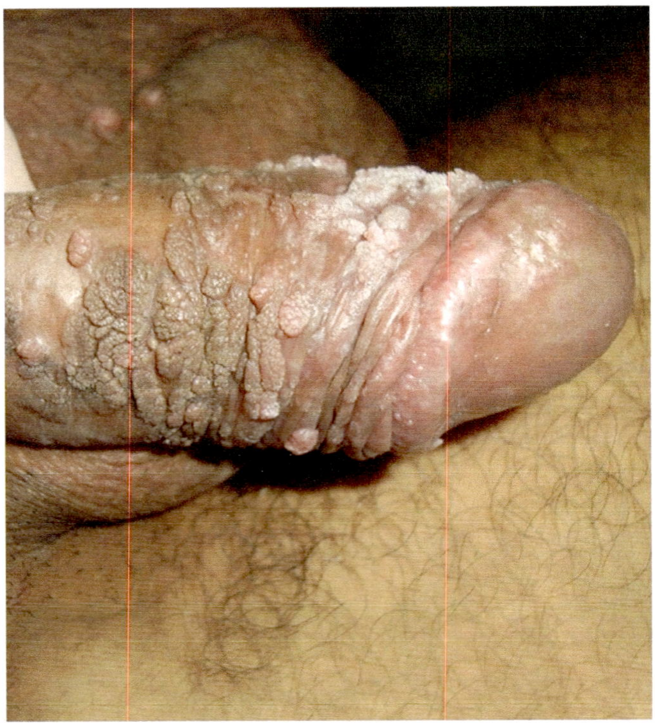

Verruca vulgaris like anogenital warts: Verruca vulgaris-like anogenital warts. Hyperkeratotic papules on the keratinised skin of penis.

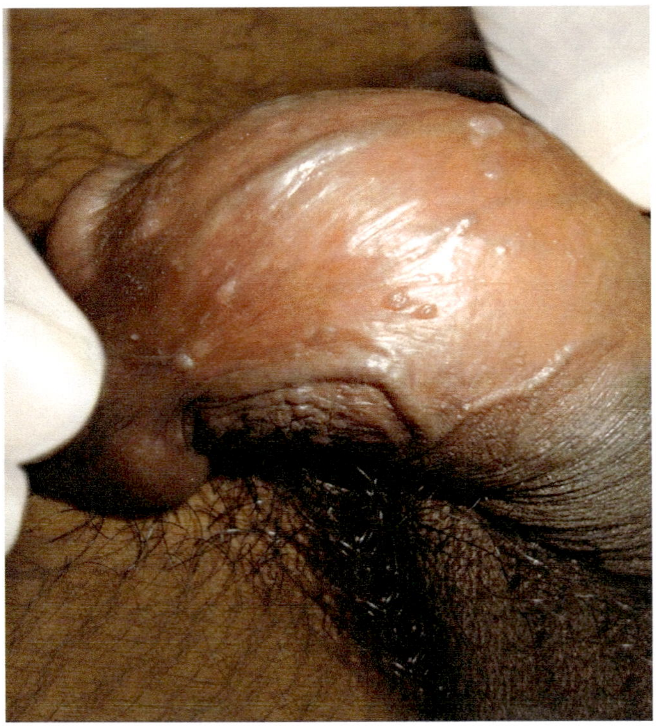

Papular variant of anogenital warts: Small papules, skin colored to hyperpigmented on keratinised skin.

Laboratory Investigations

Laboratory investigations generally not required.

Biopsy

- ***Indications:*** Confirmation of diagnosis. And to rule out malignancy in:
  - *Atypical lesions:* Large fungating exophytic masses, verrucous plaques with indurated base and macerated plaques.
  - *Premalignant lesions:* Bowenoid papulosis, Buschke-Lowenstein tumor.
  - *HIV positive patients.*
- ***Histopathology:*** Features include hyperkeratosis, papillomatosis, acanthosis, parakeratosis. And typically koilocytes[1] in epidermis. Multiple dilated capillaries in dermis.

Other tests

- ***HPV DNA testing:***
  - FDA approved tests like Hybrid capture HPV DNA test very sensitive and specific.
  - PCR.
- ***Serology:*** Of limited or no value.

TREATMENT

- Treatment aimed at removal of lesions, not removal of HPV infection.
- Warts may spontaneously resolve in few months. Or persist. Also may recur without re-exposure.
- Treatment may (or may not) reduce transmission.

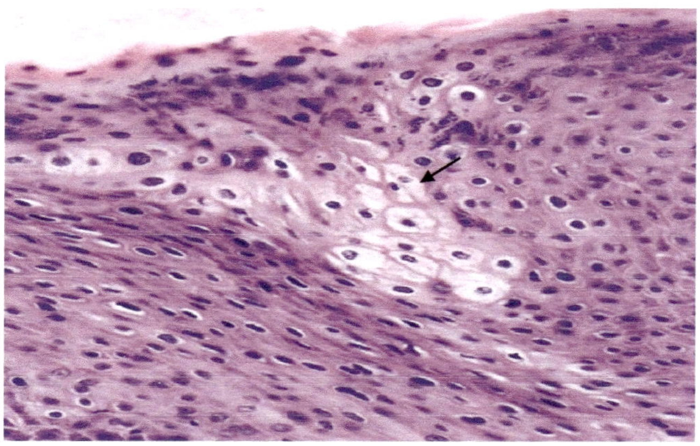

Histopathology of anogenital warts: Shows koilocytes which are epidermal cells with hyperchromatic irregular nuclei and a perinuclear halo.

Counseling

- Most sexually active adults HPV-infected, but lesion free.
  - In most, infection clears spontaneously.
  - In some, infection progresses to AGW; fewer to neoplasia.
- Correct and consistent use of male condom lowers transmission of genital HPV, but not fully protective.
- AGW may recur after treatment, especially in 1st 3 months.
- Women with AGW need not get Pap tests more frequently.
- HPV testing unnecessary in sexual partners of persons with AGW, but patient and sex partner to be screened for other STIs. However, presence of AGW not marker for infidelity.
- Persons with AGW to inform current sex partner(s) because warts sexually transmitted. Preferable to refrain from sexual activity till warts subside.

Treatments Available

AGW treated by provider-applied or patient-applied methods (Tables 9.2 and 9.3). Both associated with failures and no ideal modality.

Topical applications

- ***Podophyllin resin, 10%–25%:***
  - For warts on non-keratinized/mucosal surfaces.
  - Applied by provider with brush to individual warts after protecting surrounding area. Allowed to air-dry. And washed off after 4 hours. Application

Table 9.2: Treatment options for anogenital warts
Provider-applied regimens
• Podophyllin resin, 10%–25%
• Trichloroacetic acid (TCA), 80-100%.
• Bichloroacetic acid, (BCA) 80-90%
• Cryotherapy
• Surgery
• Radiofrequency ablation or electrocautery
Patient-applied regimens
• Podofilox, 0.5% solution or gel
• Imiquimod, 5% cream
• Sinecatechins, 15% ointment

[1]Koilocytes: Epidermal cells with enlarged (2-3 times normal) hyperchromatic irregular nuclei with a perinuclear halo.

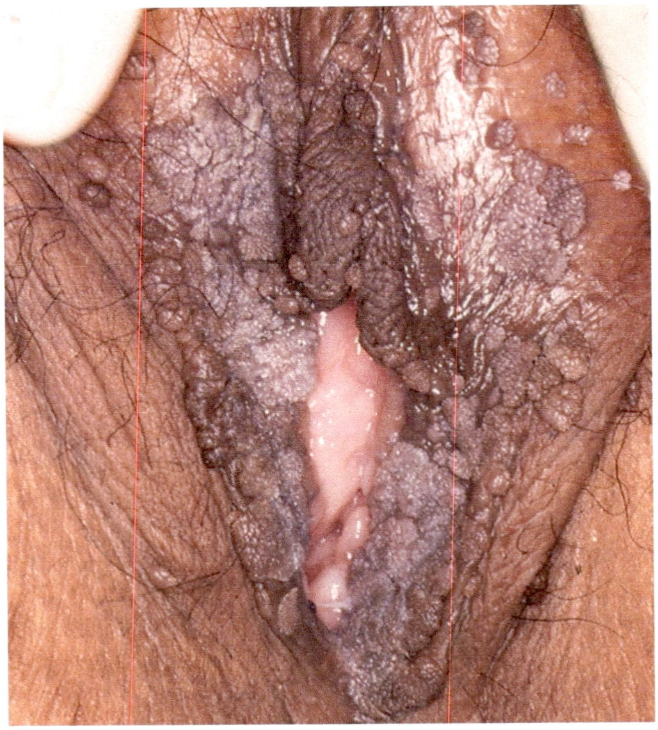

Papular variant of anogenital warts: Small papular lesions on keratinised skin.

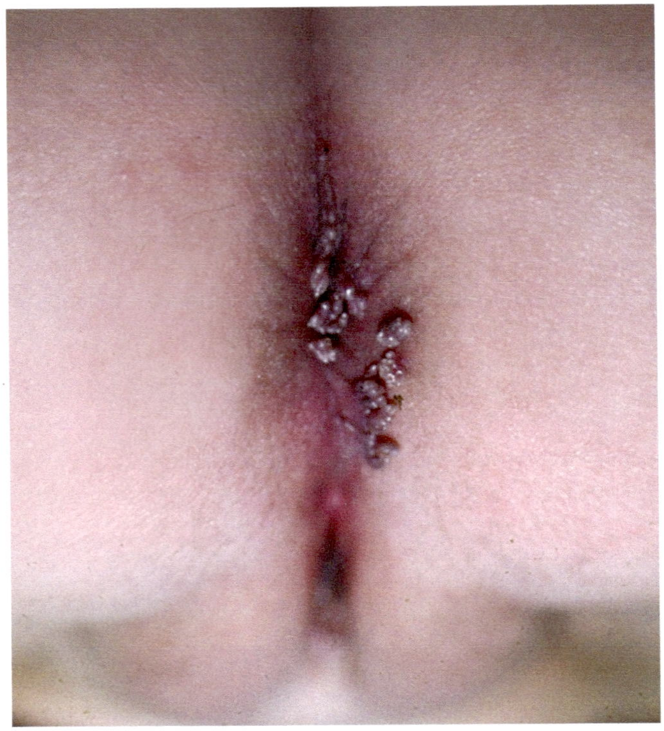

Bowenoid papulosis: Multiple 2-3 mm hyperpigmented papules, discrete, firm with velvety surface. Most frequently due to HPV 16. May sometimes regress spontaneously.

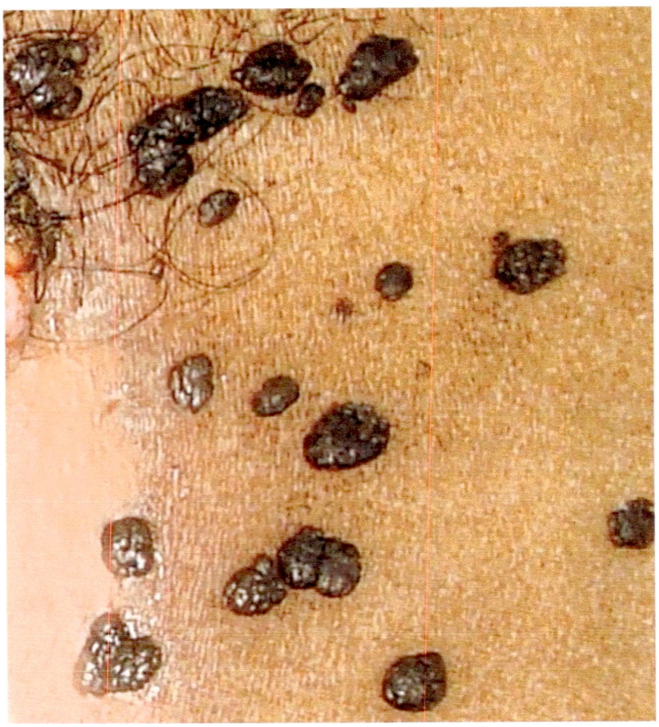

Bowenoid papulosis: Multiple, small hyperpigmented papules with a velvety surface on upper thigh. Diagnosis confirmed histopathologically-shows carcinoma *in situ*.

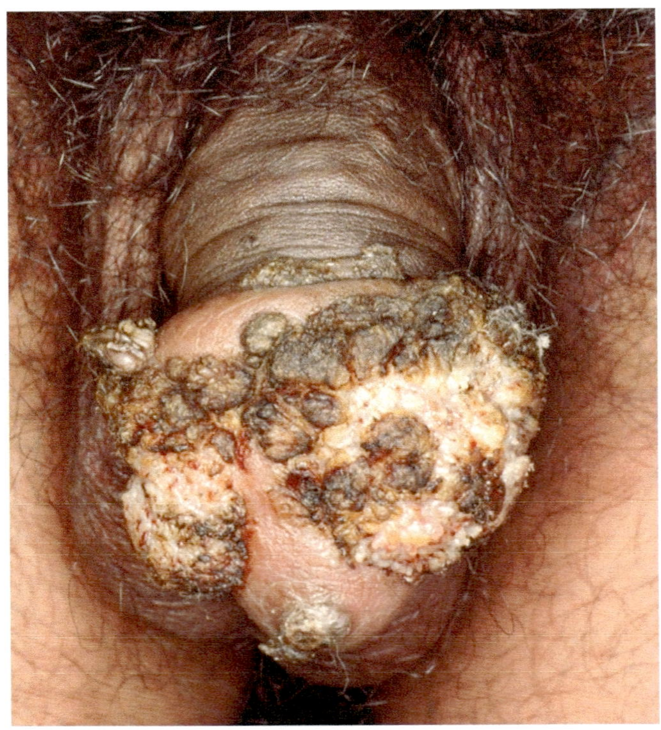

Buschke Lowenstein tumor: Large verrucous plaque with both an exophytic and deeper growth (clinically manifesting as induration). Locally invasive lesion which does not metastasize.

limited to < 0.5 mL of podophyllin or an area of < 10 cm^2 of warts/session.
- Repeated weekly for 6-8 weeks. Or till wart dissapears (whichever earlier).
- Local irritation, if excess applied. Avoid if epithelial discontinuity. Can be used in HIV-positive patients. Never in pregnancy.

❖ ***Podofilox solution/gel:***
- Applied by patient. Solution with a cotton swab. And gel with finger.
- Twice a day for 3 days, followed by gap 4 days. Cycle repeated, for up to 4 cycles. Total wart area treated < 10 cm^2, and total volume < 0.5 mL/day.
- Mild to moderate pain or local irritation may develop. Safety in pregnancy not established.

❖ ***Imiquimod:***
- Topical immune enhancer. Stimulates production of interferon and other cytokines.
- Applied by patient once daily at bedtime, 3 alternate days/week × 16 weeks. Washed off after 6–10 hours.
- Irritation (redness, induration, ulceration/erosions and vesicles) common.
- May weaken condoms, diaphragms. And safety in pregnancy not established.

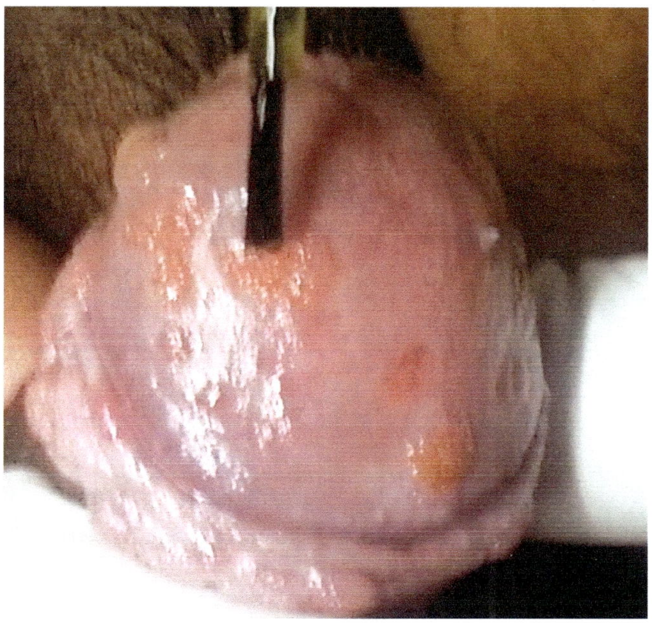

Anogenital warts: Topical application of podophyllin (using a brush) after protecting adjacent normal skin with petroleum.

❖ ***Sinecatechin ointment, 15%:***
- Green-tea extract with active ingredients (catechins).
- Applied tid till complete clearance of warts. Or for 16 weeks, whichever is earlier.
- Irritation. May weaken condoms and diaphragms. Not recommended for HIV-infected persons. Or persons with clinical genital herpes. Safety unknown in pregnancy.

Physical modalities

❖ ***Trichloroacetic acid***, 80–100%.
- Destroys by chemical coagulation of proteins.
- For warts on keratinized surfaces.
- Small amount applied only to warts and allowed to dry (appearance of white frost).
- Repeated weekly till clearance of warts.

Cryotherapy

- ❖ Destroys by cytolysis.
- ❖ Using cryogen. Or cryoprobe.
- ❖ Immediate reactions (blistering and pain). Later hypo or depigmentation.

Surgical therapy

- ❖ Eliminates warts at a single visit.
- ❖ For large warts. And intraurethral warts. And failure to other therapy.
- ❖ Tangential scissor excision, tangential shave excision, curettage.

Radiofrequency ablation

- ❖ Eliminates warts in single visit.
- ❖ For warts on keratinized skin (mons pubis, inner aspect of thighs and buttocks).
- ❖ Use cutting and coagulation mode.

Treatment Protocols for Special Sites

Treatment selected based on size, number of lesions and also co-morbidities (pregnancy, HIV). Combination of different modalities may also be used.

Cervical warts

- ❖ Rule out malignancy by biopsy.
- ❖ Treatment in consultation with gynecologist.

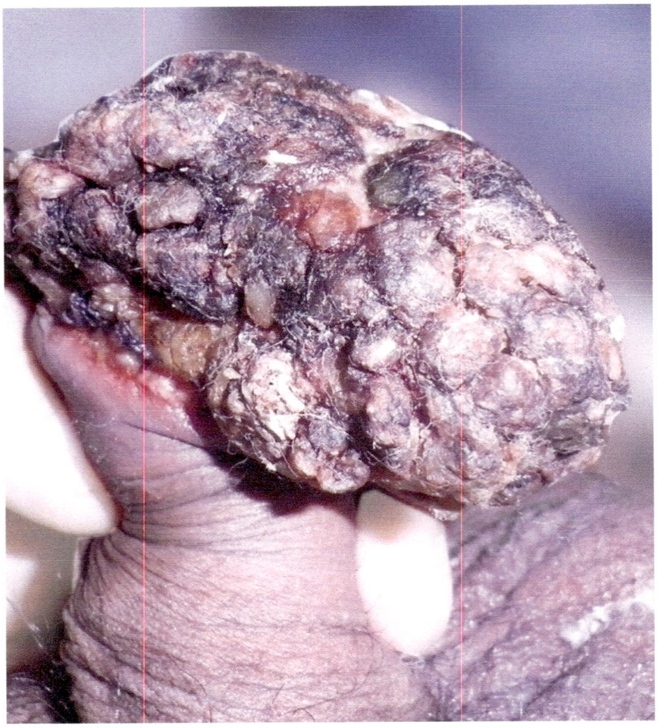

Buschke Lowenstein tumour: Due to HPV 6 and 11. It is a locally invasive lesion which does not metastasize. It may transform to squamous cell carcinoma in HIV positive.

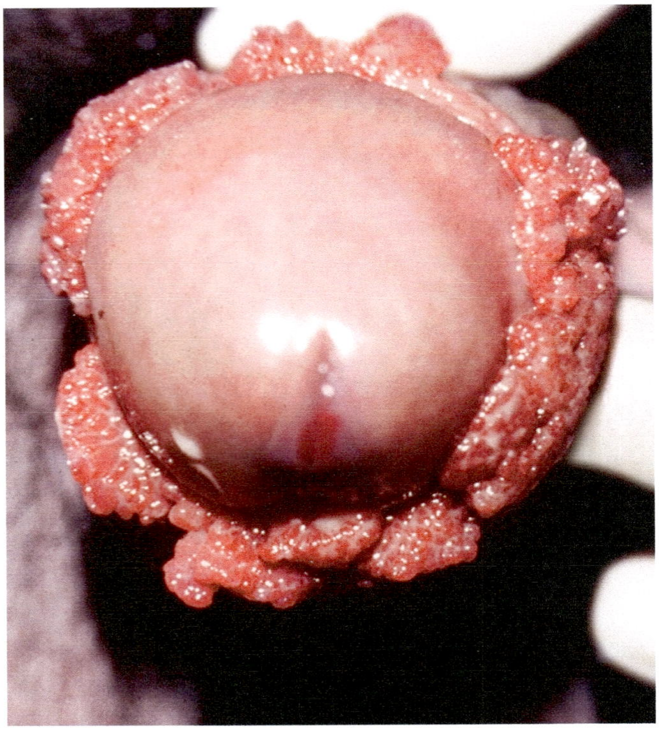

Anogenital warts in an HIV positive patient: Condyloma acuminata: Fleshy, verrucous plaque with hemorrhagic spots, present circumferentially around glans.

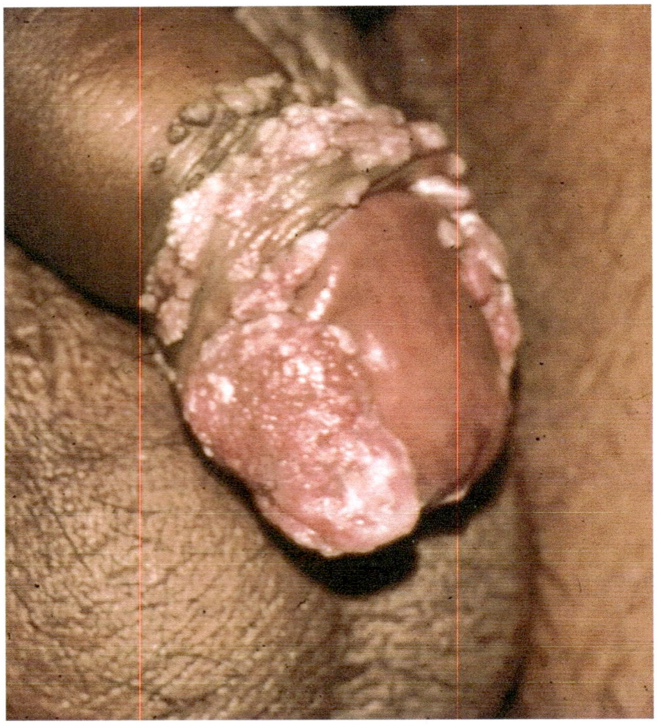

Anogenital warts in an HIV positive patient: Extensive involvement of prepuce with multiple well-defined, verrucous papules and plaques. The large lesion is indurated. There is an enhanced potential of malignant transformation of AGW in HIV positive patients, warranting a biopsy.

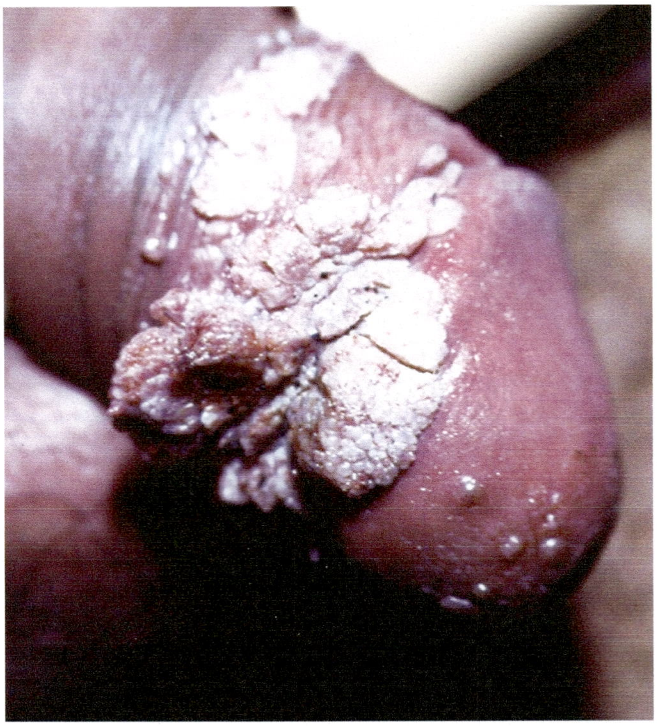

Anogenital warts in an HIV positive patient: Verrucous confluent plaques on prepuce with induration. Distal verrucous papules can be seen on glans.

Table 9.3: Treatment guidelines for anogenital warts

CDC 2010	WHO 2003	NACO 2007
Provider administered		
• Cryotherapy **OR** • Podophyllin resin **OR** • TCA **OR** • BCA (80%–90%) **OR** • Surgical removal	• Podophyllin resin **OR** • Trichloroacetic acid (TCA) or Bichloroacetic acid (BCA) 80%–90% **OR** • Cryotherapy **OR** • Surgical removal	• Podophyllin resin
Patient applied		
• Podofilox 0.5% solution or gel **OR** • Imiquimod 5% cream **OR** • Sinecatechins 15% ointment	• Podofilox 0.5% solution or gel **OR** • Imiquimod 5% cream	

Vaginal warts

- TCA application weekly.
- Cryotherapy **NOT** recommended because of risk of vaginal perforation and fistula formation.

Meatal warts

- Podophyllin applied by provider.
- Cryotherapy with liquid nitrogen.
- Limited data on use of podofilox and imiquimod for distal meatal warts.

Anal warts

- ***Perianal warts:***
  - TCA application weekly.
  - Cryotherapy with liquid nitrogen.
  - Surgical removal.
- ***Intra-anal warts:*** Managed in consultation with gastroenterologist.

Vaccines

- Two HPV vaccines available:
  - Bivalent protects against high risk HPV (type 16 and 18) which cause 80% of cervical cancers.
  - Quadrivalent protects against both high risk HPV (type 16 and 18) and low risk HPV (6 and 11) which cause most of AGW.
- Vaccines most effective when all doses administered before sexual contact.
  - *In females:* Either vaccine for 11-12 year olds but can be given upto 13-26 years.
  - *In males:* Quadrivalent vaccine in males 9-26 years.

Chapter 10

Genital Molluscum Contagiosum

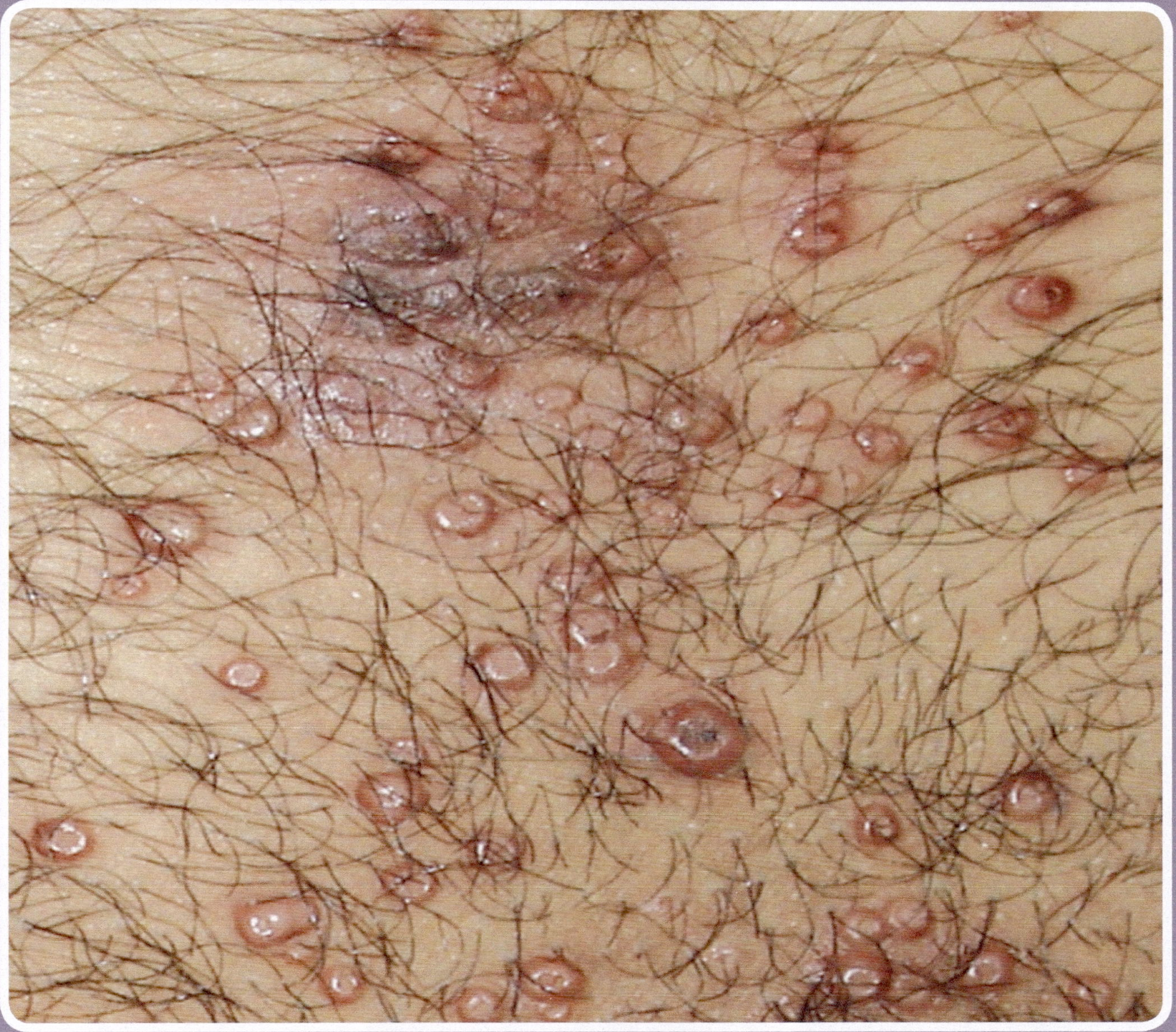

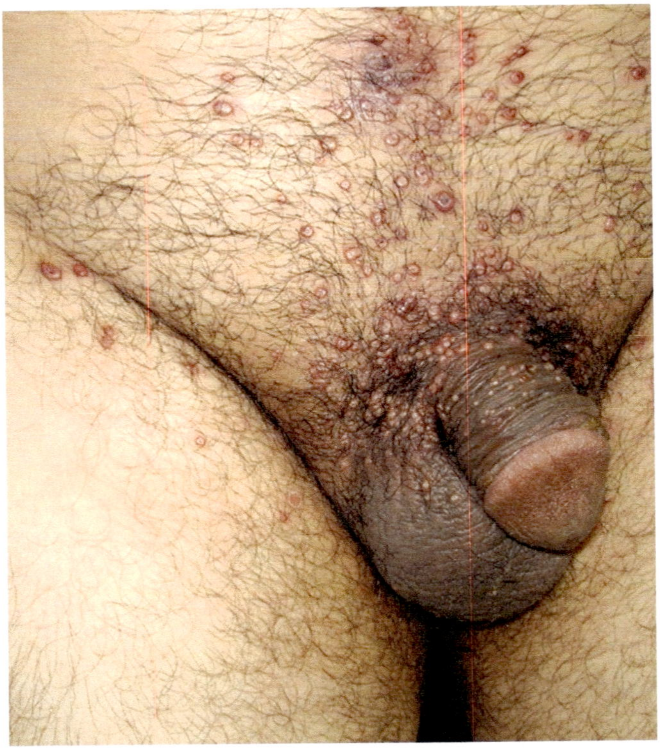

Genital molluscum contagiosum: Multiple dome-shaped papules with central umbilication aggregated on root of penis and extending on to lower abdomen and scrotum.

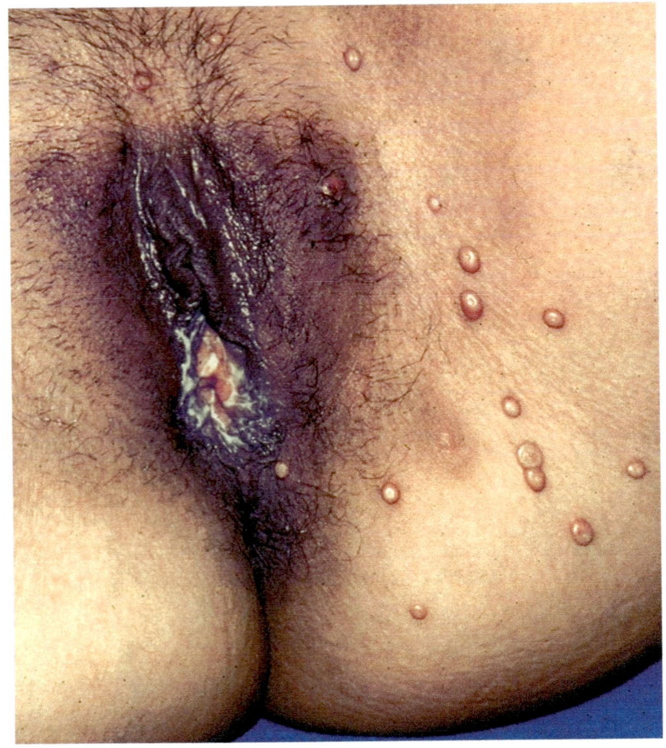

Genital molluscum contagiosum: Multiple skin-colored, dome shaped papules with central umbilication on vulva.

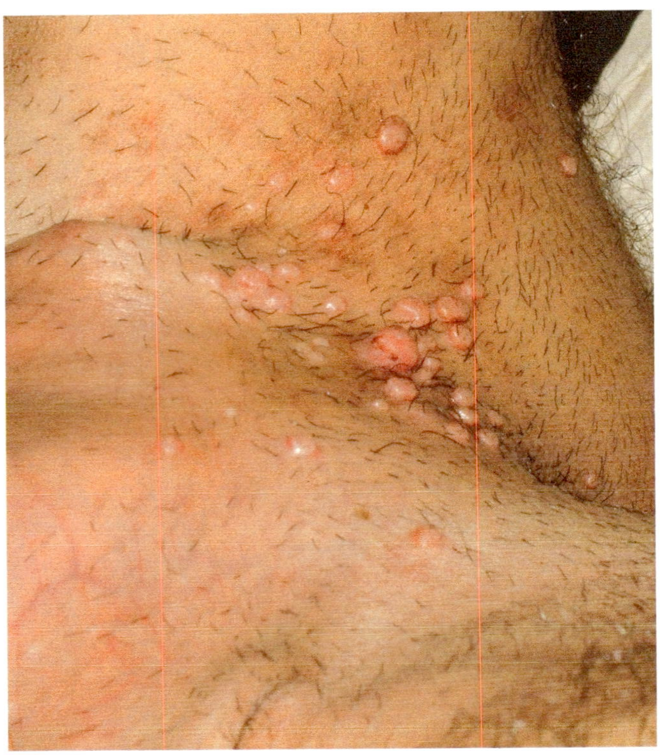

Genital molluscum contagiosum: Multiple, discrete, skin-colored papules with umbilication in the genital area.

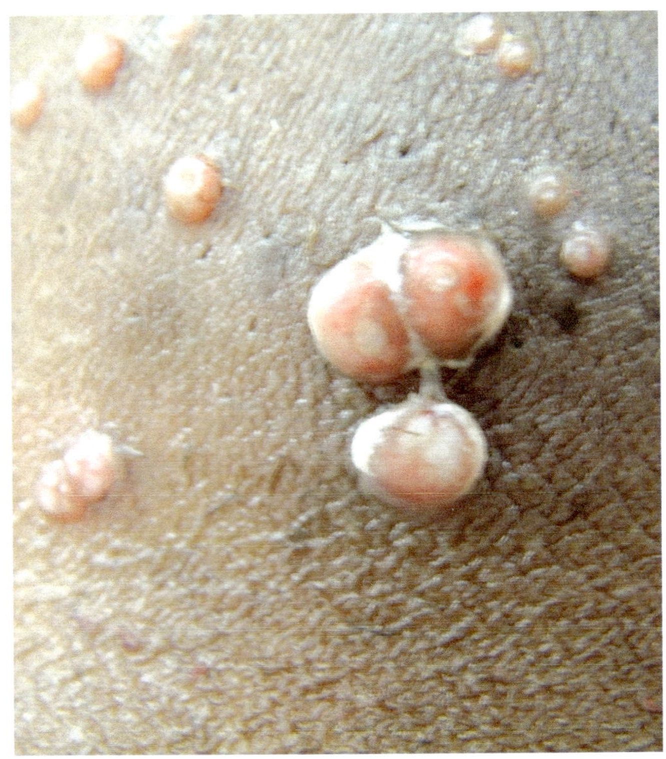

Genital molluscum contagiosum: Close up: Multiple dome-shaped papules with central umbilication. Some closely aggregated-a clue to look for underlying immunodeficiency.

ETIOLOGY

Etiological Agent

- Molluscum contagiosum virus (MCV), a virus of pox family:
- Four types—MCV 1 to 4. MCV-2 most frequently sexually transmitted.

Transmission

- ***Sexual contact:*** Leading to genital lesions. Condoms probably not (? partially) protective.
- ***Autoinoculation:*** By scratching.

EPIDEMIOLOGY

Geographic Distribution

- Varying prevalence worldwide. Three percent of all STD clinic attendees. And 6% of adolescents and young adults STD clinic attendees.
- Higher incidence in tropics, orphanages. And HIV-infected.

Demographic Distribution

- Equal in males and females.
- Extragenital MC commoner in children. Genital MC commoner in adults.

CLINICAL FEATURES

Incubation Period

Few weeks-2 months.

Morphology

- Pearly white skin colored, umbilicated, dome-shaped papules, 2-5 mm in size.
- Giant lesions in HIV-positive patients.

Sites of Lesions

- Penis, scrotum, vulva, perineum, lower abdomen and thighs in genital molluscum. Involvement of other parts of body considered extragenital.
- Molluscum localized to perianal area seen only in homosexual men. Upto 6% of MSM have perianal MC.

Variants

- **Giant molluscum contagiosum:** Larger lesions with central umbilication. Often closely aggregated. Suspect HIV infection.

COMPLICATIONS

- ***Infection:*** Secondary pyogenic infection manifesting as erythematous halo.
- ***Molluscum dermatitis:*** Ring of dermatitis (erythema, crusting, scaling) around individual papules of MC.

MOLLUSCUM CONTAGIOSUM IN HIV

- MC more frequent and numerous in HIV.
- Atypical lesions-giant lesions, verrucous indurated plaques.
- Resistance to conventional therapy. Response improves once antiretroviral treatment started.

DIAGNOSIS

Based on Clinical Features

Discrete pearly white papules with central umbilication.

Laboratory Investigations

Diagnosis made clinically. Investigations only in larger atypical lesions, in immunocompromised individuals (to rule out deep fungal infections).

- ***Crush smear:*** Extirpated core material crushed and stained with Giemsa. Shows multiple keratinocytes with intracytoplasmic pinkish ovoid bodies (Henderson-Patterson bodies) pushing the nucleus to the periphery (signet ring appearance).

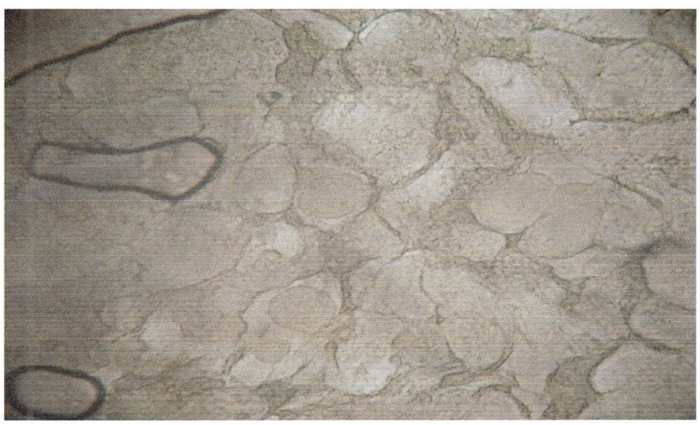

Crush smear of molluscum body: Extirpated papule mounted with normal saline shows multiple ballooned up keratinocytes stuffed with round intracytoplasmic molluscum bodies.

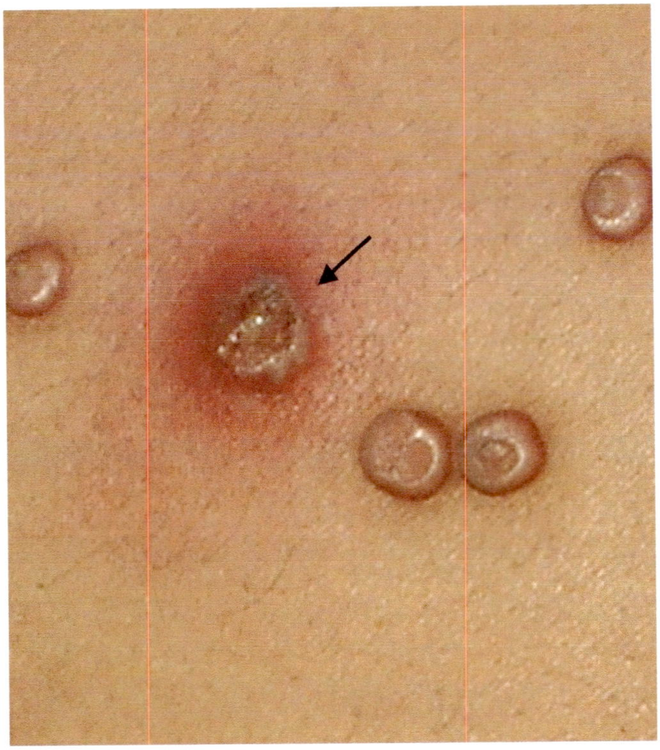

Molluscum contagiosum: With secondary infection manifesting as erythematous halo around the lesion.

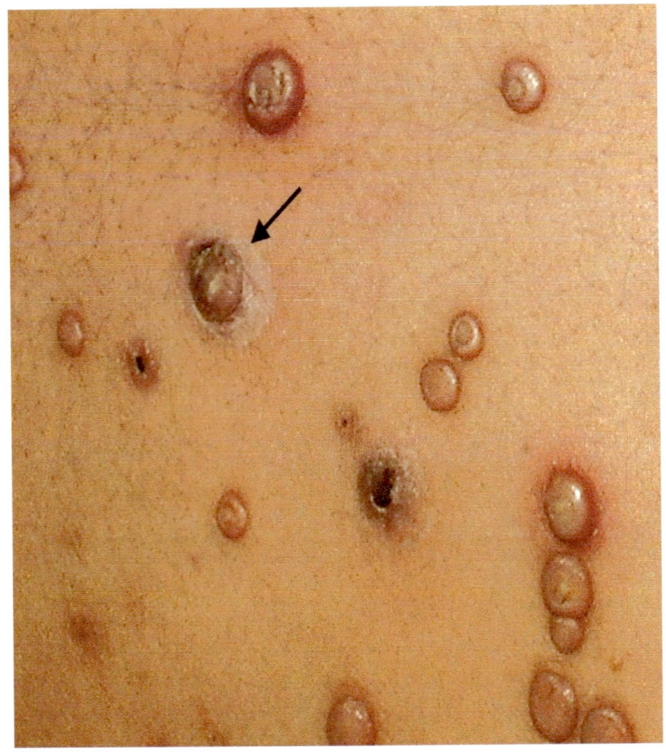

Molluscum dermatitis: Manifesting as erythema, scaling and crusting around the lesion.

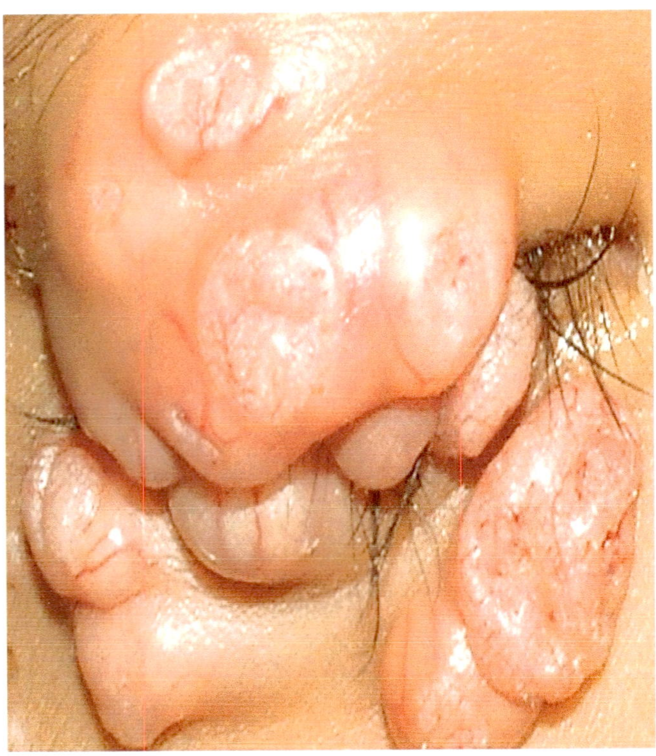

Molluscum contagiosum in an HIV-positive patient: Giant lesions with telangiectasia and clustering of lesions around the eye.

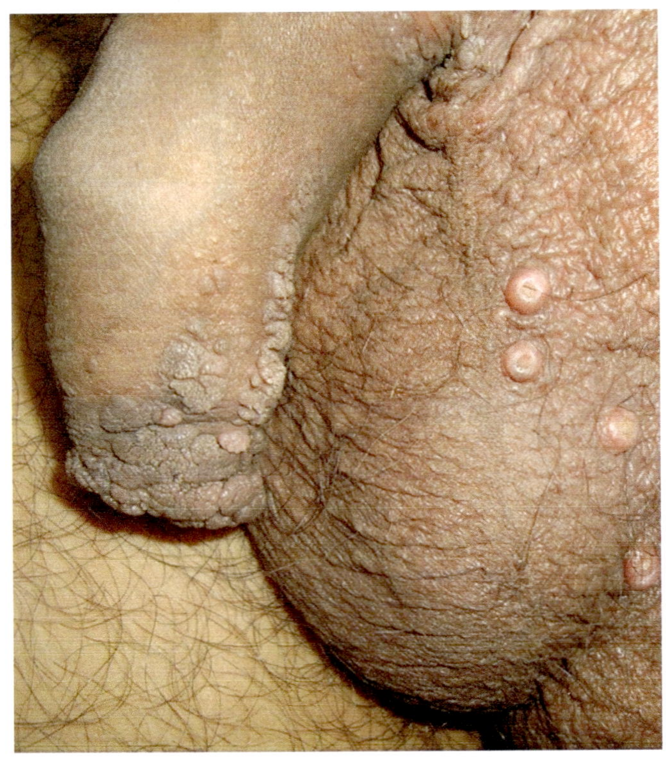

Molluscum contagiosum: In presence of one sexually transmitted disease, its important to rule out others. This patient has both anogenital warts and molluscum contagiosum.

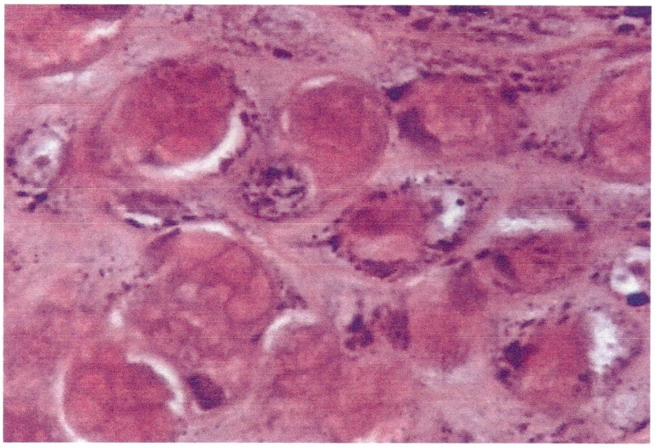

Crush smear of molluscum contagiosum: Showing pinkish ovoid intracytoplasmic bodies (Henderson-Patterson bodies) pushing the nucleus to periphery (signet ring appearance).

- ***Skin biopsy:*** Intracytoplasmic eosinophilic molluscum bodies in epidermis.
- ***Dermoscopy:*** Better visualization of umbilication. Vascular and punctiform patterns observed.

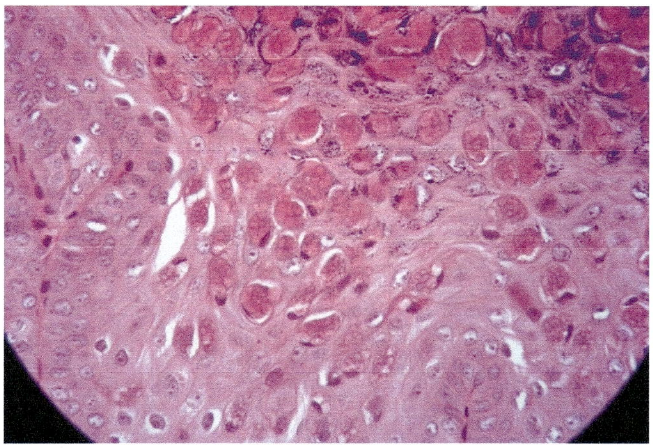

Histopathology of molluscum contagiosum: Showing eosinophilic intracytoplasmic bodies in epidermis.
Courtesy: Dr S Singh, Department of Dermatology, AIIMS.

TREATMENT

- Generally self-limiting (may take 6 months to 5 years to resolve).
- Treat to prevent sexual transmission. And for cosmetic purpose.
- Treatment options aim to destroy individual lesions (Table 10.1). Often destruction of few lesions leads to subsidence of rest due to immune stimulation.

Other Treatment Considerations

- Test for syphilis, HIV and HBV at initial visit.
- If negative, retest at 3 months.
- Evaluate for other STIs. Often several STIs transmitted together.

Table 10.1: Treatment options for molluscum contagiosum
Needle extirpation
Needle extirpation followed by trichloroacetic acid (25%) application
TCA (20-30%) application
Cryotherapy
Imiquimod (5%)
Curettage
Cidofovir (3%)

CHAPTER 11

Human Immunodeficiency Virus Infection and Acquired Immunodeficiency Syndrome

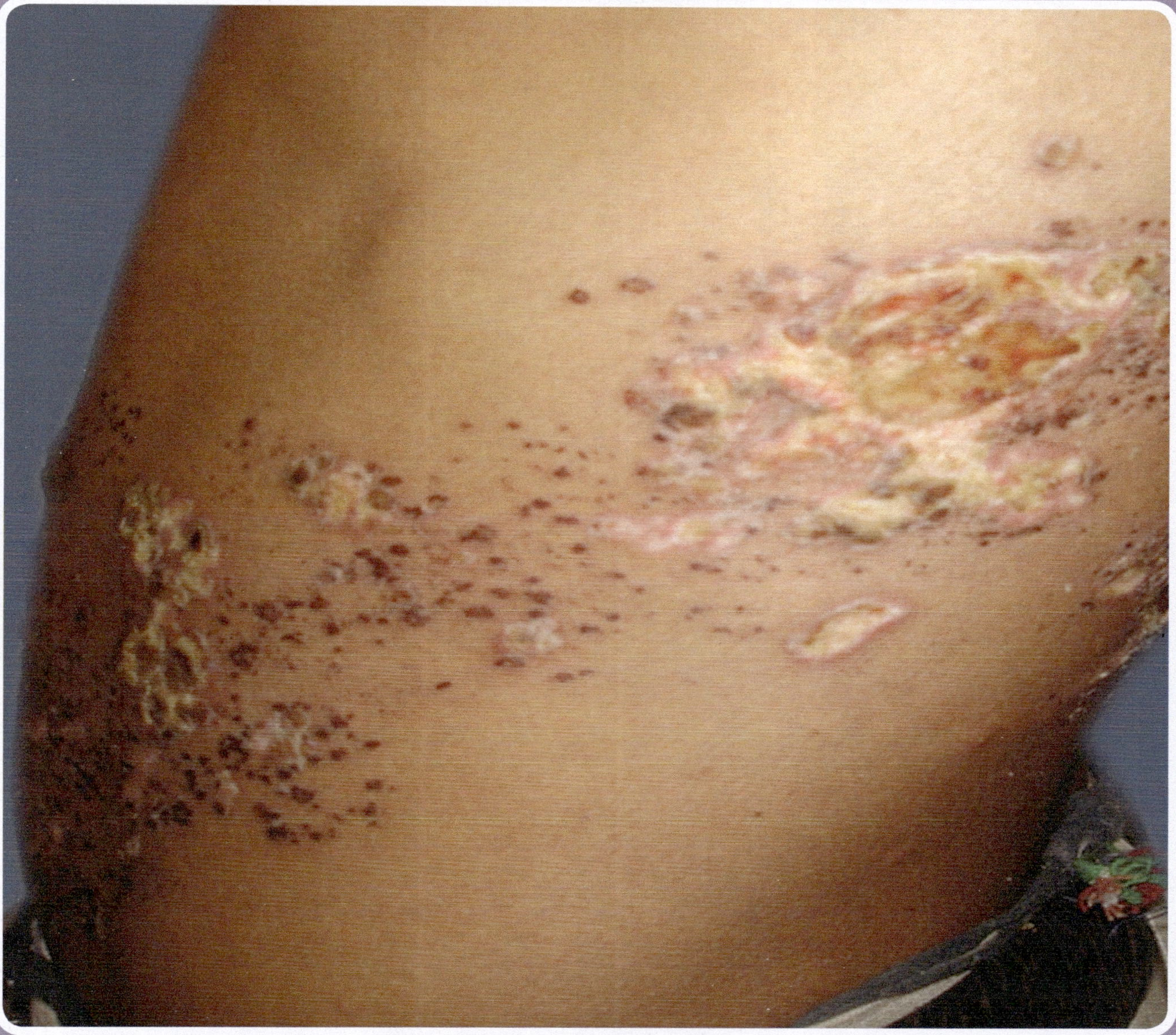

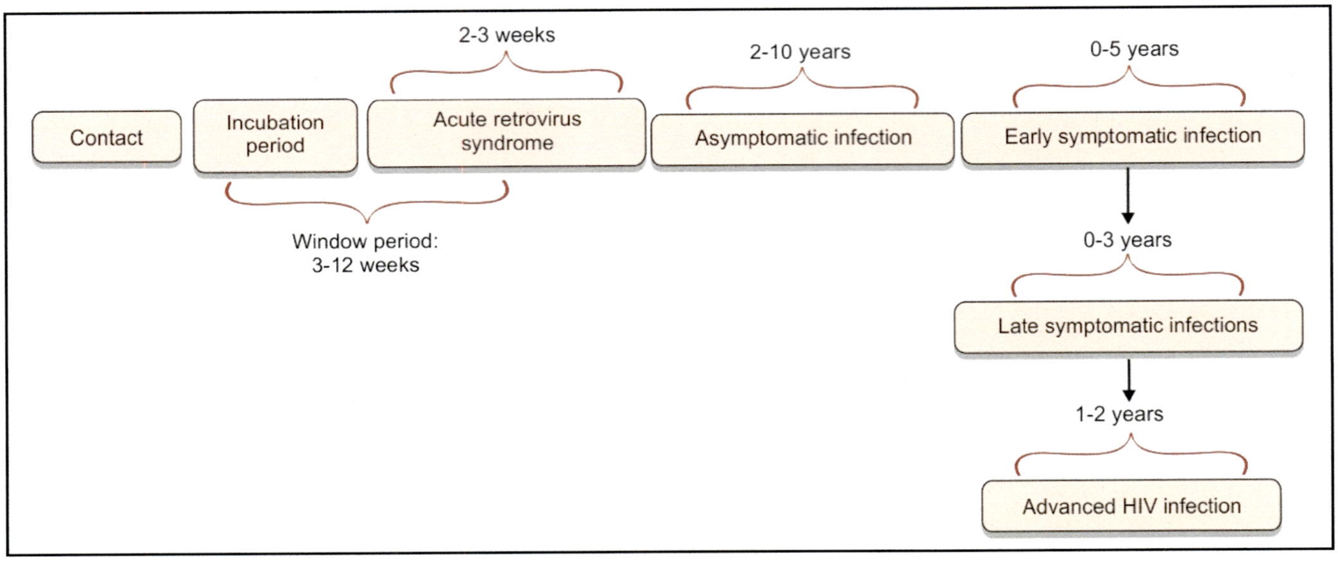

Course and stages of HIV infection

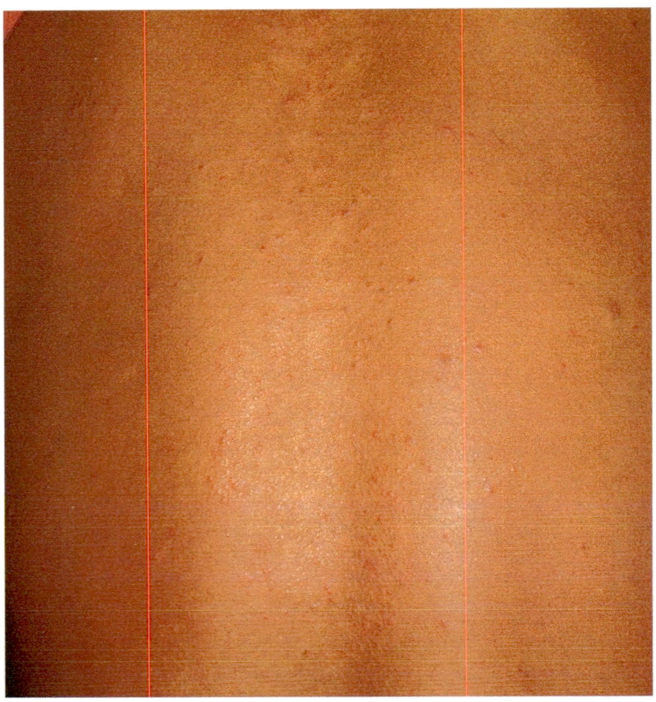

Rash of acute retroviral syndrome: A maculopapular rash is seen in 70% of patients, but is often disregarded.

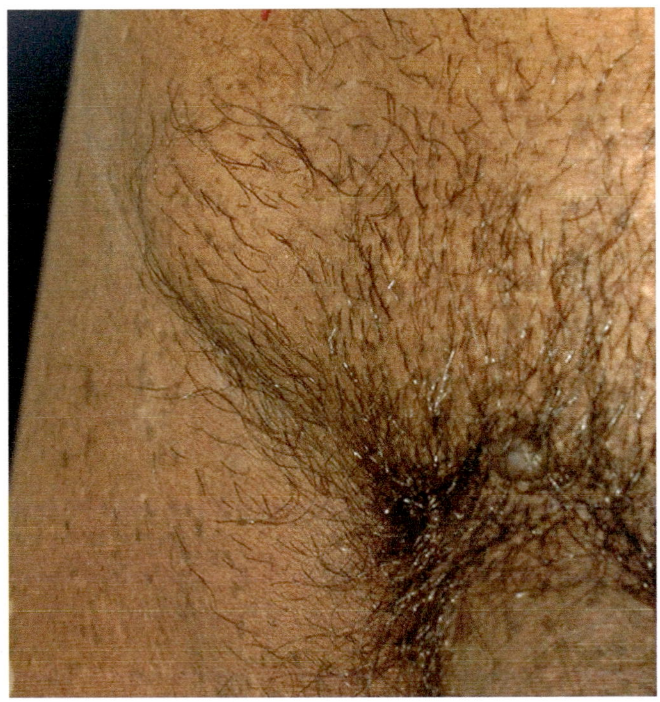

Persistent generalized lymphadenopathy in an HIV-positive patient: Enlarged inguinal lymph nodes in a clinically otherwise asymptomatic but serologically HIV-positive patient.

Acquired immunodeficiency syndrome (AIDS) and human immunodeficiency virus (HIV) infection, a major global health problem.

EPIDEMIOLOGY

Geographic Distribution

- Globally, number of people living with HIV and AIDS (PLHA) variable (Table 11.1).
- Prevalence of HIV/AIDS in high risk goups higher (Table 11.2).

Table 11.1: Number of PLHAs and prevalence of HIV infection

	PLHA in millions	Prevalence (%)
Global[1]	34.0 (2011)	0.8
India[2]	2.08 (2011)	0.29

Table 11.2: Prevalence of HIV/AIDS in high risk groups

	Prevalence
Intravenous drug users (IDU)	9.2%
Males having sex with males (MSM)	7.4%
Commercial sex workers	4.9%
STI clinic attendees	2.5%
Antenatal clinic attendees	0.49%

Demographic Distribution

- Prevalence lower in women as compared to men, but susceptibility greater in women.
- Adults more frequently affected than children.

ETIOLOGY

Etiological Agent

Caused by HIV, a lymphotropic enveloped retrovirus.

- ***Structure:*** Spherical, single-stranded, enveloped RNA virus, 120 nm in size. Consists of 2 parts:
  - *Outer envelope:* Bilipid membrane; with HIV antigens (glycoproteins[3] gp 120 and gp 41) embedded.
  - *Inner core:*
    - Bounded by 2 layers of protein coat (outer layer of p17 and inner of p24).
    - Core of 2 strands of viral RNA and 3 important viral enzymes, reverse transcriptase (RT), integrase and protease.

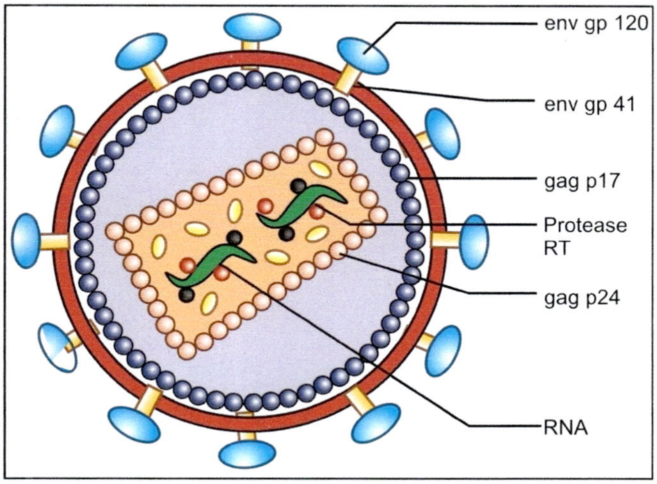

Structure of HIV

- ***Genes and proteins of HIV:***
  - *Major structural genes:*
    - Gag: coding for nuclear proteins p17 and p24
    - Pol: coding for reverse transcriptase (RT), protease and integrase.
    - Env: coding for envelope proteins gp120 and gp41.
  - *Regulatory genes:* rev, tat and nef, and other small accessory genes (vif, vpu, vpr) important for infection.
- ***Types:*** Two types—HIV-1 and HIV-2 with several differences in epidemiology and manifestations (Table 11.3).

Table 11.3: Differences between HIV-1 and HIV-2

	HIV-1	HIV-2
Prevalence	Higher	Lower
Incubation period	Shorter	Longer
Progression to AIDS	Higher, faster	Lower, slower
Natural history	Clearly defined	Not yet clear/may not have phase of acute retroviral syndrome
Lab diagnosis	Easily diagnosed	Difficult to diagnose
Response to ART	Commonly used drugs effective	Nucleoside molecules and few protease inhibitors viricidal

[1]**Globally:** Sub-Saharan Africa and Caribbean region most afflicted.

[2]**In India:** States with high prevalence—Maharashtra, Andhra Pradesh, Karnataka, Tamil Nadu and Manipur.

[3]**Glycoproteins:** Responsible for attachment of virus to CD4 receptors of host cells and subsequent fusion of virus envelope with host cell membrane.

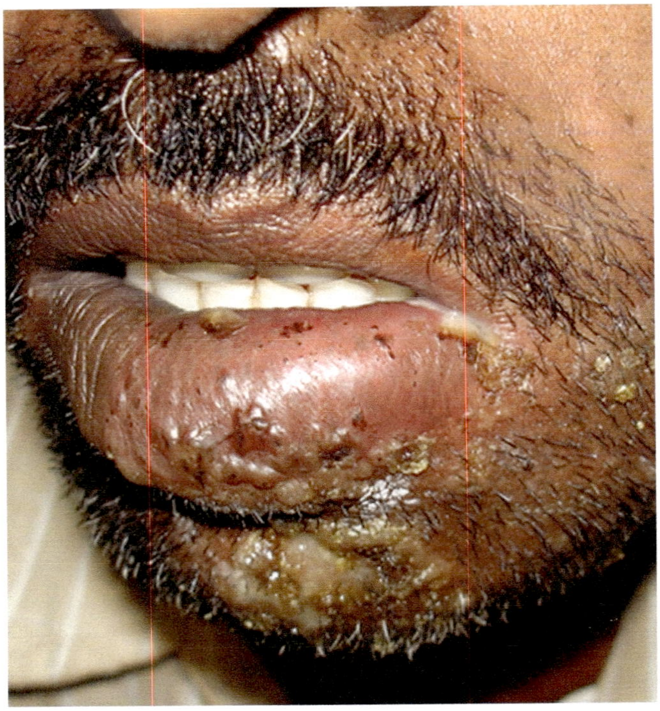

Herpes zoster in an HIV-positive patient: Involvement of mandibular division of V cranial nerve. Zoster occurs when CD4+ count $< 500/mm^3$

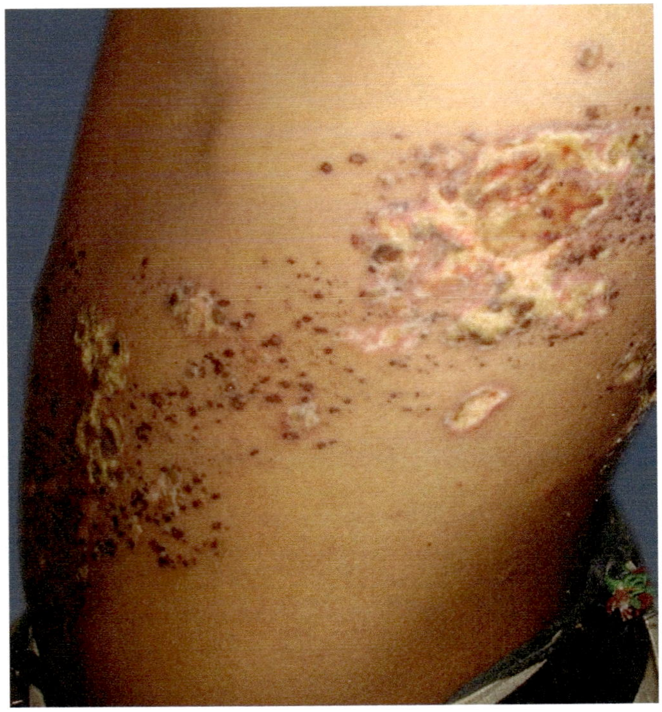

Herpes zoster in an HIV-positive patient: Involvement of trunk in dermatomal pattern. Deeper ulcers with necrotic slough a clue to test for underlying HIV infection.

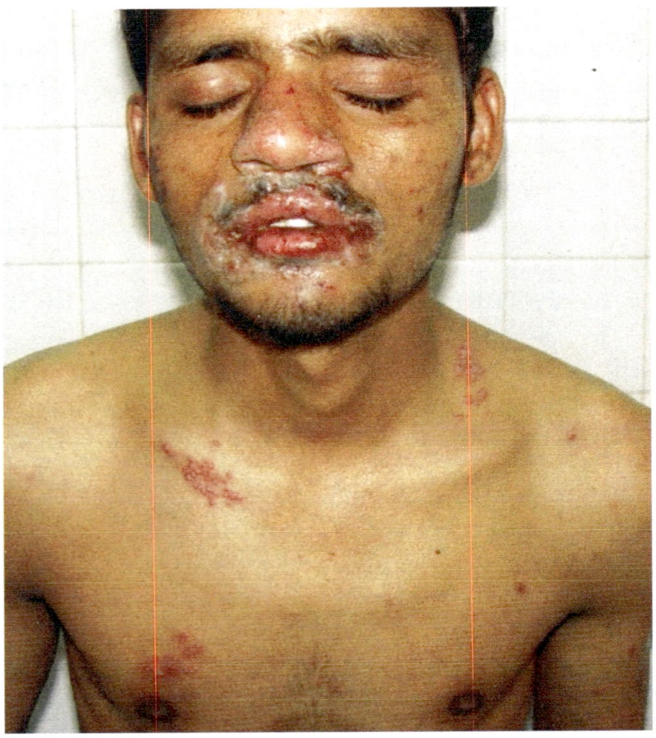

Herpes zoster in an HIV-positive patient: Multidermatomal and bilateral involvement with dissemination. Such widespread distribution suggestive of HIV-positive state. Herpes zoster often seen in early symptomatic HIV infection.

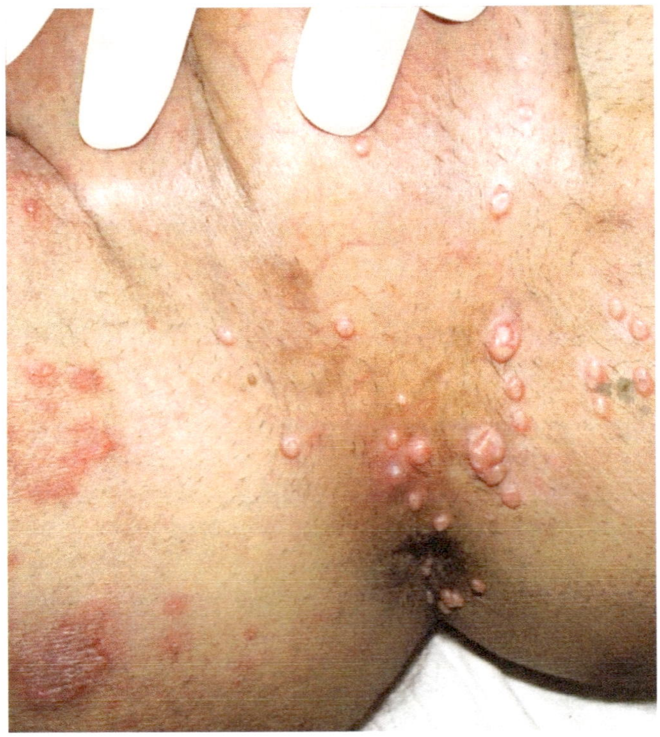

Molluscum contagiosum in an HIV-positive patient: Multiple lesions, some large. Multiple lesions occur when CD4 counts $< 250/mm^3$

- *HIV 1:* Classified into a major or M group. And an outlier or O group. Group M consists of clades (subtypes) A to N. Different geographic distribution of subtypes: India: subtype C, along with subtypes A, B and E. Africa: subtypes A, C and D. Other parts of World: subtype B.
- *HIV 2:* HIV-2 less frequently encountered; initially identified in West Africa; now spread to many parts of Asia, including India.

Transmission

Humans main reservoir of HIV. Transmission from HIV infected person to uninfected person by several routes:

- ***Sexual:*** Unprotected sexual intercourse:
  - *Heterosexual:* Risk of transmission higher from female to male (0.5%) *vs* male to female (0.2%). In India, commonest (87.1%) mode of transmission.
  - *Homosexual:* In MSM (risk of transmission, 2%)
- ***Vertical:*** From HIV positive mother to child, antenatally, perinatally or postnally (lactation). Risk of transmission 25%. Commonest mode of transmission in India, after hetrosexual exposure.
- ***Transfusion:*** From infected blood and blood products, transplantation of organ/tissue and through artificial insemination.
- ***Use of contaminated needles:*** Mainly in intravenous drug users.
- ***Nosocomial infection:*** Due to accidental needle stick injury or sharp instrument cuts from an HIV-positive patient. Rare, if universal precautions adopted.
- **No transmission through:** Arthropod bites; fomites. Or by physical touch.

Pathogenesis

HIV replication cycle

HIV an enveloped retrovirus.[4]

- ***Entry into target cells:*** HIV capsid (along with HIV RNA and enzymes) enters target cell (CD4+ T cells and macrophages) by:
  - Binding of HIV surface glycoproteins to CD4 receptors on target cells.
  - Fusion of viral envelope with cell membrane of target cells.
- ***Reverse transcription:*** RT copies single-stranded RNA genome into a complementary DNA (cDNA) strand.[5]

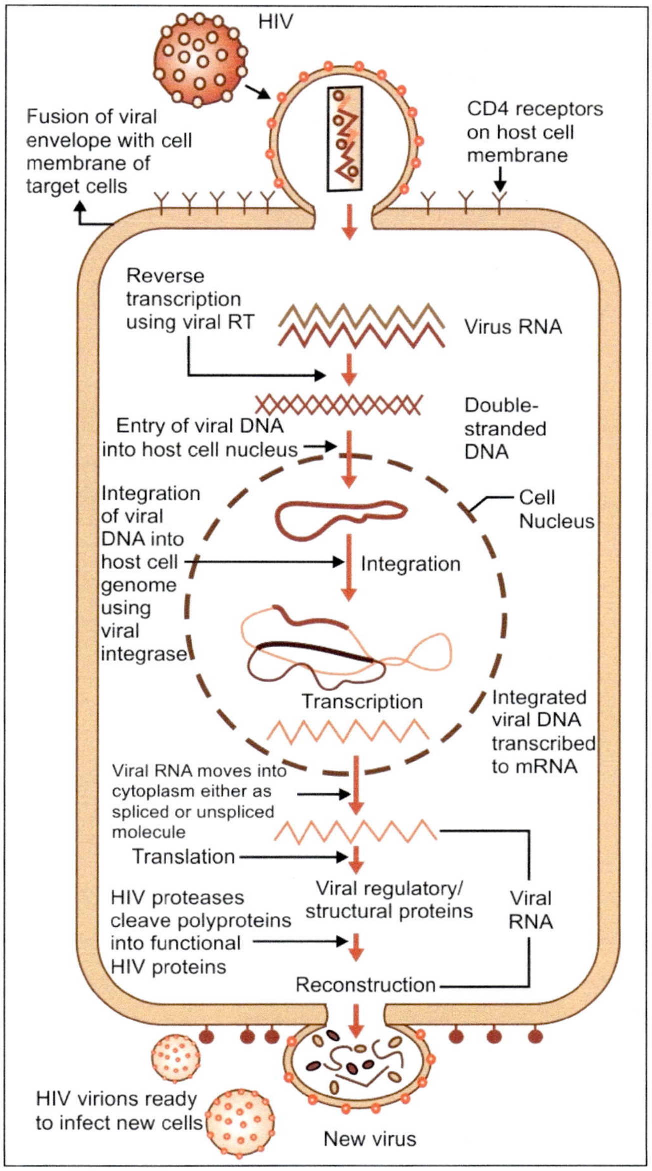

Replication of HIV

A sense DNA strand is created from this antisense cDNA to form double-stranded viral DNA, which is transported into host cell nucleus.

- ***Integration into host cell genome:*** On entering host cell nucleus, viral DNA integrated into host cell's genome (using viral enzyme integrase), a step inhibited by integrase inhibitors.
- ***Viral replication:*** Integrated viral DNA may lie dormant (in latent HIV infection). Or replicate (as infection progresses). During viral replication

[4]**Retroviruses:** So named because of an unusual step in life cycle-synthesis of DNA from RNA template, using enzyme reverse transcriptase.

[5]**Process of reverse transcription:** Extremely error-prone, resulting in mutations—responsible for evasion from host's immune system as also development of drug resistance.

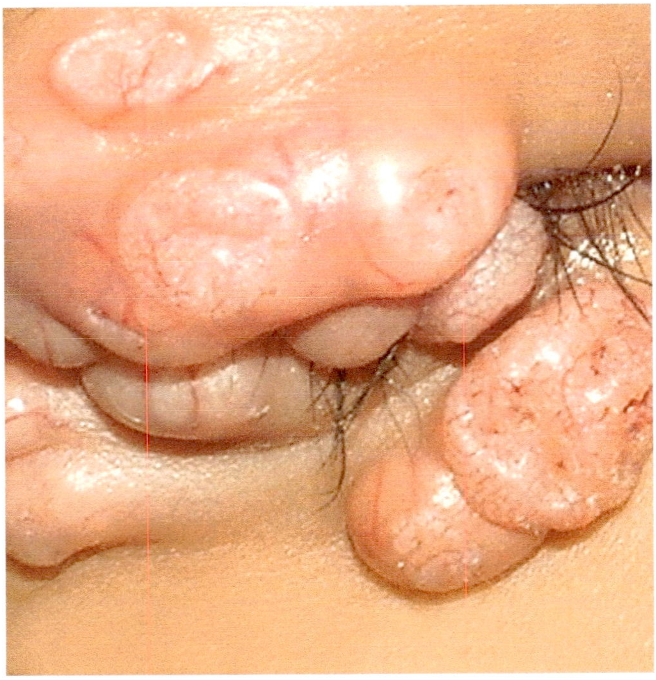

Molluscum contagiosum in an HIV-positive patient: Giant, closely aggregated lesions on the face. Giant lesions surrogate marker of low CD4 count (< 50/mm^3)

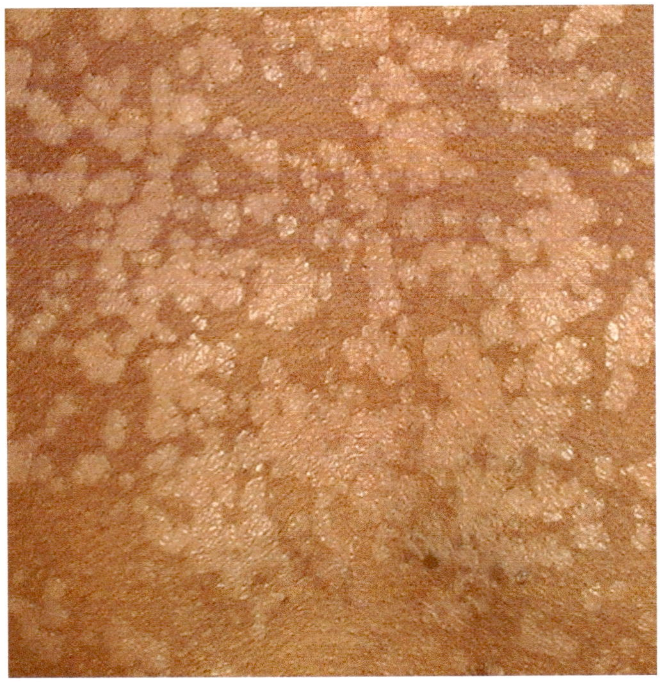

Human papilloma virus infection in an HIV-positive patient: Extensive pityriasis versicolor-like lesions, similar to those seen in epidermodysplasia verruciformis.

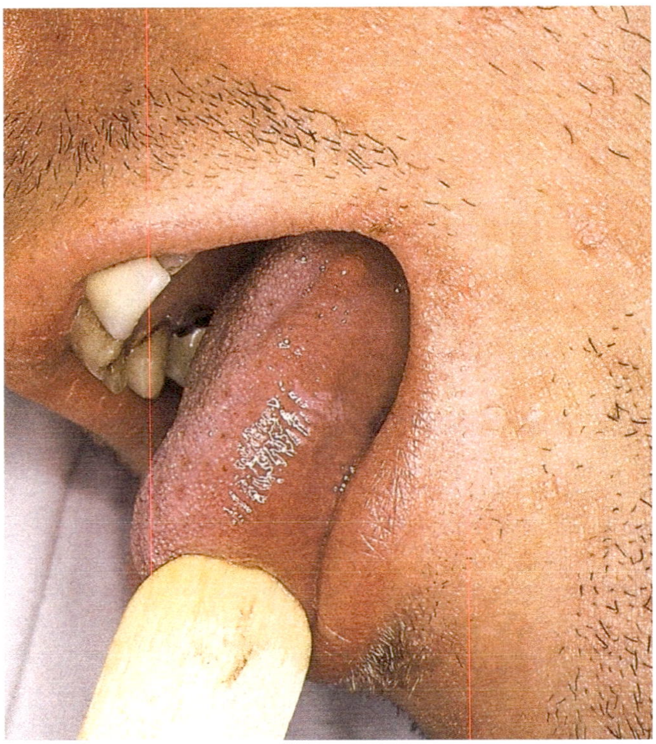

Oral hairy leukoplakia in an HIV-positive patient: Due to *Epstein Barr virus*. Manifests as asymptomatic, white plaques with characteristic vertical corrugations on lateral aspect of tongue.

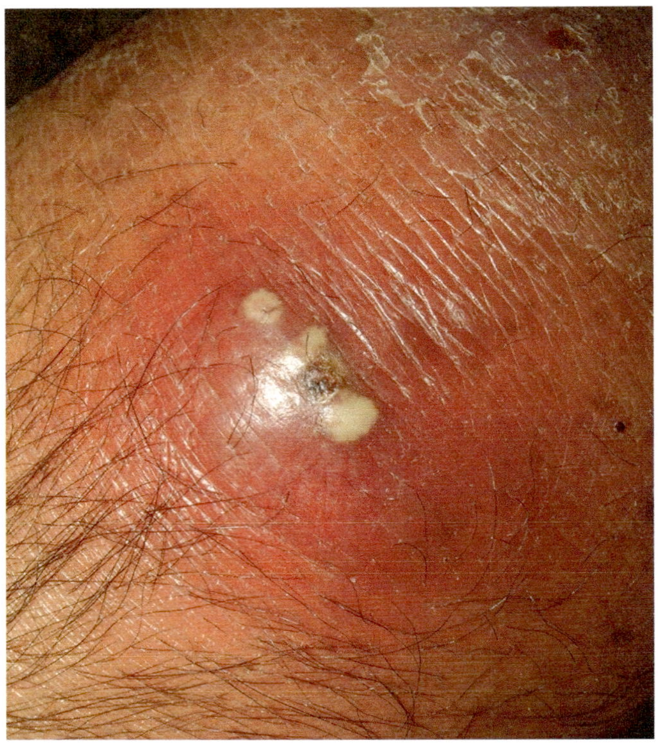

Pyogenic infections in an HIV-positive patient: Cutaneous pyogenic (especially *Staphylococcus aureus*) infections common. Sometimes resistant to treatment.

integrated DNA provirus transcribed into mRNA. May be spliced (into smaller pieces) or remain unspliced. Both move into cytoplasm → translated proteins.

- Spliced viral RNA → translated into regulatory proteins Tat and Rev.
- Unspliced RNA → translated into structural proteins Gag and Env which help in packaging of new virus particles.

❖ ***Assembly and release:*** Occurs on plasma membrane of host cell.

- Components of HIV move towards plasma membrane. And virion buds develop from host cell.
- Maturation of virion occurs either in forming buds or in the immature virion after it buds off from the host cell.
- During maturation, HIV proteases cleave polyproteins into individual functional HIV proteins (a step inhibited by protease inhibitors).
- On maturation, virion able to infect another cell.

Host's response

❖ Initially, though some virions are killed, HIV continues to multiply rapidly, infecting more CD4 cells. Antibodies against HIV absent (patient seronegative, albiet falsely) but highly infectious (window period).[6]

❖ After 3-12 weeks, patient mounts serological response and viral load decreases.

❖ Clinical manifestations depend on effects on immune system:

- In early period of immune destruction, clinical latency, *i.e.* no clinical symptoms, but serological positivity, viral load low and CD4+ counts normal.
- Later, as immunosuppression progresses, patient becomes symptomatic. Viral load increases and CD4+ count decreases.

CLINICAL FEATURES

Course

❖ Primary HIV infection at the end of which acute retroviral syndrome occurs (indicating seroconversion) 2-4 weeks after infection→ 2-10 years of asymptomatic period → symptomatic phases (early, late and advanced) → death in 1-3 years (without ART).

Stages of Disease

❖ ***Acute retroviral syndrome (ARS):***

- *Incidence:* Up to 50-90% develop ARS. Commoner if infection sexually acquired.
- *Lasts:* 2-3 weeks.
- *Manifestations:*
  - Fever, lymphadenopathy, pharyngitis, arthralgia, myalgia, neck stiffness.
  - And in 70%, maculopapular rash and mucosal ulcers.
  - Trunk, palms and soles.

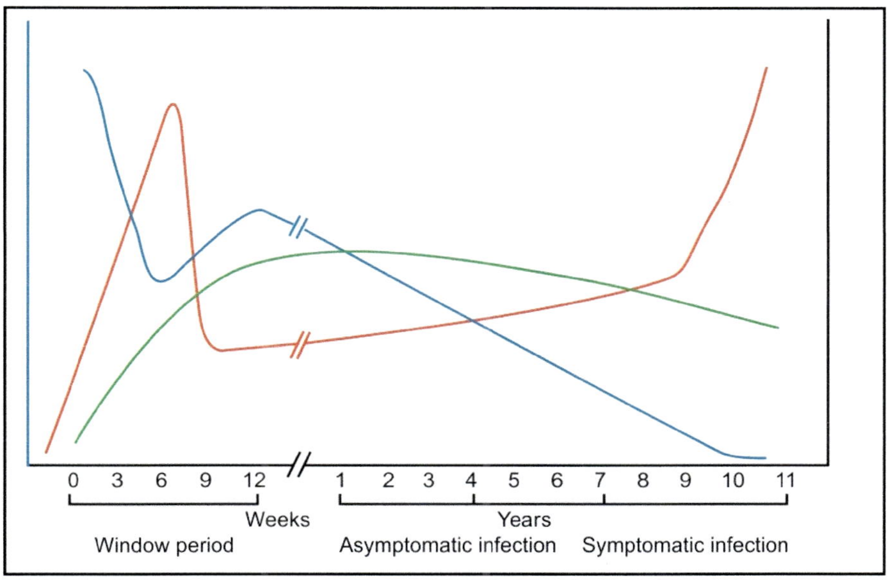

Relationship of HIV load (red), HIV antibodies (green) and CD4 counts (blue) as HIV infection progresses.

[6]**Window period:** Variable; shorter for transfusion acquired infection. Diagnosis of HIV infection during window period by detection of p24 antigen. Or using nucleic acid-based assays.

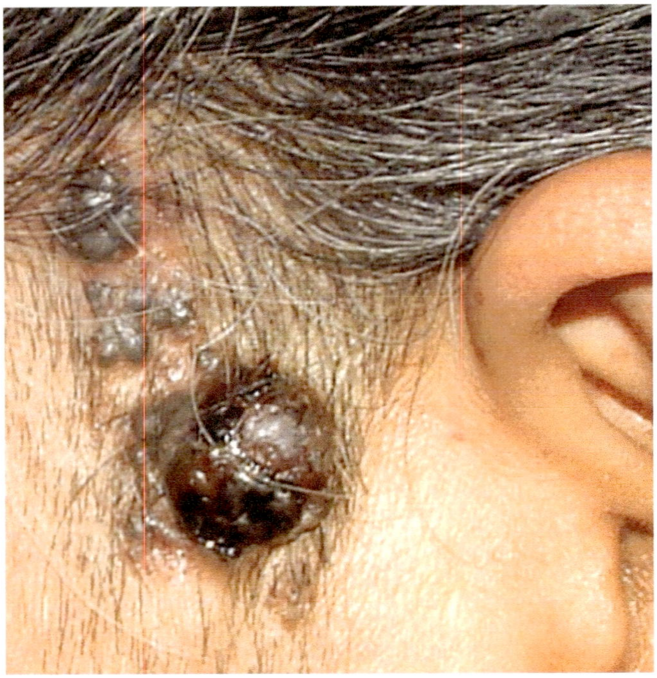

Bacillary angiomatosis in an HIV-positive patient: Multiple (sometimes solitary) pyogenic granuloma-like nodules. Local lymphadenopathy frequent.

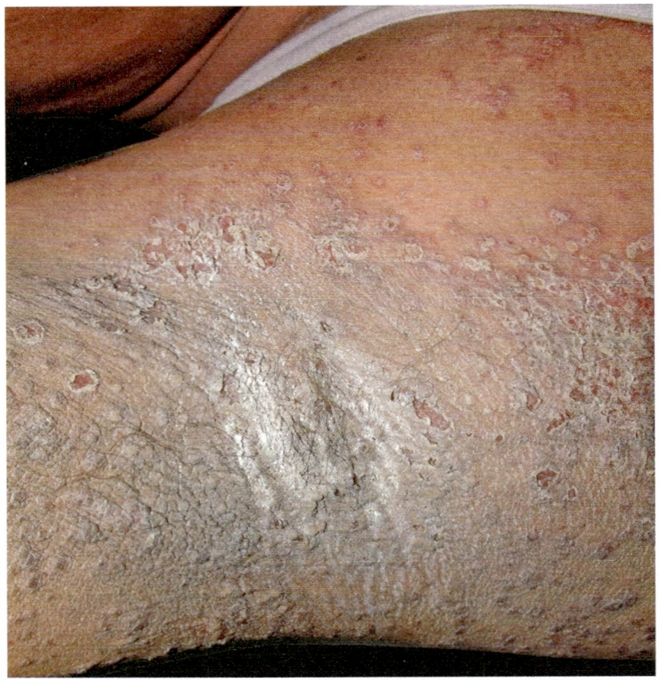

Candidiasis in an HIV-positive patient: Most common cutaneous infection. Often severe, extensive and indicative of disease progression.

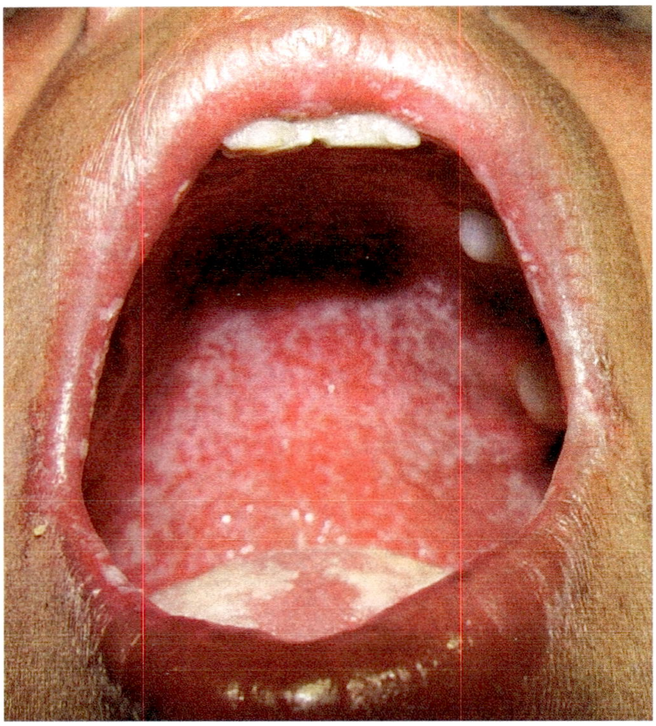

Oral candidiasis in an HIV-positive patient: Extensive, recurrent oropharyngeal infections. Associated dysphagia a clue to esophageal involvement, an AIDS defining criteria.

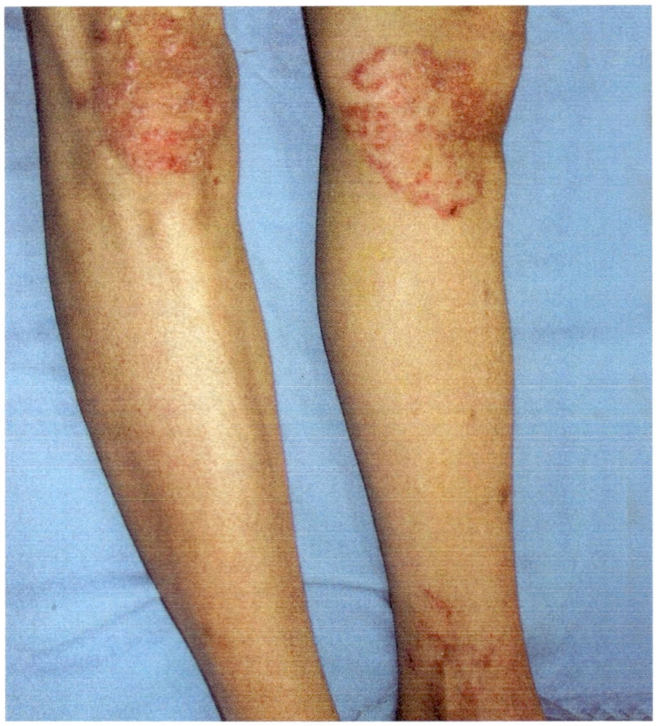

Dermatophyte infection in an HIV-positive patient: Tinea corporis, multiple extensive, recurrent lesions.

- *Treatment:* Antiretroviral treatment (ART) given during ARS may ? delay/abort progress to AIDS.

- ***Asymptomatic HIV infection:*** WHO clinical stage 1.
  - *Incubation period:* 2-10 years.
  - *Lasts:* 2-10 years.
  - *Manifestation:* Clinically asymptomatic. But persistent generalized lymphadenopathy often present.
- ***Early symptomatic disease:*** WHO clinical stage 2.
  - *Lasts:* 0-5 years.
  - *Manifestations:* Moderate unexplained weight loss (< 10% of presumed or measured body weight), recurrent respiratory tract infections (sinusitis, tonsillitis, otitis media and pharyngitis). And cutaneous manifestations (herpes zoster, onychomycosis, angular cheilitis, recurrent oral ulcerations, seborrhoeic dermatitis).
- ***Late symptomatic disease:*** WHO clinical stage 3.
  - *Lasts:* 0-3 years.
  - *Manifestations:*
    - Constitutional symptoms: Progressive. Include unexplained severe weight loss (> 10% of presumed/measured body weight), unexplained chronic diarrhoea (> 1 month) and unexplained persistent fever (> 1 month).
    - Infections: Persistent oral candidiasis, oral hairy leukoplakia, pulmonary tuberculosis, severe bacterial infections (pneumonia, empyema, pyomyositis, bone/joint infections, meningitis or bacteremia), acute necrotizing ulcerative stomatitis, gingivitis or periodontitis.
    - Hematological manifestations: Unexplained anemia (< 8 g/dl), neutropenia (< 0.5 x 109/l), chronic thrombocytopenia (< 50 x 10^9/l).
- ***Advanced HIV:*** WHO clinical stage 4.
  - *Lasts:* 1-2 years.
  - *Manifestations:*
    - HIV wasting syndrome.
    - Infections: AIDS defining opportunistic infections like *Pneumocystis* pneumonia, recurrent bacterial pneumonia, chronic herpes simplex infection, *Cytomegalovirus* infection (retinitis or infection of other organs), esophageal candidiasis, extrapulmonary cryptococcosis (including meningitis), disseminated coccidioidomycosis and histoplasmosis, extrapulmonary tuberculosis, disseminated non-tuberculous mycobacterial infections chronic isosporiasis. And cryptosporidiosis, atypical leishmaniasis recurrent non-typhoidal *Salmonella* bacteremia.
    - Neoplasms: Kaposi's sarcoma, lymphoma (cerebral or B-cell non-Hodgkin). Or other solid HIV-associated tumors.
    - Symptomatic HIV-associated nephropathy. Or symptomatic HIV-associated cardiomyopathy. Or neurological changes like HIV encephalopathy, progressive multifocal leukoencephalopathy.

Cutaneous Manifestations

Skin involvement invariable in HIV-infected; generally not life threatening. Often distinct helping in early recognition of disease and recognizing progression.

Infections

Viral infections

- ***Herpes zoster:*** Initially normal course. Later, multidermatomal involvement, dissemination (involvement of > 3 contiguous dermatomes, > 20 lesions outside initial dermatome or systemic involvement) and hemorrhagic. Also severe postherpetic neuralgia. Always treat with antivirals.
- ***Molluscum contagiosum:*** Initially typical presentation. Later atypical - larger (also giant), aggregated, progressive, persistent. Extragenital lesions (on face) of adult warrants ruling out HIV infection. Also excellent marker of HIV disease progression, number of lesions correlate inversely with CD4 cell count. Treatment response erratic often resistant to standard therapy. May respond to antiretroviral therapy (ART). Topical and systemic cidofovir helpful.
- ***Human papilloma virus:*** Normal presentation. Or warts extensive, numerous, exuberant. May present as a pityriasis versicolor—like eruption akin to epidermodysplasia verruciformis. Greater oncogenic potential. Anogenital lesions exuberant. May contribute to causation of Bowen's disease, erythroplasia of Queyrat and bowenoid papulosis.
- ***Oral hairy leukoplakia:*** Due to *Epstein Barr virus*. Asymptomatic white plaques with characteristic vertical corrugations. On lateral aspect of tongue. May occur even with CD4+ counts > 500/mm^3.

Bacterial infections

- ***Pyogenic infections:*** Cutaneous and systemic pyogenic (especially *Staphylococcus aureus)* infections common. Sometimes resistant to treatment.
- ***Tuberculosis:*** (And ? leprosy) get reactivated.

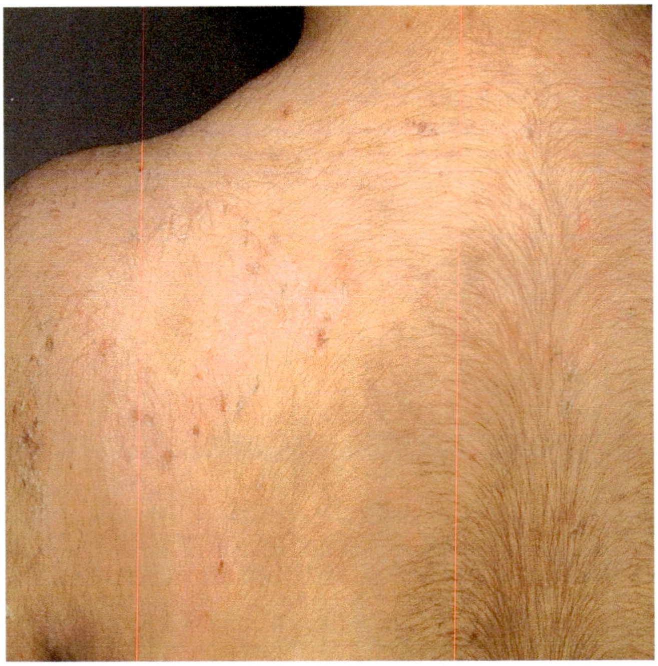

Dermatophytic infection in an HIV-positive patient: Tinea incognito. Ill defined lesions with diffuse scaling. Diagnosis confirmed by potassium hydroxide mount which shows innumerable dermatophyte hyphae.

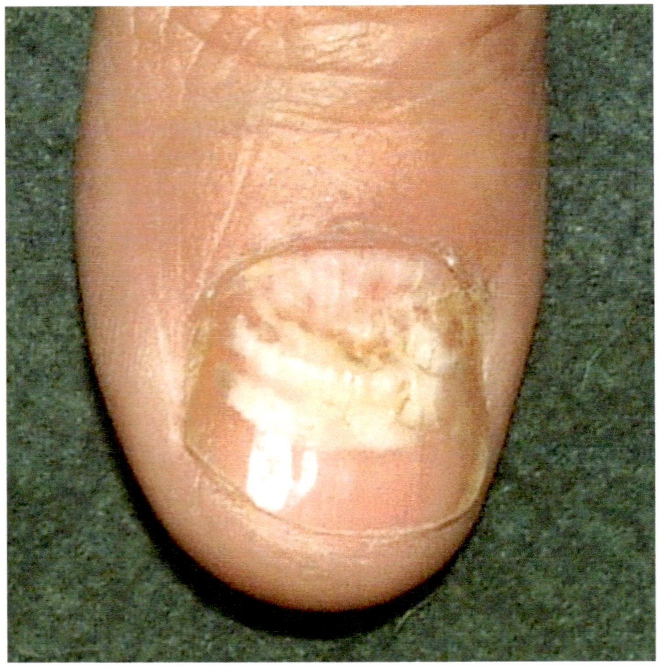

Onychomycosis in an HIV-positive patient: Proximal subungual onychomycosis. Characterized by presence of whitish discoloration in proximal nail plate with only minimal thickening of nail. This type of onychomycosis typically present only in an HIV-positive patients.

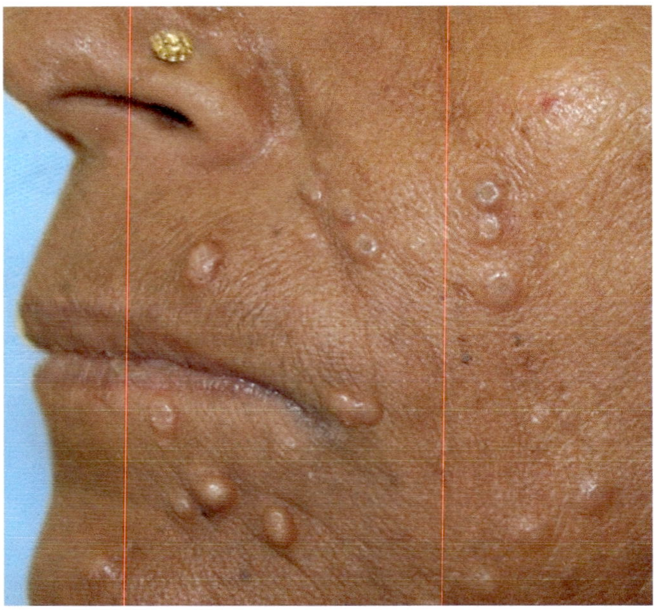

Cryptococcosis in an HIV-positive patient: Multiple skin colored papules with umbilication, resembling molluscum contagiosum on the face. Confirmed on biopsy.

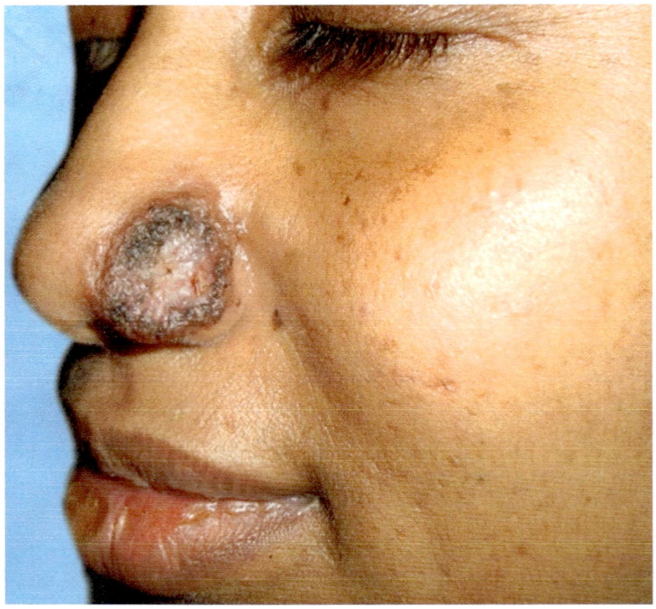

Histoplasmosis: Well-defined erythematous scaly nodule which on biopsy revealed histoplasmosis.

- ***Bacillary angiomatosis:*** *Bartonella henselae* infection. Typical pyogenic granuloma-like papules and nodules. Or Kaposi's sarcoma-like plaques. Occurs when CD4+ counts < 250 mm^3. Responds to erythromycin.

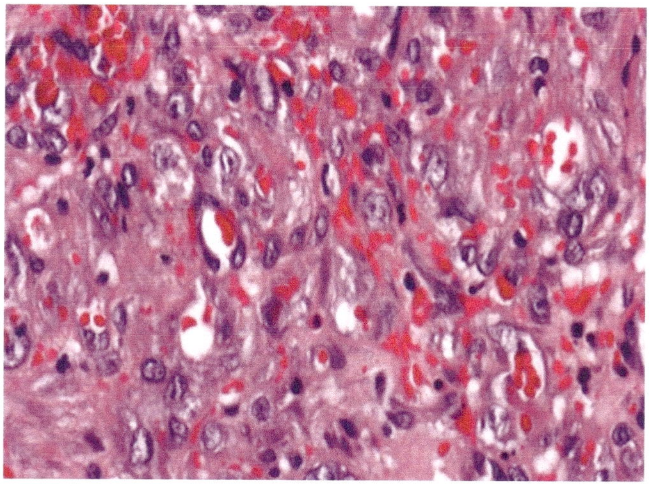

Bacillary angiomatosis: *Is a reactive vascular proliferation triggered by Bartonella henselae.* Histopathologically shows abundant vessels lined by plump endothelium with clear cytoplasm, mild atypia, and occasional mitotic figures and polymorphs in interstitium.

Fungal infections

- ***Candidiasis:*** Most common cutaneous infection. Manifests in oropharynx, esophagus, bronchi, genitalia and nail folds. Severe and recurrent. Indicates progression of HIV disease. Esophageal candidiasis (when CD4 cell count < 100/μL), an AIDS-defining illness.
- ***Dermatophytic infections:*** Very common. Usually typical lesions. Later chronic, recurrent, extensive. Or tinea incognito.[7]
- ***Onychomycosis:*** Usually of proximal subungual type which occurs only in HIV-infected.
- ***Deep fungal infections:*** Disseminated cryptococcosis, and histoplasmosis—develop with CD4 count 50-150/μL.
  - *Cryptococcosis:* Usually presents as papules and nodules. Sometimes umbilicated molluscum contagiosum-like lesions.
  - *Histoplasmosis:* Manifests as umbilicated skin colored, crusted papules and nodules usually on face. Or as cellulitis, panniculitis, palpable purpura and ulcers. Relapses common, even after adequate antifungal therapy.

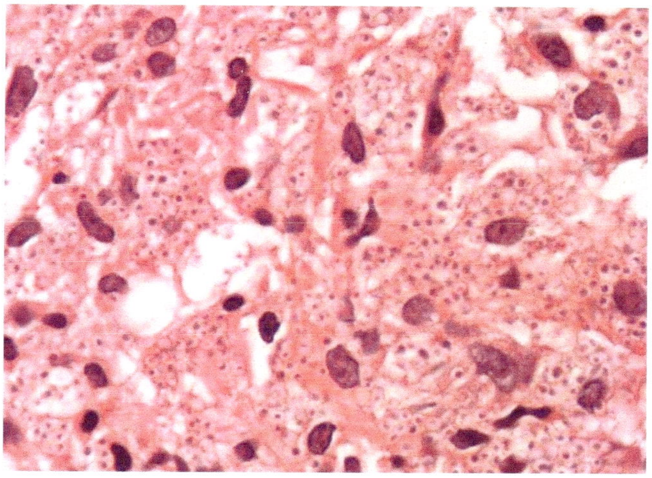

Histoplasmosis: Presence of intracytoplasmic budding yeast cells in macrophages.
Courtesy: Prof. M. Ramam, Department of Dermatology, AIIMS, New Delhi.

Infestations

- ***Leishmaniasis:*** With progress of HIV disease, florid cutaneous or visceral leishamaniasis may develop. Relapses frequent.
- ***Scabies:*** In advanced HIV disease, pruritus subtle. Or severe. May present with classical disease. Or Norwegian (crusted) scabies or erythroderma.

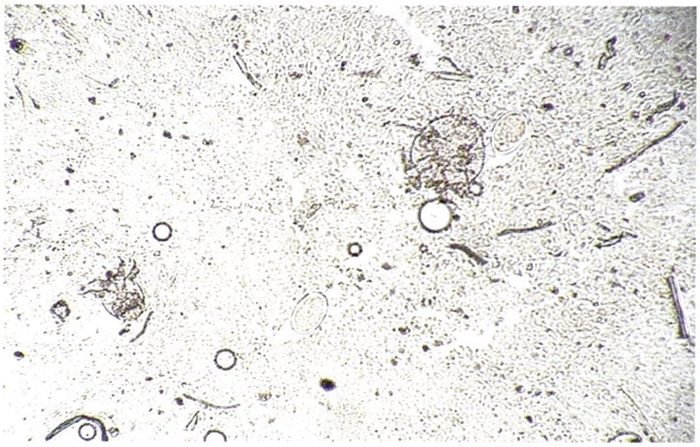

Potassium hydroxide mount: From an HIV-positive patient showing multiple mites.

[7]**Tinea incognito:** Does not have classical lesions.

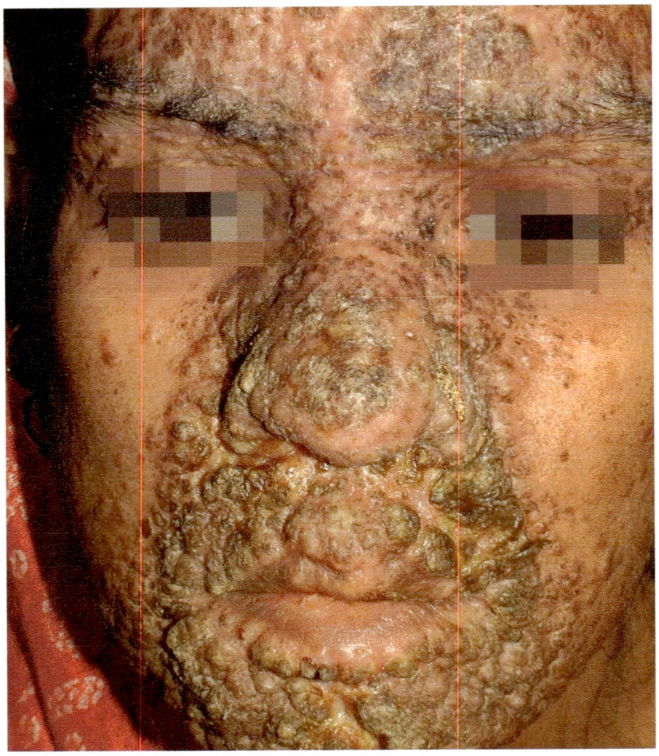

Histoplasmosis in an HIV-positive patient: Multiple crusted nodules and plaques. Diagnosis often made histolopathologically.

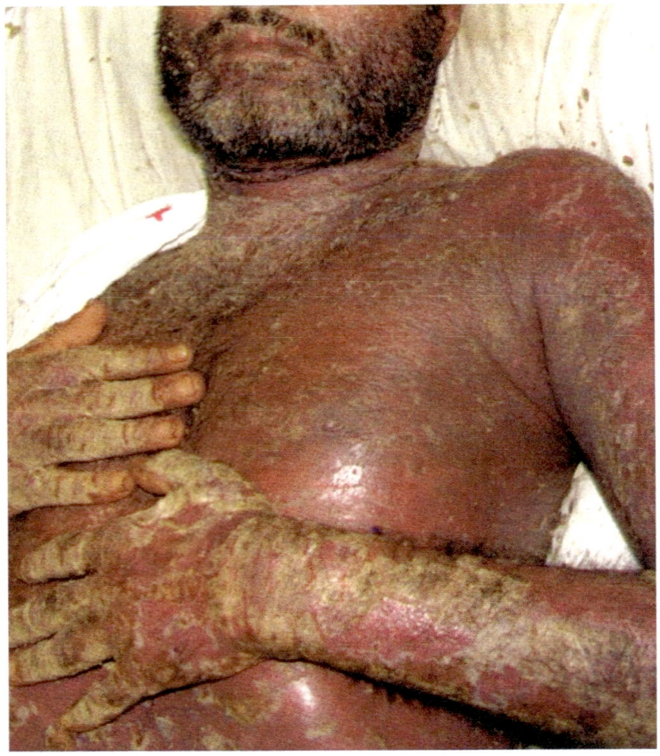

Scabies in an HIV-positive patient: May manifest as classic disease. Or as crusted (Norwegian) scabies presenting as hyperkeratotic, crusted plaques or as erythroderma. Often not diagnosed clinically.

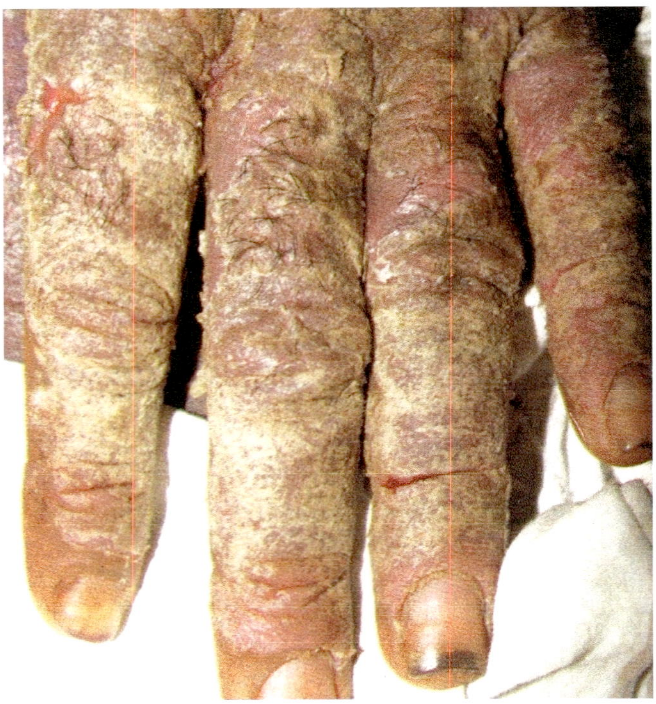

Crusted scabies in an HIV-positive patient: Presenting as hyperkeratotic, crusted plaques. Often diagnosed on scraping or biopsy.

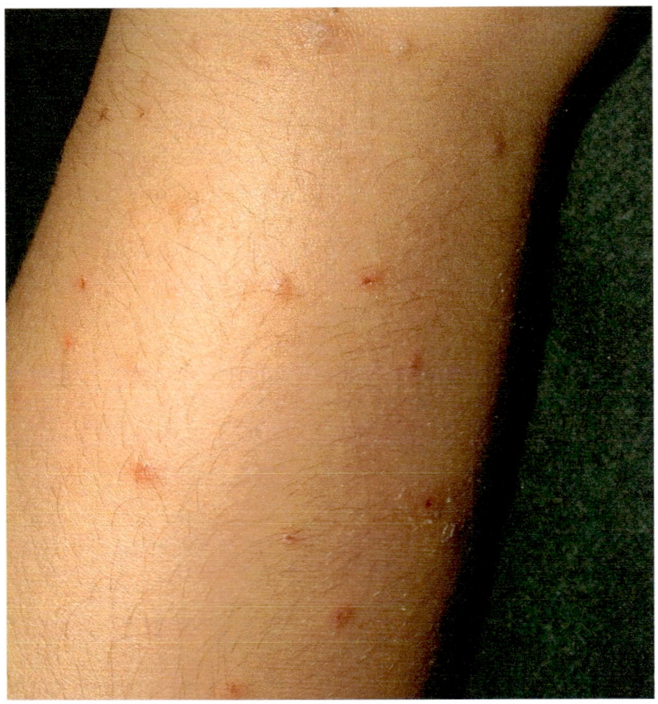

Insect bite hypersensitivity in an HIV-positive patient: Excoriated papules on exposed parts-extremities and face. Presence of such lesions in adults warrants HIV testing.

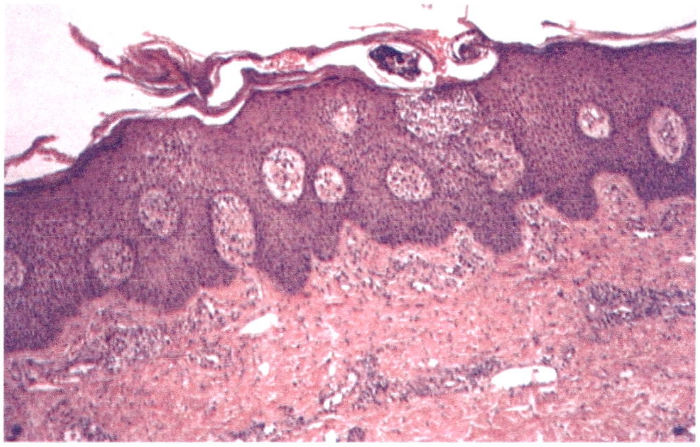

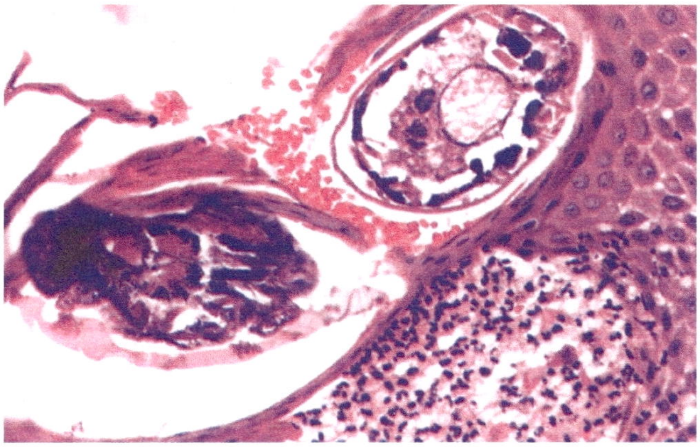

Norwegian scabies: Histopathology reveals multiple mites in hyperkeratotic acanthotic epidermis and inflammation in dermis.

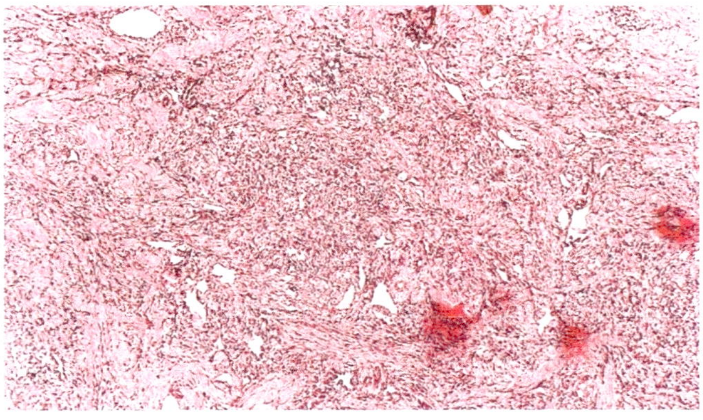

Kaposi's sarcoma: Areas of sarcomatous fascicles intermingled with vascular channels.

Diagnosed often on potassium hydroxide mount. Or on biopsy. Response to conventional therapy with permethrin/ivermectin adequate.

- ***Insect bite hypersensitivity:*** Initially seasonal, later persistent; excoriated papules on exposed sites. Such lesions, especially if extensive and persistent and in adults warrant HIV testing.

Non-infectious cutaneous manifestations

Skin rashes

- Several types described in ARS.
- Also a manifestation of drug reaction, which are more frequent in HIV-infected.

Seborrhoeic dermatitis

- Most common cutaneous manifestation in HIV infected.
- May be mild-moderate. Or florid and extensive with intense erythema, thick scales and involving unusual sites. And extensive.
- Responds to antiretroviral therapy.

Eosinophilic folliculitis

- In spectrum of pruritic papular eruption of HIV disease.
- Etiology unknown. Seen with low CD4 counts.
- Severely itchy, chronic follicular papules and pustules.
- Upper trunk, head and neck.
- Responds to topical steroids and phototherapy.

Psoriasis

- Can present as extensive lesions. Or as atypical lesions.
- Difficult to treat. May need oral retinoids/phototherapy (methotrexate avoided as immunosuppressive).

Reiters syndrome

- Post chlamydial or salmonella infections
- Mucocutaneous lesions: Rupioid/pustular lesions, keratoderma blenorrhagicum, circinate balanitis, oral lesions.
- Extracutaneous lesions: Severe, often mutilating sacroiliitis and lower limb arthritis. And eye involvement.
- Often resistant to treatment.

Kaposi's sarcoma

- Probably due to human herpes virus 8 which is sexually cotransmitted; most frequently seen in HIV infection acquired homosexually.
- Single or multiple. Asymptomatic brown to dusky red-purple macules or plaques. On ankles and shins, face, trunk and mucosae involved.

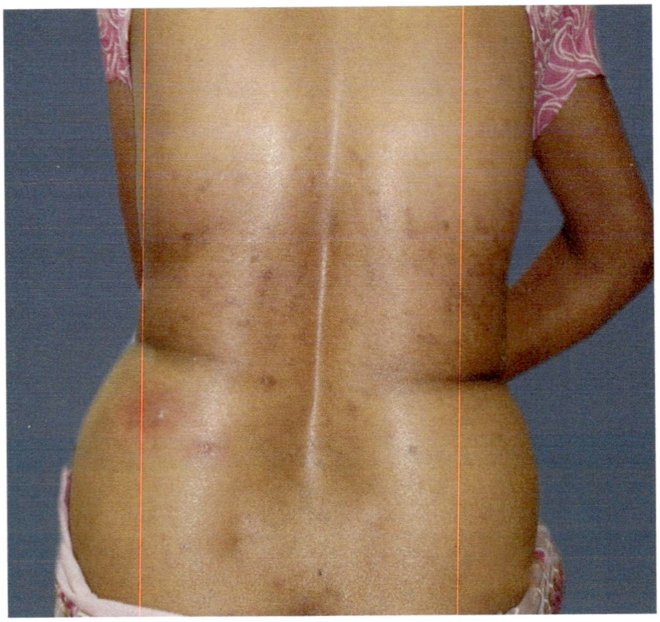

Insect bite hypersensitivity: Exposed area on waist involved with excoriated erythematous papules with sparing of area covered by garments. Lesions may be persistent and extensive.

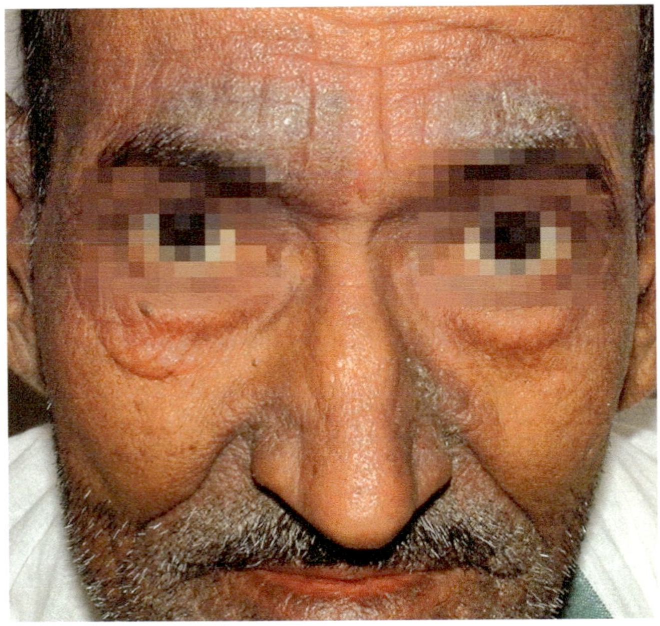

Seborrhoeic dermatitis in an HIV-positive patient: Erythematous plaques with greasy scales on the eye brows and nasolabial folds. Sudden onset of extensive lesions in elderly warrants ruling out underlying HIV infection.

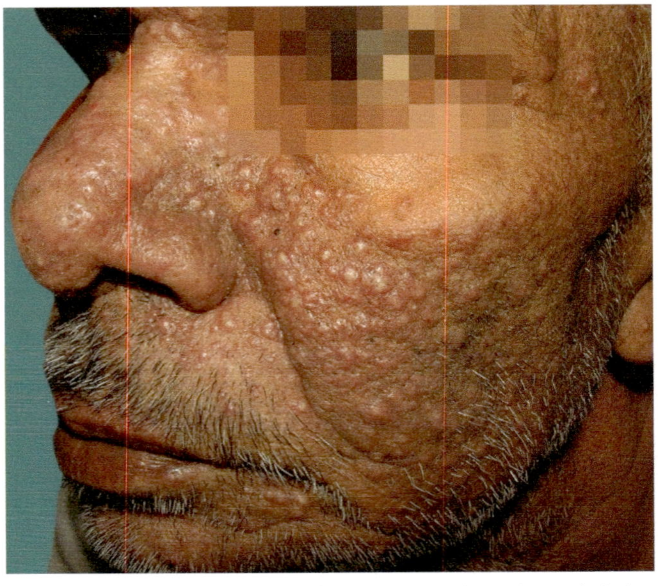

Eosinophilic folliculitis in an HIV-positive patient: Severely itchy, chronic follicular papules and pustules on the face. Eosinophilic folliculitis in the spectrum of pruritic papular eruption of HIV disease.

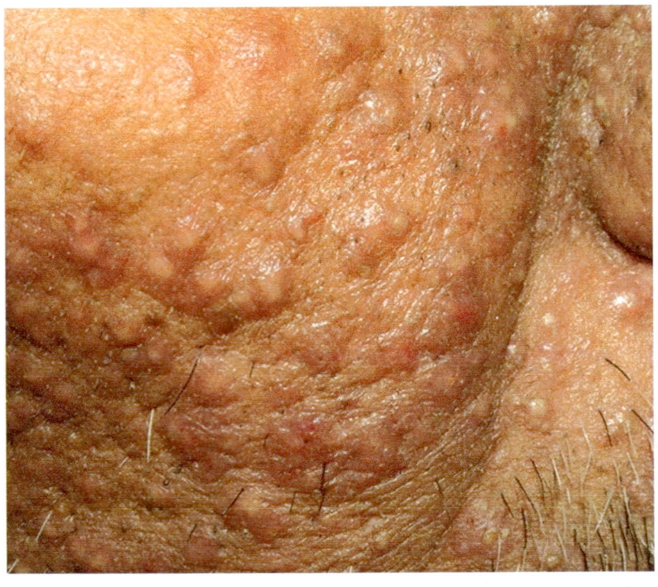

Eosinophilic folliculitis in an HIV-positive patient: Severely itchy, chronic follicular papules and pustules in neck, upper trunk and face. Treated with topical steroids and phototherapy.

- Treatment includes radiofrequency desiscation, mechanical curettage, excision, interferon therapy, radiotherapy and chemotherapy.

Others

Xerosis and acquired ichthyosis common. Long eyelashes (trichomegaly) and photosensitivity reported.

HIV and STIs

Effect of STIs on HIV

- ***STIs associated with genital ulcerations:*** Amplified transmission of HIV 10-fold, due to epithelial breach, concentration of inflammatory cells (like CD4 cells which are target cells for HIV) in genital mucosa.
- ***STIs associated with discharges:*** Amplified transmission of HIV 4-fold due to microfissures in epithelium, concentration of inflammatory cells (like CD4 cells which are target cells for HIV) in genital mucosa.

Effect of HIV on STIs

- ***Syphilis:***
  - Usually manifestation and course of syphilis in HIV unaltered, especially if no immune depletion. So also serological and therapeutic response.
  - Less frequently atypical presentation. Include:
    - Chancre: Slow healing of chancre, multiple chancres, phagedenic lesions and large painful ulcers.
    - Secondary syphilis: Lues maligna.
    - Neurosyphilis: Rapid progress to neurosyphilis even in secondary stage. More frequent occurrence.
    - Serology: Aberrant response. So other tests (dark ground microscopy, biopsy) needed.
- ***Chancroid:*** In early HIV infection course similar. With immunosuppression atypical features seen:
  - Atypical ulcers: More in number, larger, extragenital lesions.
  - Reduced response of chancroid to therapy, so single dose regimens avoided.
- ***Lymphogranuloma venereum:*** No effect generally noted.
- ***Donovanosis:*** In early HIV-infection course similar. Treatment regimens same as in non-HIV individual. But treatment failure and slower response. Then consider adding parenteral aminoglycosides.
- ***Genital herpes:***
  - In early HIV infection, course similar. Later, prolonged and severe episodes of genital, perianal or oral herpes. Chronic nonhealing ulcers, lasting more than a month and with herpetiform margins in perianal area characteristic of GH in HIV infected.
  - Lesions atypical—verrucous plaques, chronic non healing ulcers, pseudogranulomatous herpes.
  - Increased asymptomatic shedding.
- ***Anogenital warts (AGW):***
  - AGW more frequent in HIV-positive.
  - More numerous lesions, extensive involvement and larger nodules. Also multiple clinical types.
  - Higher prevalance of carcinoma *in situ* in cervix, vulva and anal canal. So regular monitoring of these areas.
  - More resistant to treatment. And more recurrences.
- ***Molluscum contagiosum:***
  - MC more frequent and numerous in HIV.
  - Atypical lesions–giant lesions, verrucous indurated plaques.
  - Resistance to conventional therapy. Response improves once ART started.
- ***Candidal genital tract infection:***
  - Increased prevalence.
    - Also of non-albicans candidal infection.
    - Increased severity and extent.
    - Fluconazole prophylaxis often recommended. But sometimes resistant to treatment.
- ***Non gonococcal genital tract infections:*** Probably no alteration.
- ***Bacterial vaginosis:*** Clinical presentation of bacterial vaginosis in HIV negative and positive patients probably similar.
- ***T. vaginalis:*** Probably no change.

DIAGNOSIS

Tests for Diagnosis of HIV infection

Several tests available (Table 11.4). And different tests used for different stages due to varying senstivity (Table 11.5).

- ***Serological tests:*** Tests to detect antibodies against HIV.
- ***Virological tests:*** Tests to detect components of HIV.

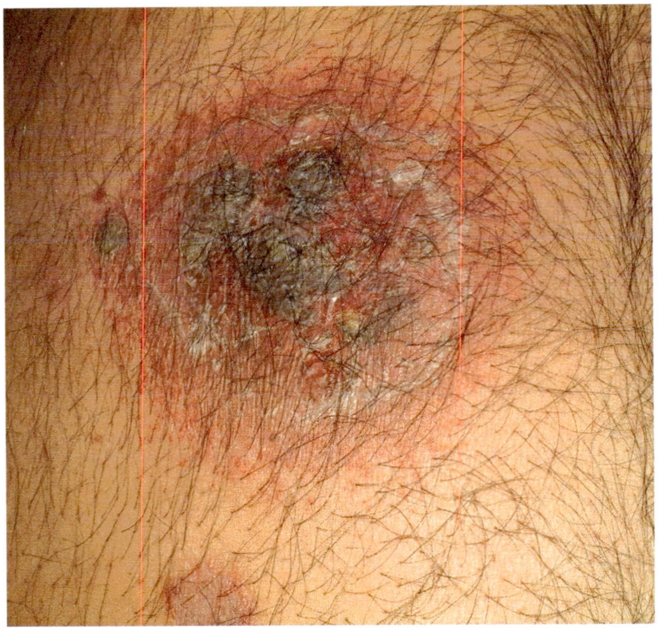

Psoriasis in an HIV-positive patient: Can present as extensive lesions. Or as atypical lesions with intense erythema.

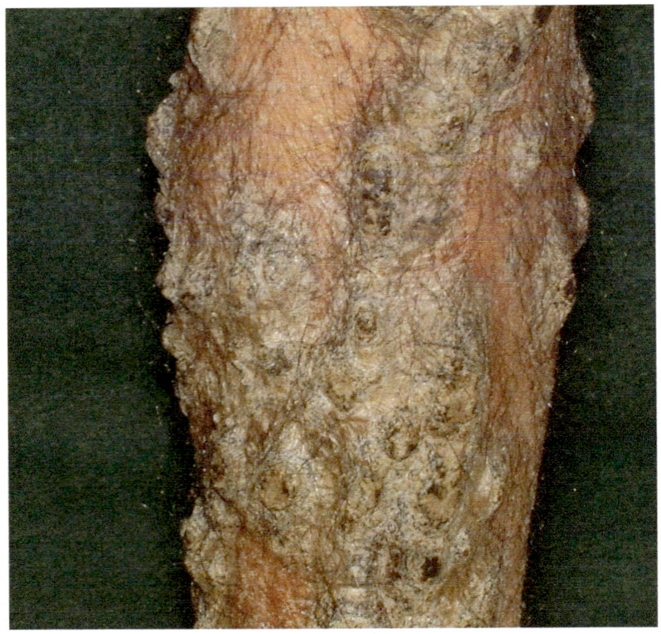

Reiter's syndrome in an HIV-positive patient: Hyperkeratotic lesions some conical resembling a limpet-the so called rupioid lesions. Many of have a central cupping, similar to an oyster shell.

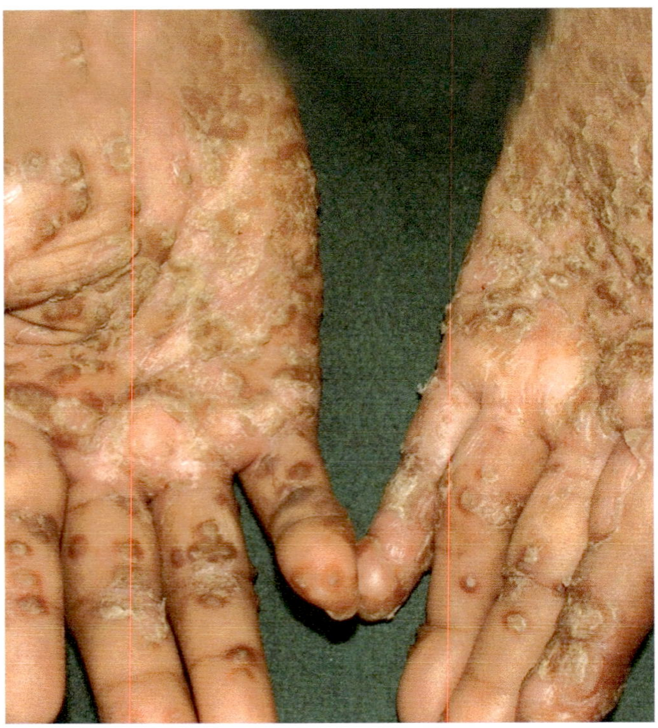

Keratoderma blenorrhagicum in an HIV-positive patient: Erythematous hyperkeratotic plaques on palms (and soles).

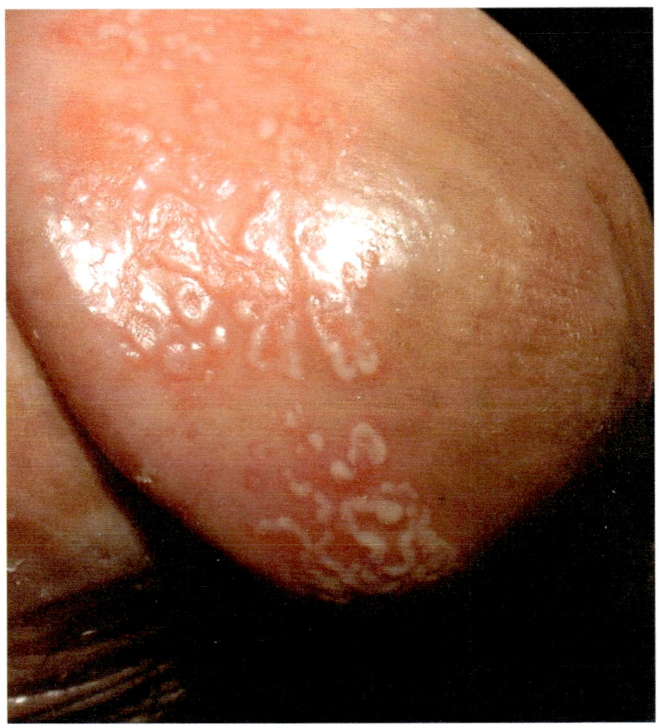

Circinate balanitis in an HIV-positive patient: Moist annular plaques with serpiginous margin.

Table 11.4: Diagnosis of HIV infection	
Serological tests	**Virological tests**
• Screening tests: – ELISA – EIA • Supplemental: – Western blot – Immunofluorescence – Line immunoassay	• Viral RNA • p24 antigen • Viral culture

Table 11.5: Laboratory tests for diagnosis of HIV infected patients in different clinical stages

Clinical stage	HIV serology	P24 antigen assay	PCR	Plasma viral load
Window period	-	-/+	+	++
Asymptomatic HIV infection	+	-/+	+	-/+
Early and late symptomatic infection	+	+	+	+
Advanced HIV	+	++	+	+++

Serological tests

Two types of serological tests for HIV infection:

- Screening tests.
- Supplemental test.

Screening tests

- ***Features:*** Rapid, inexpensive. Highly sensitive, may not be very specific (i.e. false positives occur), so are presumptive and not confirmatory tests.
- ***Types:*** Of 2 types:
  - *Lab-based tests:* Include ELISA or EIA. Are the most frequently used tests.
  - *Point of care tests:* Available at point of contact of physician and patient. Most use color change

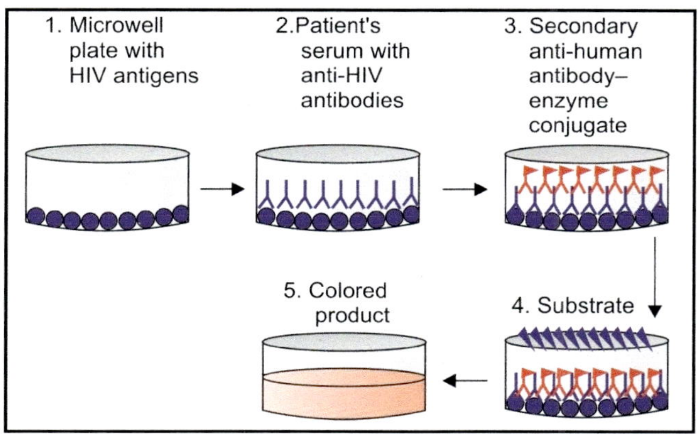

Principle of EIA

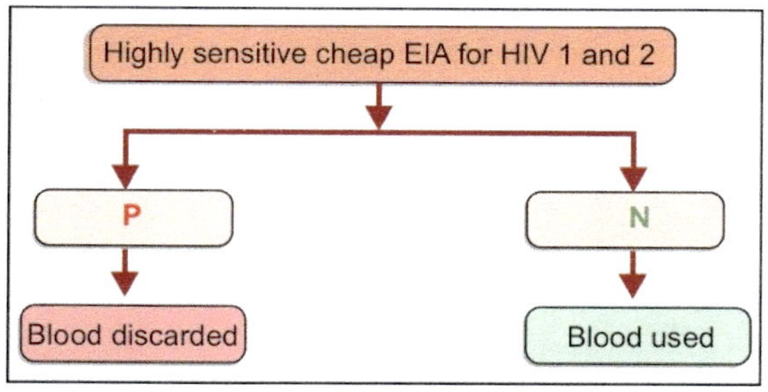

HIV serological testing strategy for screening donors

(immunochromatographic assays) or particle agglutination. Some do not require blood samples as can be done on saliva (oraquick and orasure) or urine.

- ***Indications and interpretation of screening tests:***
  - *Screening donors:*
    - Is unlinked, anonymous sampling, without pre-test counseling because patient not informed about HIV status.
    - Uses single, highly sensitive, reliable, cheap enzyme immunoassay (EIA) for HIV-1 and HIV-2.
    - Positive samples discarded; negative samples used.
  - *Serosurveillance:* Epidemiologically for sentinel serosurveillance:
    - Is unlinked, anonymous sampling, so pretest counseling not needed.
    - Samples tested 1st with highly sensitive, reliable, cheap EIA for HIV-1 and HIV-2.
    - Positive samples need confirmation by a specific EIA based on another antigen; negative samples considered negative.

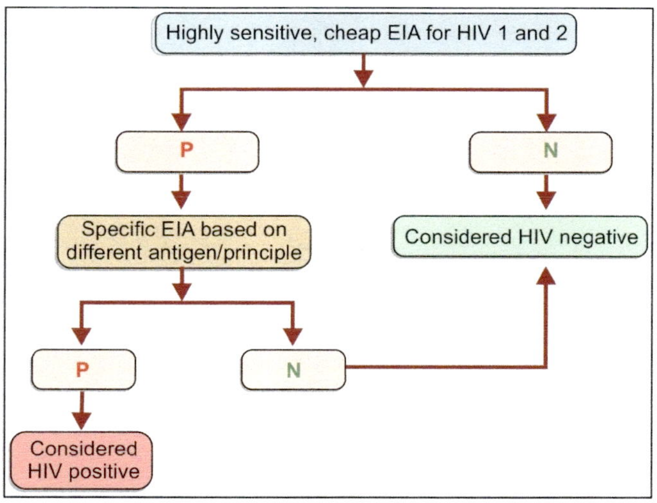

HIV serological testing strategy for diagnosis of HIV for serosurveillance

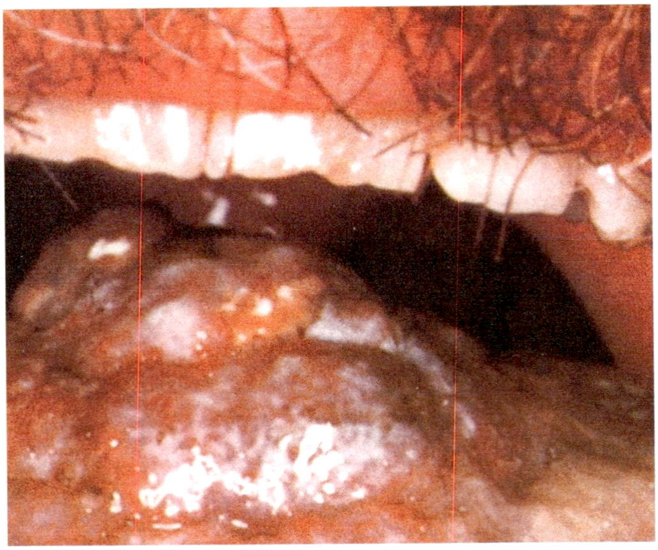

Kaposi's sarcoma in an HIV-positive patient: Intraoral lesion manifesting as single dusky erythematous-violaceus plaques. Other sites of predilection include ankles, shins, face and trunk.

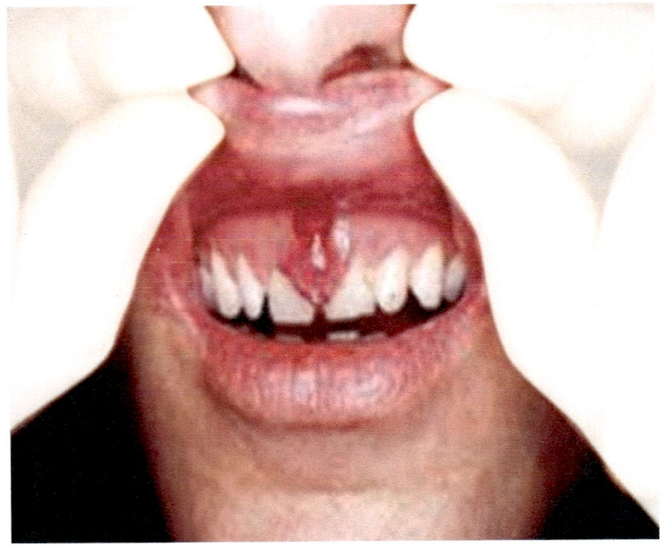

Kaposi's sarcoma in an HIV-positive patient: Manifests as a dusky violaceus plaques. Kaposi's sarcoma in HIV-infected can occur both with CD4 counts $> 300/mm^3$ (with a longer median survival) and also in advanced HIV infection (with a shorter median survival). May respond to HAART. Or may need treatment with cryotherapy (if few lesions) or radiotherapy/chemotherapy if extensive.

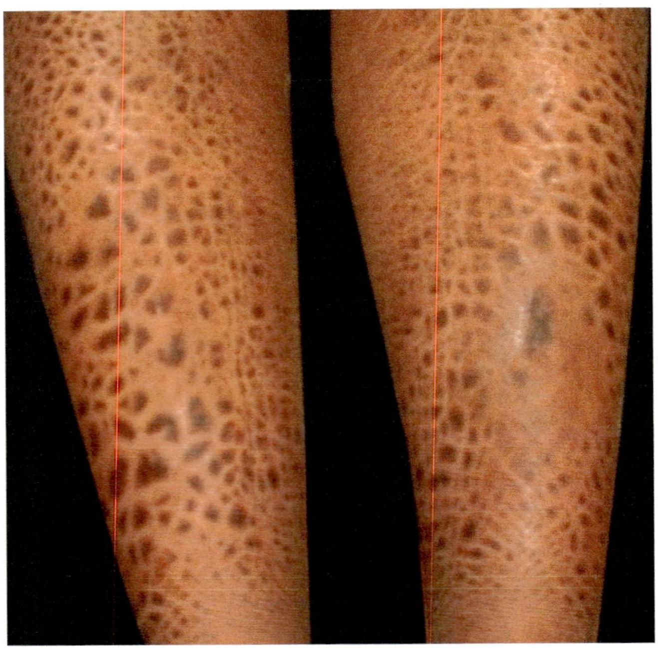

Acquired ichthyosis in an HIV-positive patient: Lesions of acquired ichthyosis resemble ichthyosis vulgaris. Appearance of ichthyosis in later life warrants search for an underlying disease including an HIV infection. Ichthyosis in HIV-infected generally occurs in advanced HIV infection.

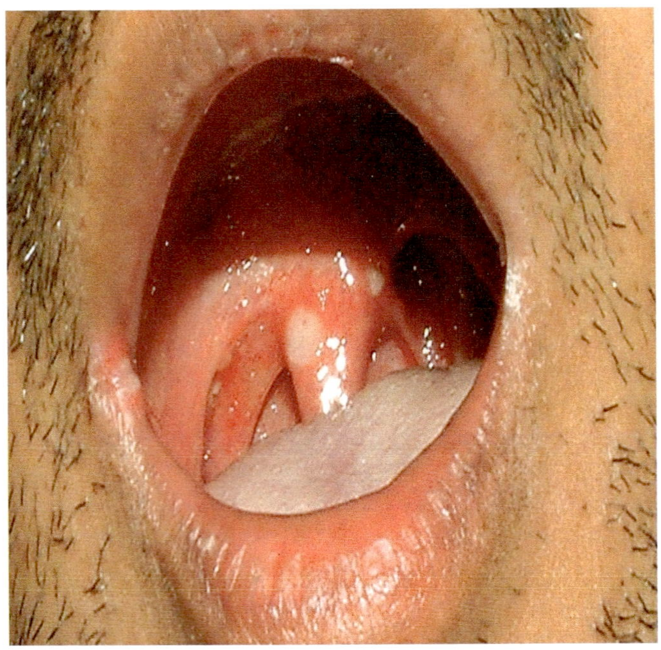

Oral aphthae: Ulcers with central necrotic slough and halo of erythema. Occur when CD4+ count $< 100/mm^3$.

- *Diagnosis of HIV infection:* Pretest counseling mandatory. And strategy used depends on whether patient is asymptomatic or symptomatic.
  - If asymptomatic: samples 1st tested with sensitive EIA; if positive→ Repeat tested with 2nd specific EIA (based on a different antigen or principle). If positive, further confirmed with 3rd (both specific and sensitive) EIA. Negative samples from 2nd test considered negative.

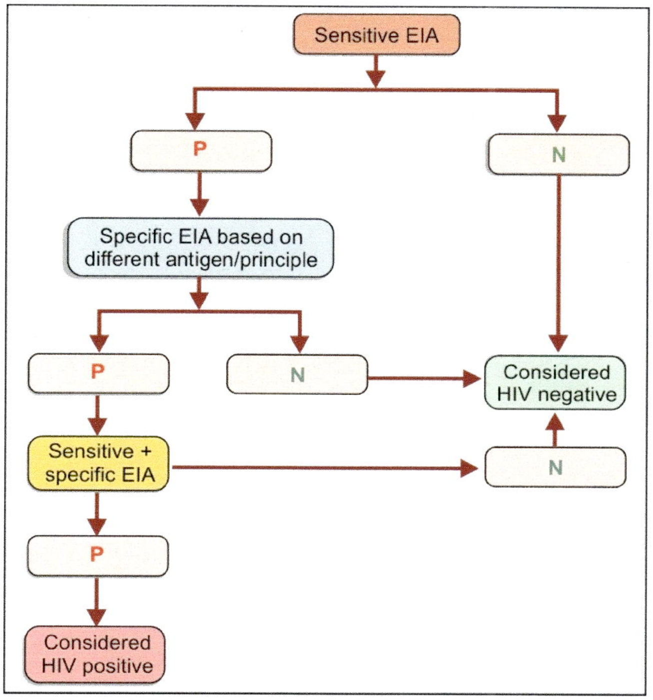

HIV serological testing strategy for diagnosis of HIV infection in asymptomatic patients.

  - If symptomatic: samples 1st tested with highly sensitive, reliable, cheap EIA for HIV-1 and HIV-2. Positive samples need confirmation by a specific EIA based on another antigen; negative samples considered negative.

Supplemental tests

- Done to validate the positive tests of screening.
- Two types available:
  - Western blot (WB) assay.
  - Immunofluorescence test.
- Are expensive (Western blot) and difficult to interpret (both). So replaced by combination of 2 or > EIAs (using different principles/antigens, one highly sensitive, 2nd highly specific) now used instead of ELISA-WB combination as more reliable and less expensive.

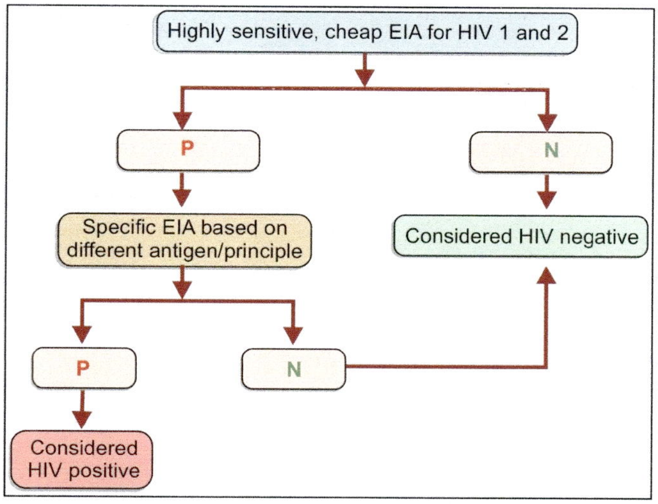

HIV serological testing strategy for serosurveillance

Virological tests

Confirmatory tests, as detect HIV antigens. So positive even in window period in seronegative patients. And confirm presence of virus in a seropositive (or serologically equivocal) patient.

Detection of viral RNA

- 1st test to become positive, so short window period (median 17 days). Expensive and resource intensive.
- Uses polymerase chain reaction (PCR). And real time PCR. Can be used to determine viral load (expressed as number of RNA copies/ml).

Detection of HIV specific core antigen (p24)

- ***Useful in:***
  - *Window period:* p24 detectable earlier than seropositivity in 30% of patients.
  - *Diagnosis of HIV infection in newborn:* Because just presence of antibodies in newborn often due to transplacental transfer of maternal antibodies.
  - *Detection of HIV in CSF.*
- Test sometimes falsely negative, if antigen complexed with p24 antibody; overcome by preliminary acid hydrolysis of serum sample.

Viral culture

- Not routinely done as resource intensive and not safe. And takes 4–8 weeks for reporting.
- But is 100% specific. And sensitivity depends on stage of infection.

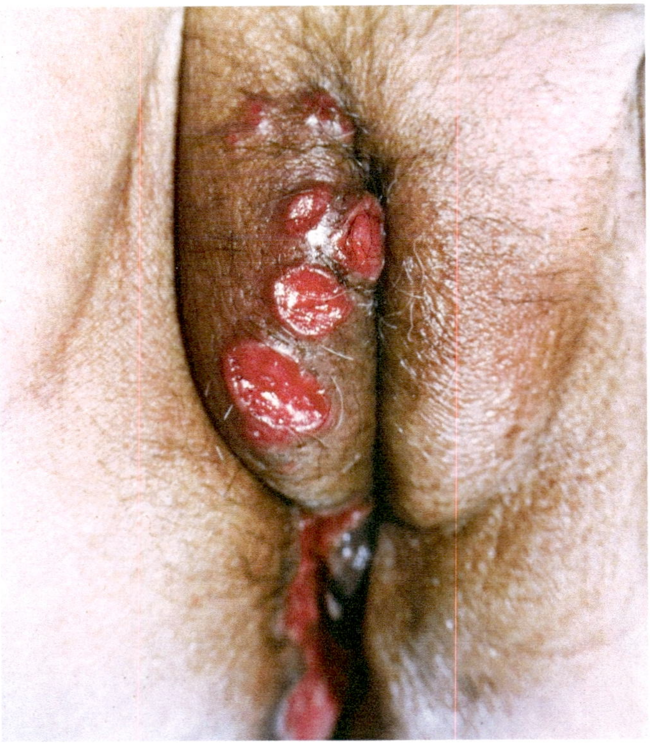

Syphilis in an HIV-positive patient: Multiple chancres. Many raised indurated ulcers with regular margins and clean base.

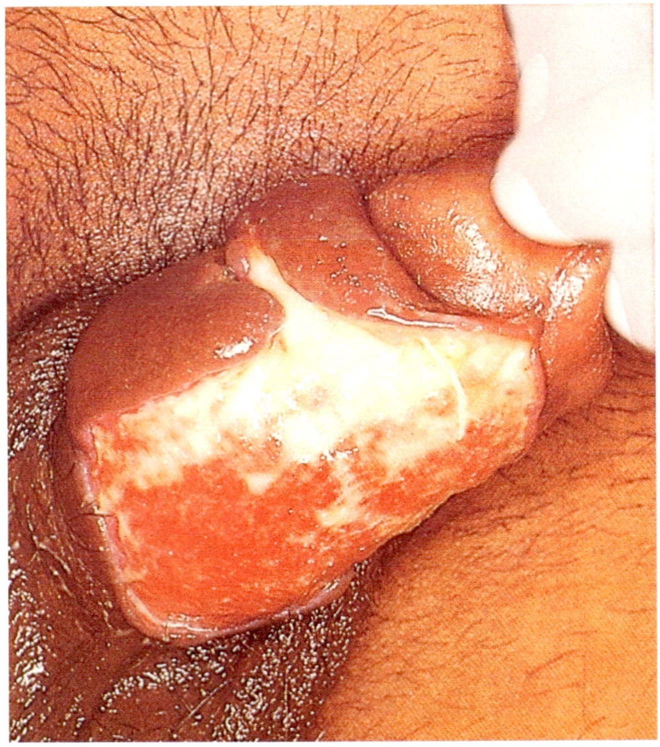

Chancroid in an HIV-positive patient: Phagedenic variant: most of the shaft of penis involved.

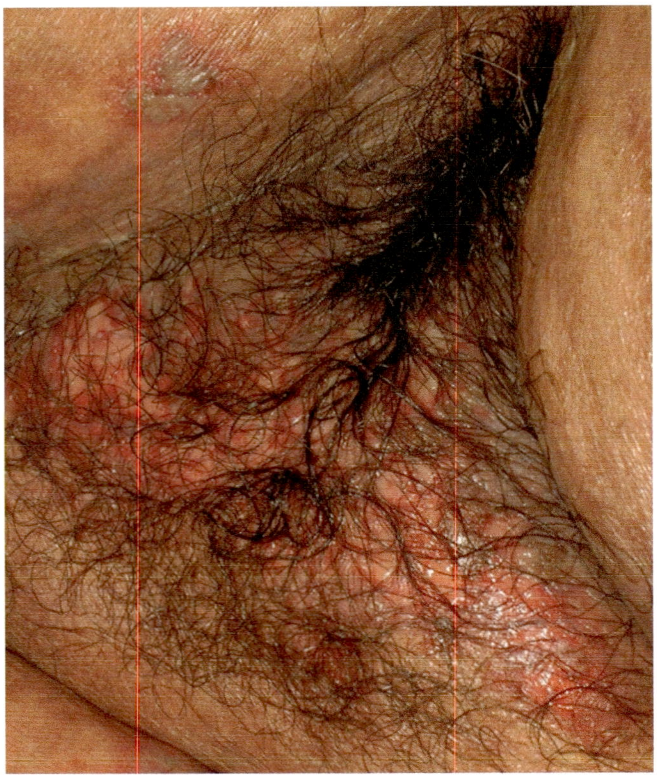

Genital herpes in an HIV-positive patient: Extensive polycyclic lesions extending from genital area onto lower abdomen.

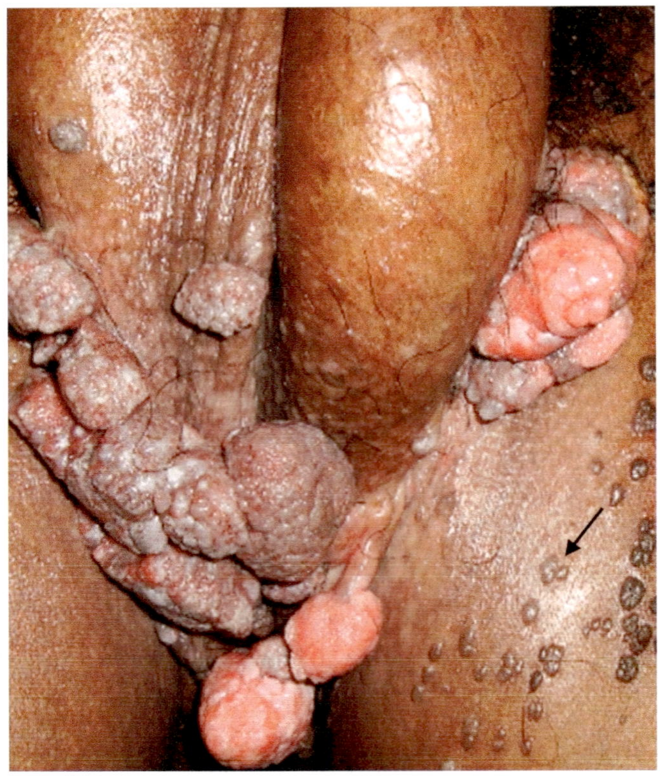

Anogenital warts in an HIV-positive patient: Large lesions of condyloma acuminata and smaller lesions of bowenoid papulosis (marked).

Other Tests

- ***Tests to monitor progress of HIV infection:***
  - *Viral load.*
  - *CD4 counts.*
- ***Tests to rule out:***
  - Opportunistic infections.
  - Development of neoplasia.
- ***Tests to monitor side effects of drugs:*** Since drugs often toxic base line and follow-up hematological and biochemical tests needed.

TREATMENT

Treatment encompasses counseling (always and repeatedly), prescribing (often providing) antiretroviral treatment (ART) when indicated, and managing complications including opportunistic infections and neoplasia.

Counseling

- In HIV and AIDS counseling a core element of holistic management.
- ***Objectives:*** 2 objectives
  - *Prevention of HIV transmission:* Spread of HIV hugely curtailed by behavior change—safe sexual practices including consistent and correct use of condoms, avoiding casual sex and intravenous drug use.
  - *Supporting of those afflicted directly and indirectly by HIV:*
- ***Types:***
  - *Pre-test counseling:* Involves providing basic information on HIV/AIDS. And risk assessment of those being HIV tested.
  - *Post-test counseling:* Depends on result:
    - If negative: basic knowledge on HIV reiterated to assist client to adopt behaviors that reduce future risk of getting infected. A repeat test is recommended after 12 weeks.
    - If positive test: client assisted to cope with result. And helped to access treatment and care. And supported to disclose HIV status to partner.
    - Follow-up counseling: to re-emphasise adoption of safe behaviors to prevent transmission of HIV infection. And assists in establishing linkages and referrals to services for care and support including ART, nutrition, home-based care and legal support.

Antiretroviral therapy

Antiretroviral drugs

- ***Objective of therapy:*** Antiretroviral treatment (ART) suppresses disease, does not eradicate virus. So reduces morbidity and mortality but does not cure.
- ***Classification:*** ART broadly classified by phase of retrovirus life-cycle inhibited (Table 11.6):
  - *Reverse transcriptase inhibitors:*
    - Nucleoside reverse transcriptase inhibitors (NRTI): compete with natural deoxynucleotides[8] for incorporation into viral DNA chain but form defective DNA which cannot extend DNA chain resulting in chain termination.
    - Nucleotide reverse transcriptase inhibitors (NtRTI): act as NRTI.
    - Non-nucleoside reverse transcriptase inhibitors (NNRTI): act as non-competitive inhibitors of reverse transcriptase (by binding to it).

Table 11.6: Classification of ART

NRTI	NtRTI	NNRTI	PI	FI	II
Zidovudine (AZT)*	Tenofovir (TDF)*	Nevirapine (NVP)*	Indinavir (INV)*	Enfuvirtide (T-20)	Raltegravir
Didanosine (ddI)*		Efavirenz (EFV)*	Ritonavir (RTV)*		
Zalcitabine (ddC)*		Delaviridine (DLV)	Saquinavir (SQV)*		
Stavudine (d4T)*		Etravirine	Nelfinavir (NFV)*		
Lamivudine (3TC)*			Lopinavir (LPV)*		
Abacavir (ABC)*			Atazanavir (ATV)*		
Emtricitabine (FTC)			Darunavir		
*Available in developing countries					

[8]**NRTIs:** Are analogues of naturally occurring deoxynucleotides which are needed to synthesize HIV DNA.

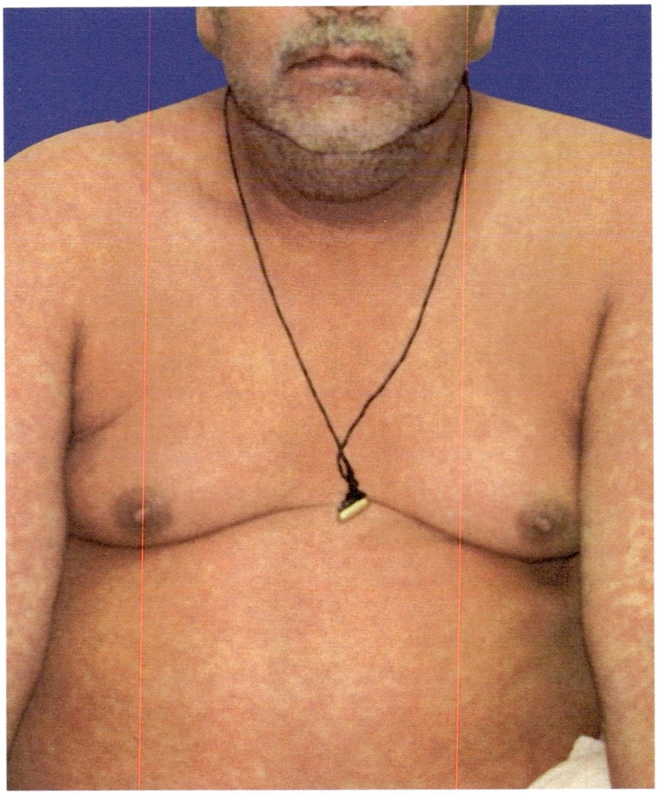

Morbilliform eruption: Generalized erythematous, maculopapular eruption due to nevirapine. Similar rash can develop with abacavir.

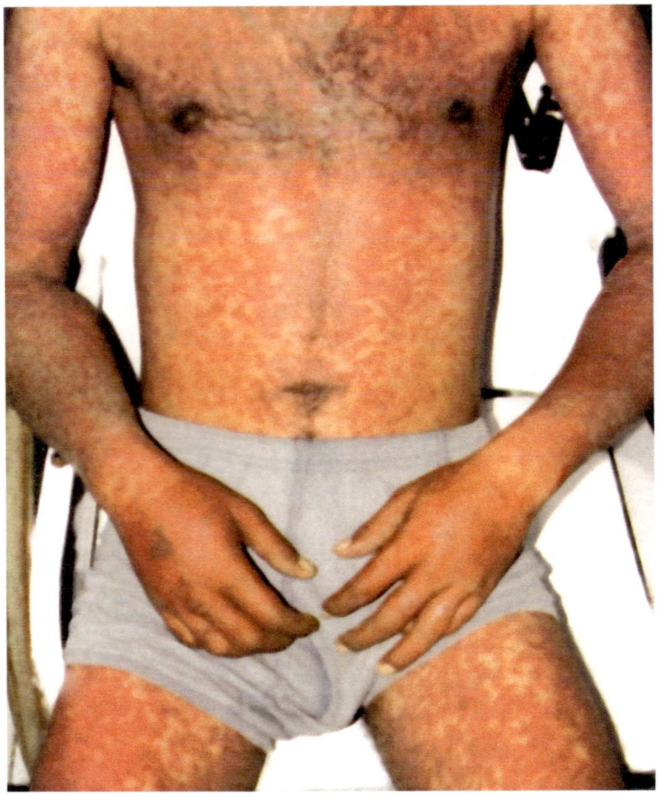

Drug hypersensitivity reaction: Generalized erythematous maculopapular eruption with peripheral edema due to nevirapine. Abacavir can also cause similar reactions.

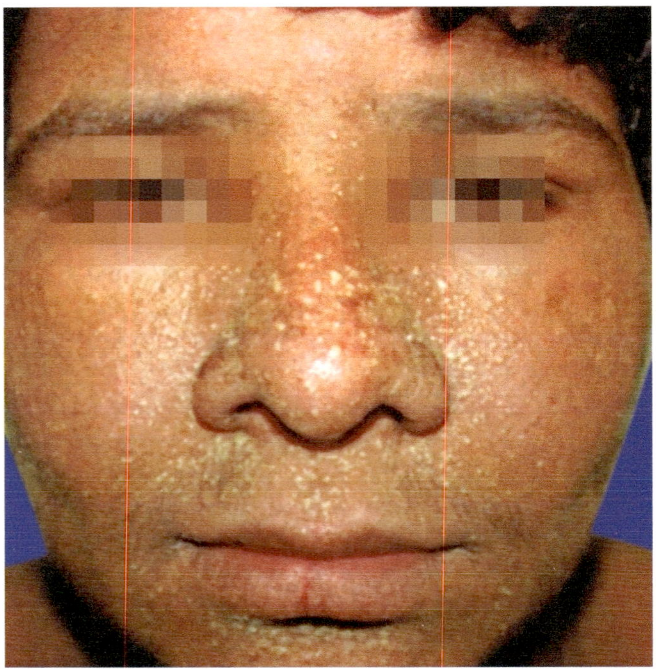

Acute generalized exanthematous pustulosis: Widespread eruption of sterile pustules due to nelfinavir.

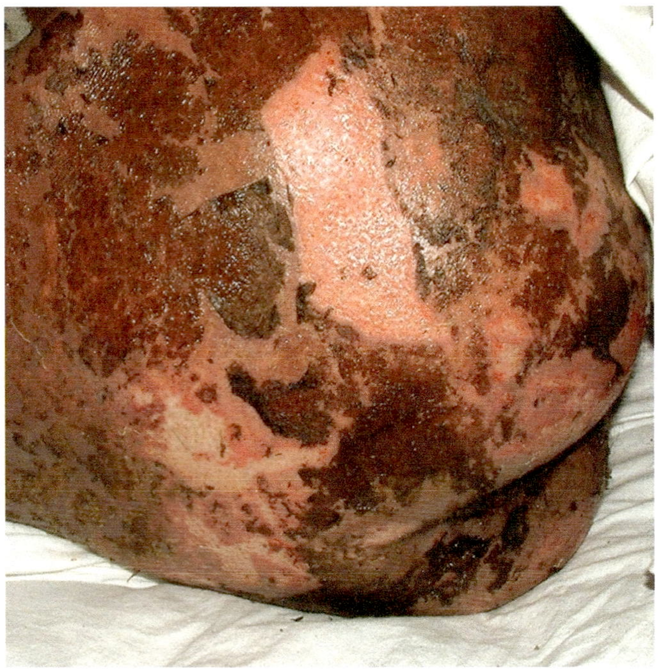

Toxic epidermal necrolysis: Large areas of sheets of dusky red skin which denude to reveal erosions. Due to nevirapine can also develop with abacavir.

- *Protease inhibitors (PI):* inhibit protease which cleaves polyproteins for final assembly of new HIV virions.
- *Fusion inhibitors (FI):* Prevents fusion of viral envelope with cell membrane of target cells.
- *Integrase inhibitors (II):* Inhibit enzyme integrase, which integrates HIV DNA into infected cell DNA.

❖ ***Side effects:*** Several side effects described with ART. Common ones include:
- *Zidovudine (AZT):* Anemia, (hemoglobin monitoring recommended) and lipoatrophy.
- *Stavudine (d4T):* Peripheral neuropathy, lipodystrophy, dyslipidemia lactic acidosis.
- *Lamivudine (3TC):* Relatively safe, but drug most prone to HIV developing resistance.
- *Tenofovir* (TDF): Nephropathy (so renal function monitoring).
- *Nevirapine (NVP):* Drug eruptions (maculopapular eruptions, Steven-Johnson syndrome-toxic epidermal necrolysis), hepatotoxicity.
- *Efavirenz (EFV):* Gastrointestinal side effects, hepatotoxicity, nephrotoxicity.? Safety in pregnancy.
- *Abacavir (ABC):* Severe hypersensitivity reaction not uncommon.
- *Protease inhibitors:* Dyslipedemia (high total and LDL cholestrol, decreased HDL cholestrol and elevated triglycerides).

Indications

ART to be initiated only if indicated (Tables 11.7 and 11.8), not only on basis of presence of HIV infection.

Table 11.7: WHO guidelines for starting ART in HIV-positive patients

Clinical scenario	Start ART if:
Asymptomatic ARV-naive individuals	CD4 count < 350 cells/mm^3
Symptomatic ARV-naive individuals	WHO clinical stage 2 and CD4 < 350 cells/mm^3 **OR** WHO clinical stage 3 or 4, irrespective of CD4 cell count
Pregnant women	CD4 < 350 cells/mm^3, irrespective of clinical symptoms **OR** WHO clinical stage 3 or 4, irrespective of CD4 cell count
HIV/TB coinfection ARV-naive individuals	Presence of active TB disease, irrespective of CD4 cell count
HIV/HBV coinfection ARV-naive individuals	HBV infection warranting treatment, irrespecive of CD4 cell count

Table 11.8: NACO guidelines for starting ART

Clinical scenario (WHO clinical stage)	CD4 test not available	CD4 test available
Asymptomatic (1)	Do not treat	Treat if CD4 < 200
Mild symptoms (2)	Do not treat	
Advanced symptoms (3)	Treat	Consider treatment if CD4 < 350 and initiate ART before CD4 drops below 200
Severe/advanced symptoms (4)	Treat	Treat irrespective of CD4 count

Drug Regimens

❖ ART given as Highly Active Antiretroviral Therapy (HAART), a combination of 3 drugs (Table 11.9):

Table 11.9: Which antiretroviral therapy to start when:

Target population	WHO, 2010 guidelines	NACO, 2007 guidelines
HIV + ARV-naive adults and adolescents	3TC/FTC+ AZT/TDF + NVP/EFV	3TC + AZT/ d4T + NVP/EFV
HIV + pregnant women	AZT +3TC + NVP	AZT + 3TC + NVP
HIV/TB coinfection	AZT/TDF + 3TC/FTC + EFV	AZT/D4T+ 3TC+EFV/NVP
HIV/HBV coinfection	TDF + 3TC (or FTC) + EFV	

Monitoring of HAART

Real challenge to monitor efficacy of ART because of immunological and virological discordancy. And to diagnose resistance to initiate. 2nd line therapy.

❖ ***Viral load estimation.***
- Most sensitive marker of efficacy. But resource intensive.
- Recommended to measure every 3-6 months.
- Expressed as RNA copies.

❖ ***Surrogate markers:*** Used individually or in combination but poorly sensitive.
- Clinical improvement.
- CD4 counts.

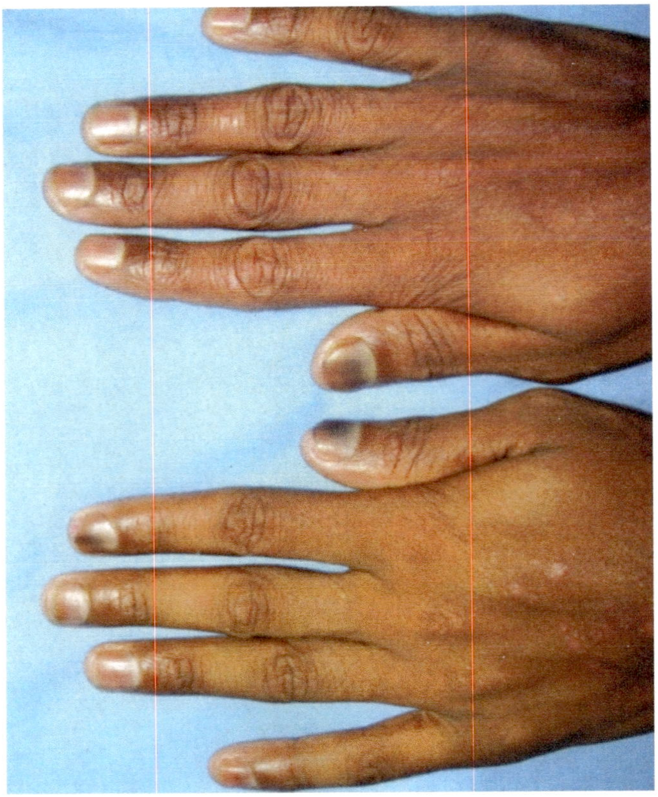

Nail pigmentation: Bluish-black nail pigmentation due to zidovudine. Pigmentation of nail may appear as early as 1 month after inititation of zidovudine.

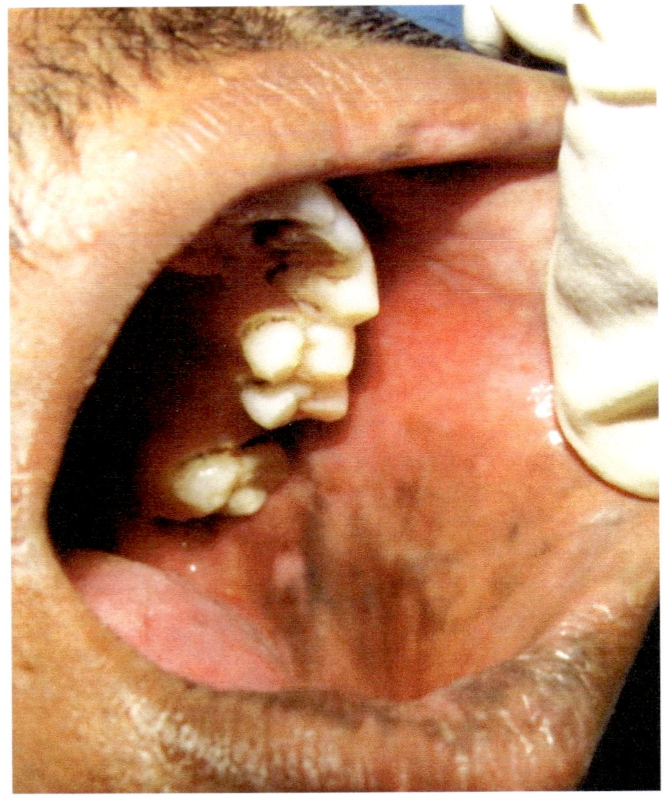

Mucosal pigmentation: Bluish-black mucosal pigmentation due to zidovudine. Zidovudine typically causes pigmentation of lateral aspect of tongue.

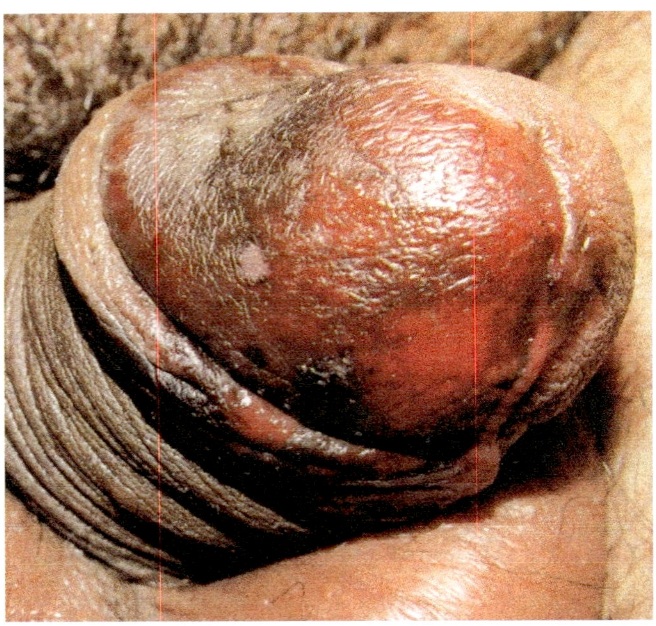

Fixed drug eruption on glans: Well-defined erythematous plaque on the glans which developed after taking cotrimaxozole for prophylaxis for pneumocytis pneumonia.

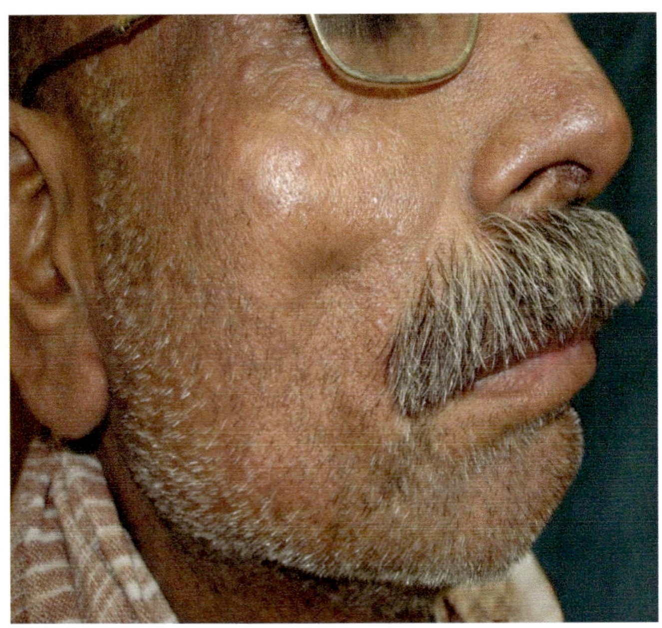

Facial lipoatrophy: Irreversible loss of subcutaneous fat began 6 months after starting therapy with zidovudine (also seen with stavudine).

Drugs for Opportunistic Infections

Various regimens recommended for prophylaxis and therapy of opportunistic infections (Table 11.10).

Table 11.10: Management of opportunistic infections in HIV patients

	Treatment (daily)	Prophylaxis	
Infections		**Indications**	**Drug regimen (daily)**
Pneumocystis Jiroveci	TMP (15 mg/kg) + SMZ* (75 mg/kg) × 3 weeks	CD4+ < 200/mm^3	TMP (2.5 mg/kg) + SMZ (12.5 mg/kg)
Toxoplasma encephalitis	Sulfadiazine (4-8 g) + Pyrimethamine (200-400 mg) × 6 weeks	Toxoplasma seropositive CD4+ < 100/mm^3	Sulfadiazine (2-4 g) + Pyrimethamine (100 mg)
Herpes simplex virus	Acyclovir 400 mg × 5 times × 2 weeks	> 6 recurrences/year	Acyclovir 400 mg bid
Herpes zoster	Acyclovir 800 mg × 5 times × 2 weeks		
M. tuberculosis	Standard therapy. Look for MDR tuberculosis. ATT initiated before HAART		
Candidiasis	Fluconazole 100-200 mg daily × 3 weeks		Fluconazole 150 mg weekly

*TMP-SMZ: trimethoprim-sulfamethoxazole

4 SECTION

MISCELLANEOUS

CHAPTER 12

Balanitis and Balanoposthitis

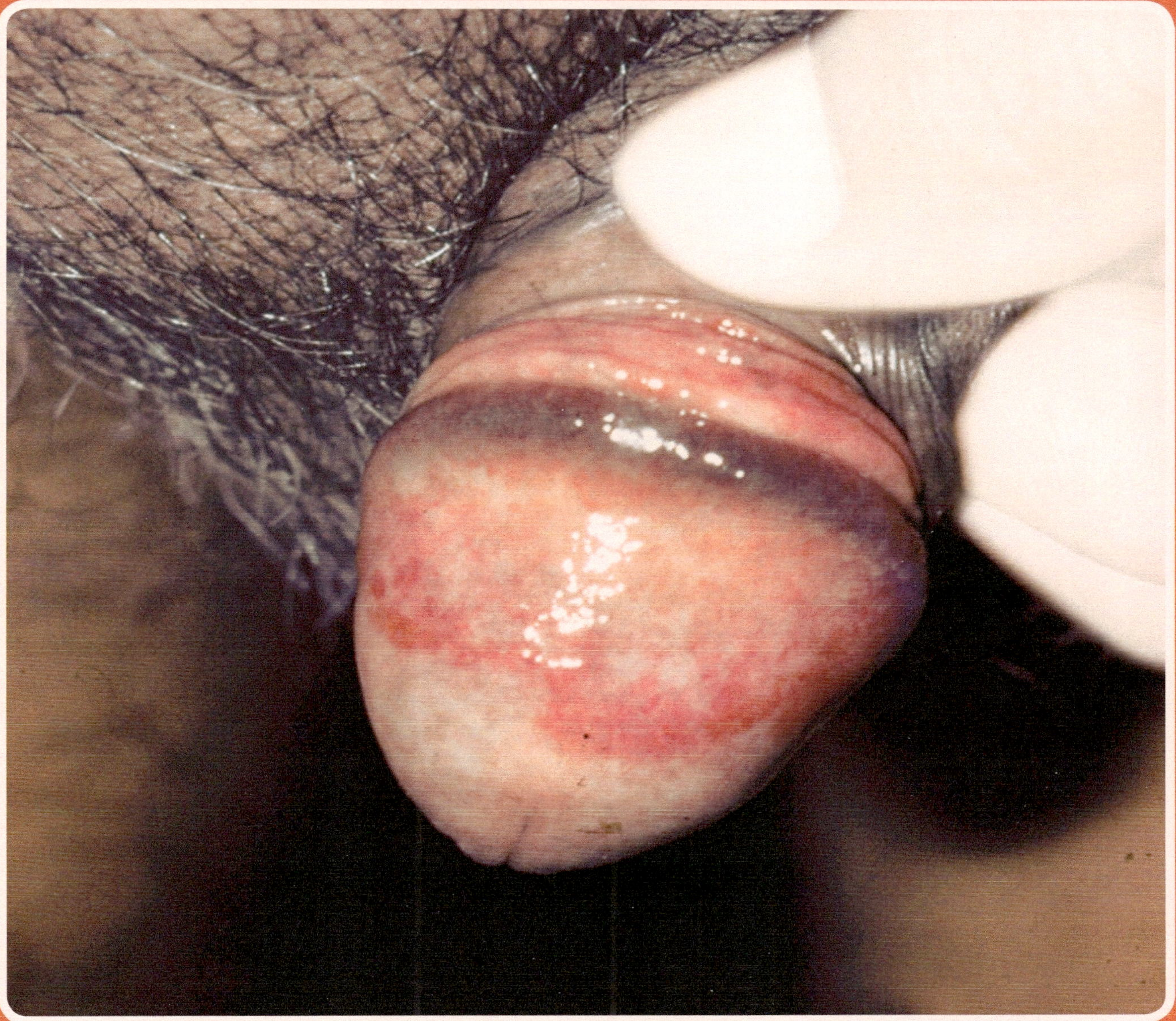

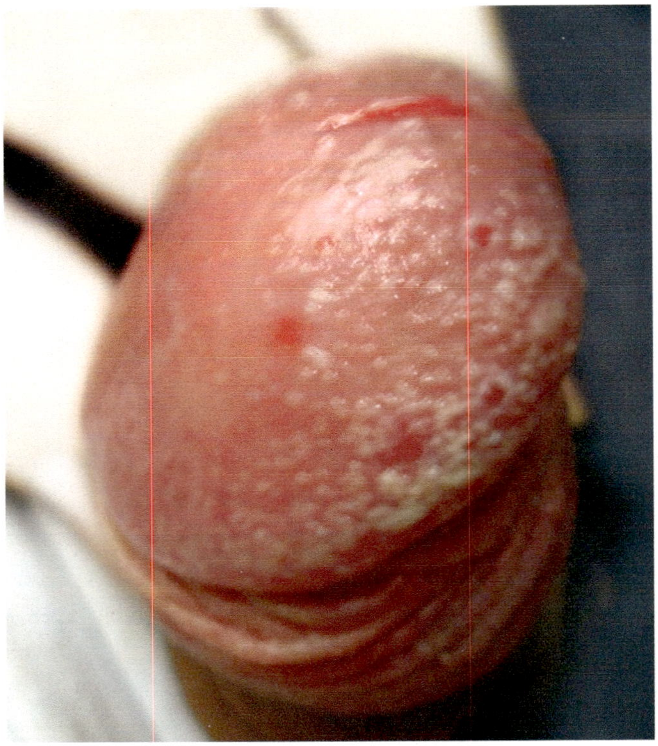

Candidal balanoposthitis: Entire glans studded with multiple tiny pustules on background of erythema.

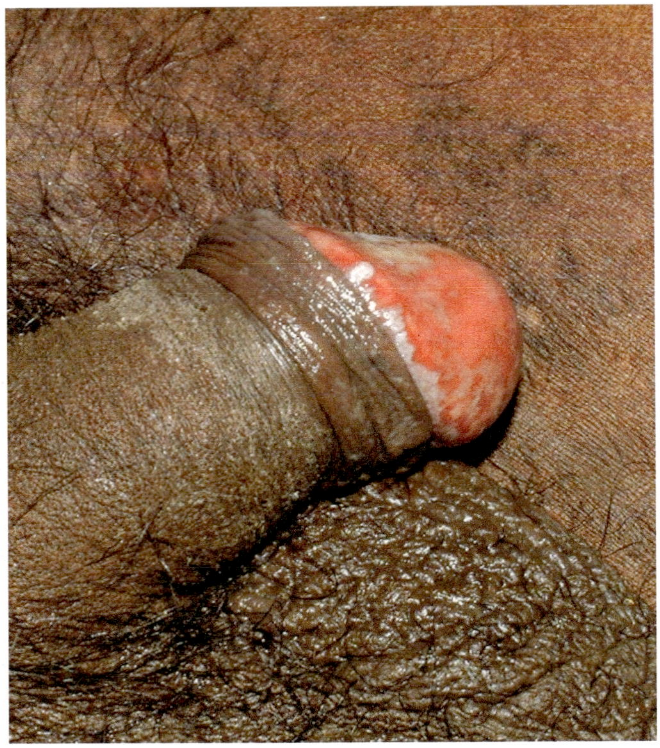

Candidal balanoposthitis: Erythematous erosions on glans with tiny pustules at the periphery.

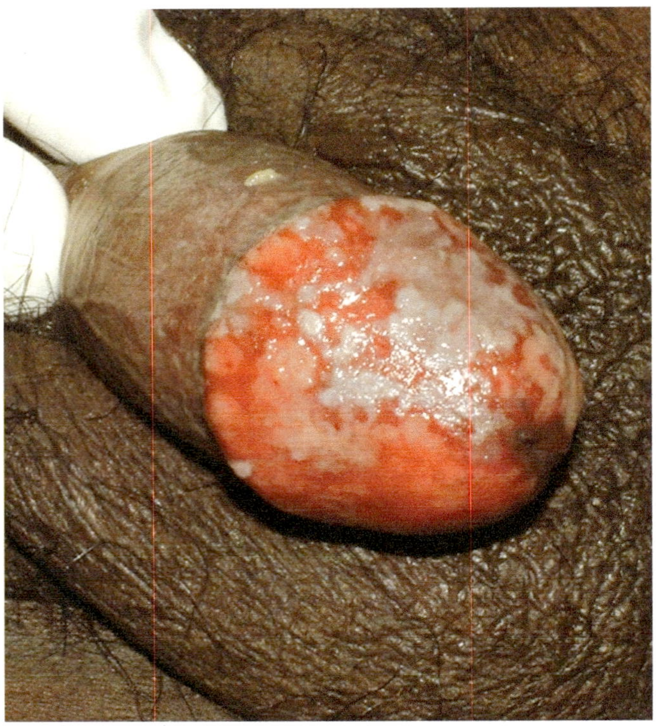

Candidal balanoposthitis: Erythematous superficial erosion on glans with coalescent pustules.

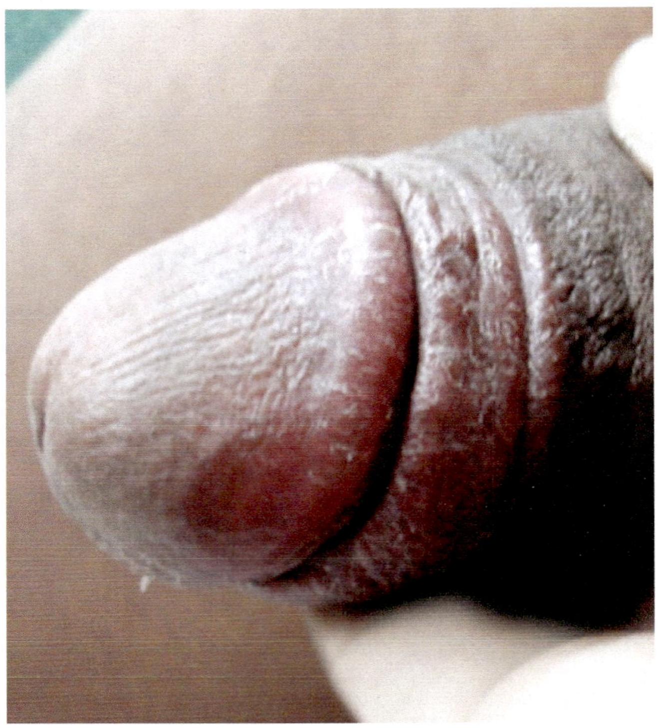

Chronic candidal balanoposthitis: Ill-defined erthematous scaly plaques on glans with marked longitudinal fissures at junction of glans and prepuce.

Balanitis inflammation of glans penis while posthitis—inflammation of mucosal surface of prepuce. Inflammation of both glans penis and prepuce—balanoposthitis. More common than balanitis or posthitis in isolation.

EPIDEMIOLOGY

Geographic Distribution

Worldwide distiribution.

Demographic Distribution

Affects adults more than children.

ETIOLOGY

Etiological Agents

Various causes of balanoposthitis, both infective and non-infective (Table 12.1).

- Infective causes commoner. Among infective causes, candidal balanoposthitis commonest.
- Cause not detectable in 30% patients.
- Recurrences in 12.7% patients.

Predisposing Factors

- Uncircumcised state.
- Poor hygiene, collection of smegma.
- Diabetes.
- HIV.
- Other immunocompromised states (malignancies).

Table 12.1: Etiology of balanoposthitis

Infective causes	Non-infective causes
• *Candida spp* • *Treponema pallidum* • *Hemophilus ducreyi* • *Neisseria gonorrhoeae* • *Gardnerella vaginalis* • *Streptococci* • *Herpes simplex virus* • *Human papilloma virus* • *Trichomonas vaginalis*	• Irritants • Trauma • Fixed drug eruption • Premalignant conditions • Malignancy: leukemia • Plasma cell balanitis • Circinate balanitis

CLINICAL FEATURES

Symptoms

- Itching, burning sensation.
- Distal dysuria, foul-smelling subprepucial discharge. Inability to retract prepuce phimosis/paraphimosis.

Signs

- ***Mild:*** Erythematous macules or plaques on glans penis and prepuce.
- ***Severe:*** Prepucial edema, phimosis, profuse sub-prepucial discharge. And erosions, fissures.
- ***Others:*** Clue to diagnosis of clinical conditions such as syphilis, chancroid, herpes genitalis, fixed drug eruption.

COMPLICATIONS

- ***Phimosis:*** Due to prepucial edema. Paraphimosis may develop.
- ***Phagedenic ulcers:*** In untreated anaerobic balano-posthitis.
- ***Malignancy:*** In high-risk HPV-associated balano-posthitis.

INVESTIGATIONS

Identification of Pathogen

- ***For Candida spp***
  - *Samples:* Scraping from affected area-pustule roof. Or scale.
  - *Potassium hydroxide mount:* Shows pseudo–hyphae and budding yeast cells.
  - *Culture:* To speciate (for *C. glabrata*) in treatment resistant cases.
- ***For Herpes simplex virus***
  - *Samples:* Scraping and swab from floor of affected area.
  - *Tranck smear:* Shows multinucleated giant cells.
  - *Others:* Direct immunofluorescent test, HSV-PCR, culture.
- ***For Treponema pallidum:*** Smear for dark ground microscopy. Also serology.
- ***For Trichomonas vaginalis:*** Wet mount preparation.

Skin Biopsy

In case of Zoon's balanitis, erythroplasia of Queyrat. And if other premalignant and malignant conditions suspected.

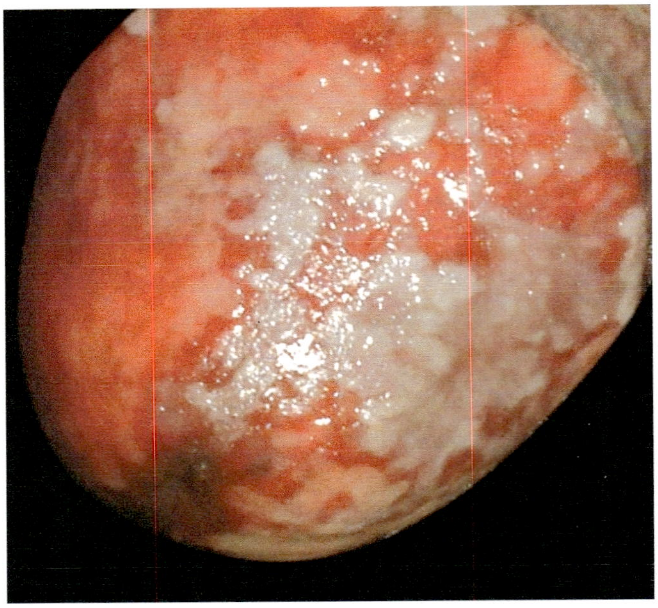

Herpetic balanitis: Polycyclic plaques with background of diffuse erythema.

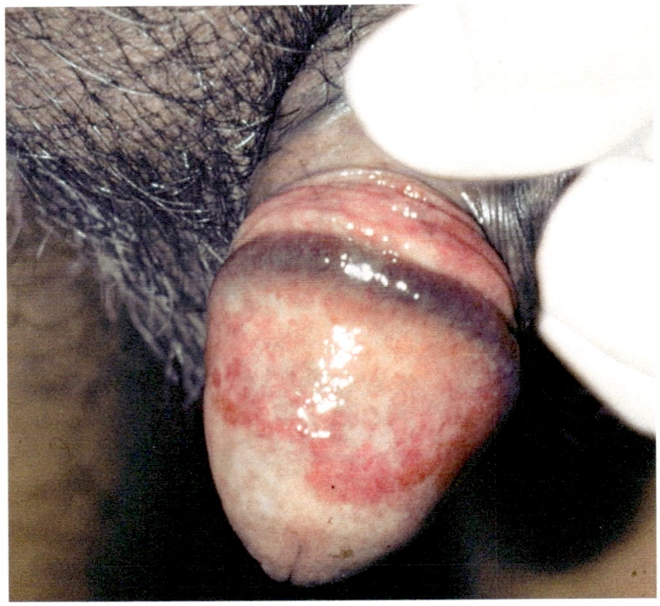

Zoon's balanitis: Well-defined erythematous plaque on glans with prominent erythematous stippling at the periphery.

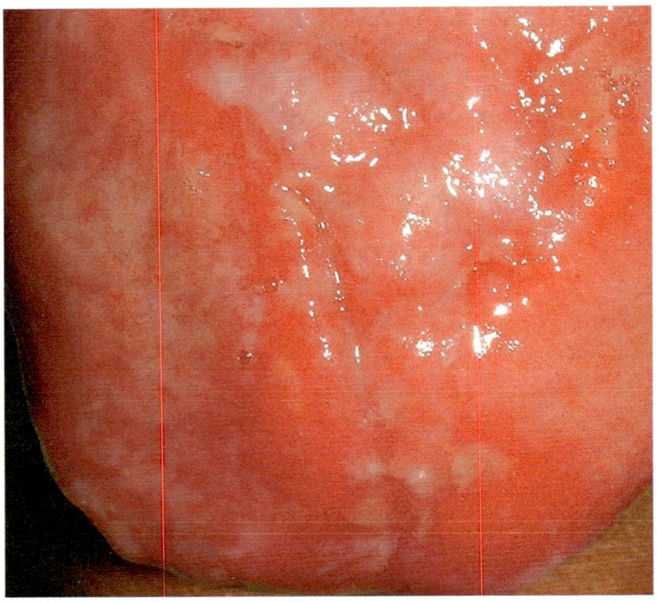

Zoons balanitis: Diffuse shiny plaque with erythematous stippling.

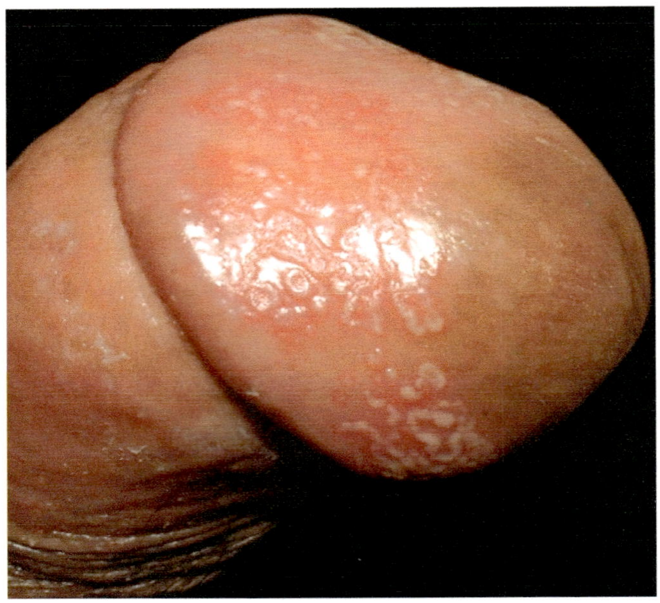

Circinate balanitis: Moist superficial plaques with serpiginous margins.

TREATMENT

- When cause found, specific therapy instituted.
- When cause not ascertained, general measures:
  - Proper hygiene.
  - Keeping area dry and aerated.
  - Symptomatic treatment for itching like antihistamines emollients.
  - Review with further investigations.

SPECIFIC DISEASES

Candidal Balanoposthitis

- Most common cause of balanoposthitis, accounting for 10-50% of cases.
- ***Transmission***
  - ***Sexually:*** From partner with candidal vulvovaginitis.
  - ***Non-sexually:*** When commensal strains overgrow in background of predisposing factors.
- ***Predisposing factors:*** Especially important in nonsexually acquired infection. Diabetes, immunosuppressed states (HIV infection), steroid intake and prolonged use of antibiotics.
- ***Clinical features:***
  - *Acute:* Marked erythema, soreness, erythematous erosions with peripheral tiny pustules.
  - *Chronic:* Scaly erythematous plaques occurring circumferentially on glans and prepuce with longitudinal fissures.

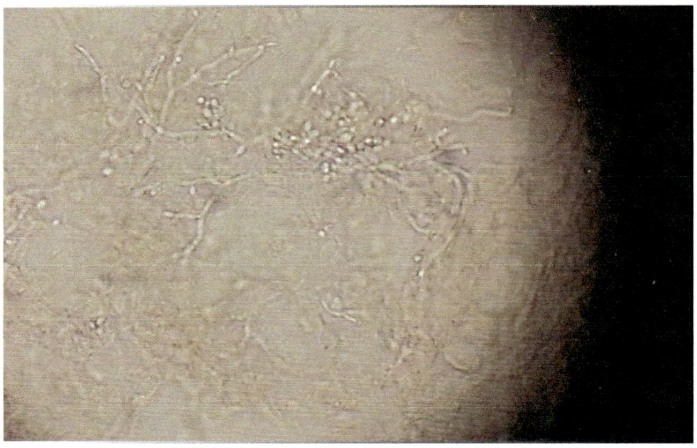

KOH mount in candidal balanoposthitis: From scales or pustules shows budding yeast cells and pseudohyphae.

- ***Recurrences:*** Common in diabetes, immunocompromised state. And if inadequate treatment of partner.
- ***Diagnostic tests.***
  - *KOH mount:* Shows budding yeast cells and pseudohyphae.
  - *Culture:* To speciate.
- ***Management:***
  - *Topical antifungal creams:* For 7 days.
  - *Systemic antifungals:* Fluconazole 150 mg weekly for 4-6 weeks. Needed for extensive disease, recurrences and in HIV positive patients.
  - Partner evaluation and treatment for vaginal discharge.
  - Investigate for underlying diabetes mellitus, HIV.
  - Condom use, till complete remission.

Zoon's Balanitis

- Also known as plasma cell balanitis, balanitis circumscripta plasma cellularis.
- Benign idiopathic chronic condition of glans.
- Occurs in middle aged to elderly, uncircumcised males.
- ***Clinical features:*** Solitary persistent well-defined superficial erythematous plaque. Shiny and glazed surface with erythematous stippling (cayenne-pepper appearance).
- ***Histopathology:*** Epidermal edema, dense upper dermal band of chronic inflammatory cells, with many plasma cells, dilated capillaries, extravasated red blood cells, and hemosiderin deposition.
- ***Treatment:*** Response to topicals (corticosteroids, tacrolimus, pimecrolimus) variable and temporary. Circumcision offers long term remission. So also carbon dioxide laser.

Circinate Balanitis

- Seen in patients with reactive arthritis (Reiter's syndrome).
- Appears as moist superficial erythematous plaques with serpiginous margins. On glans.
- Associated with spondyloarthropathy, conjunctivitis, psoriasiform skin lesions and keratoderma blennorrhagicum.

CHAPTER 13

Vaginal Discharge

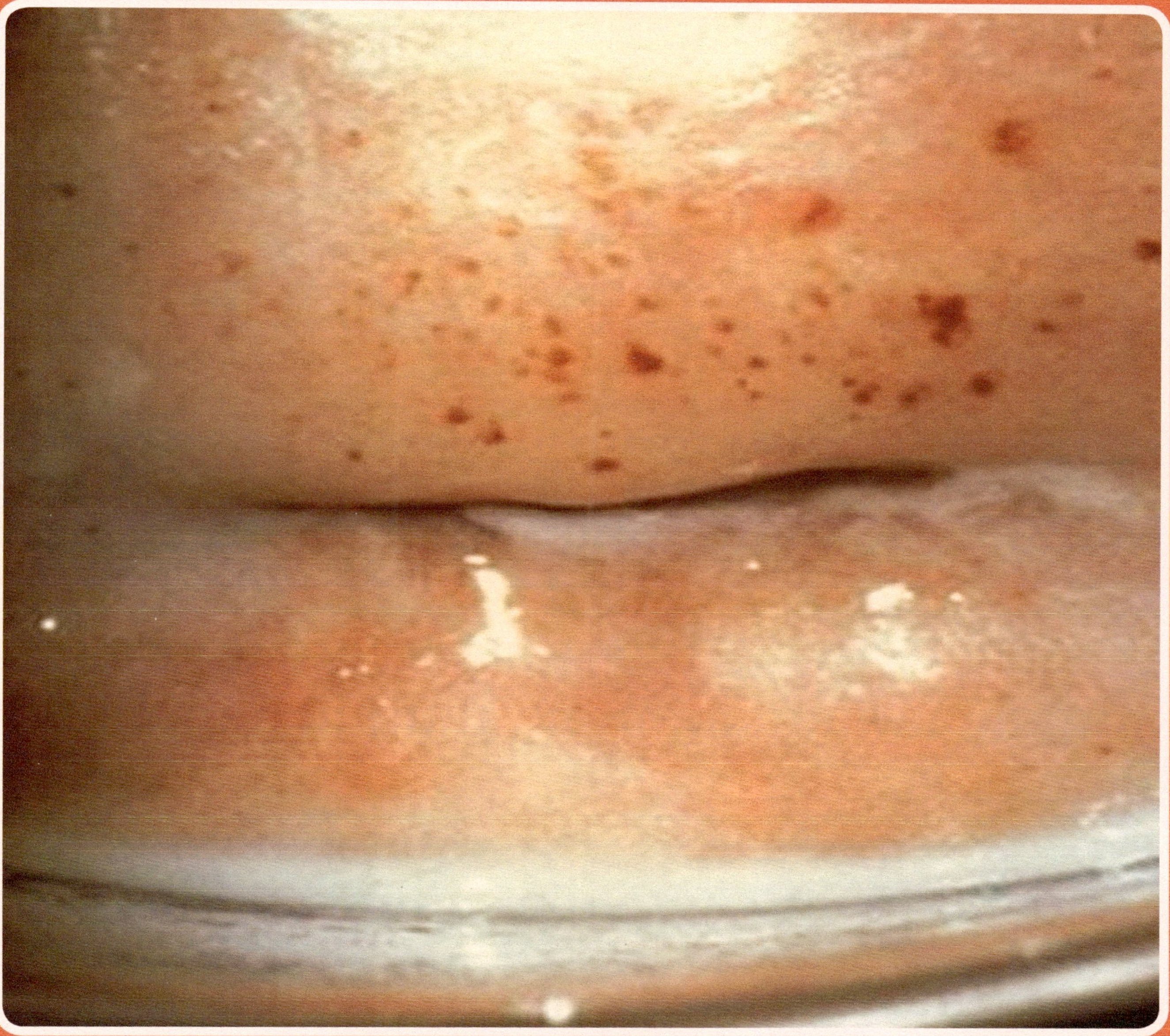

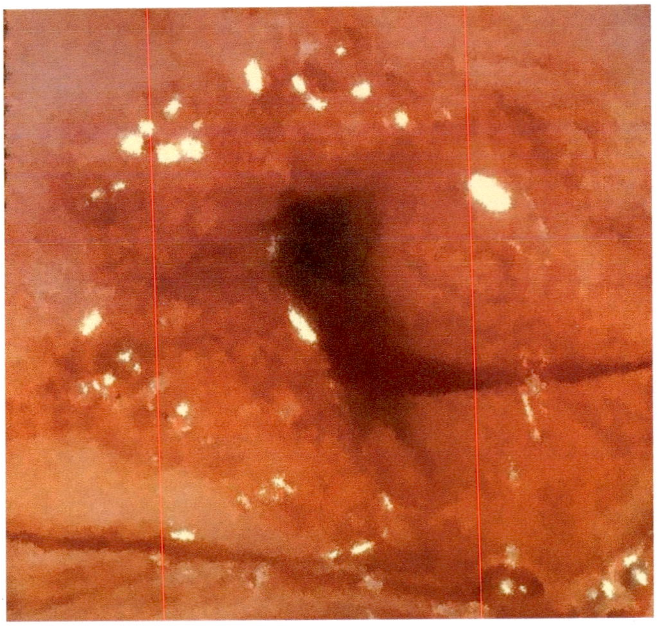

Vaginal discharge due to chlamydial cervicitis: Minimal mucopurulent cervical discharge. Such a patient may be asymptomatic. Or may have dysuria or post coital bleeding. Only infrequently presents with vaginal discharge. Discharge with *U. urealyticum* and *M. genitalium* infections also minimal.

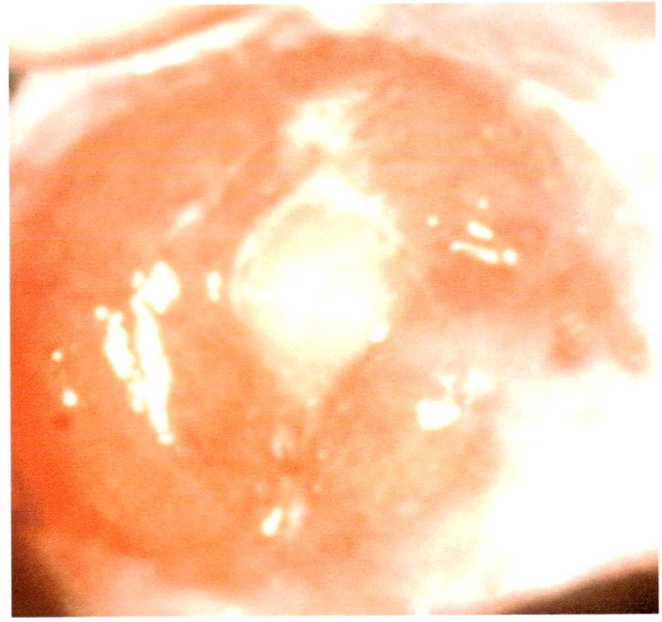

Vaginal discharge due to gonococcal cervicitis: Profuse mucopurulent cervical discharge. Patient may be symptomatic (vaginal discharge, dysuria or post coital bleeding) but is often asymptomatic.

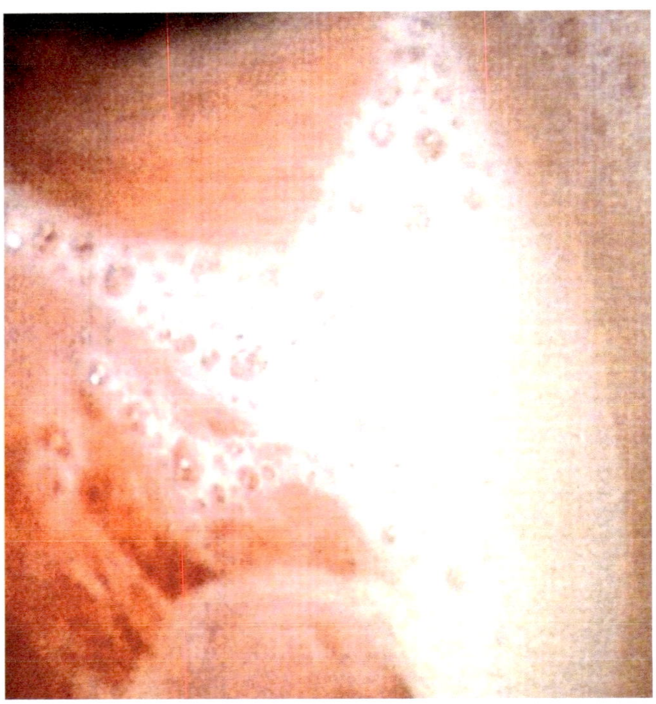

Vaginal discharge due to *T. vaginitis*: Discharge is profuse, white, homogenous, frothy and is associated with vulvar dermatitis and strawberry (erythematous stippling) cervix.

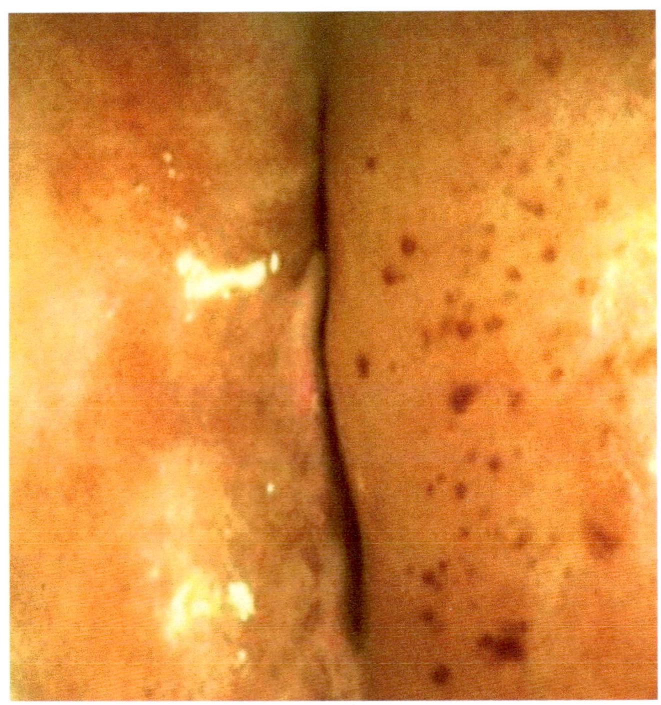

Vaginal discharge due to *T. vaginalis:* Strawberry cervix visible on per speculum examination as erythematous, hemorrhagic stippling around cervical os.

Vaginal discharge considered pathological if not associated with menstruation (pre, mid and post-period) and is:

- Increased in amount.
- Foul-smelling.
- Yellowish.
- Associated with itching.

EPIDEMIOLOGY

Geographic Distribution

- Worldwide distribution.

Demographic Distribution

- Most common sexually transmitted syndrome affecting females.
- Self reported history of genital discharge in previous 12 months in 3% of population, with half seeking treatment.

ETIOLOGY

Several infective and non-infective causes of vaginal discharge (Table 13.1).

CLINICAL FEATURES

History

Following history important:

- ***Risk assessment:***[1]
  - Is used as surrogate marker of cervicitis.
  - Sensitivity and positive predictive value significantly lower than per speculum (P/S) examination, but useful tool where P/S examination not possible.
  - *Positive predictors of high risk include:*
    - Symptomatic partner?
    - Recent new partner?
    - Multiple partners?
    - Spouse/partner returning home after long stay away from home?
- ***Symptoms:***
  - Itching, burning sensation, dyspareunia, pelvic pain.
  - Character of discharge per vagina.

Table 13.1: Etiology of abnormal vaginal discharge

Infective	Non-infective
Cervicitis • *Neisseria gonorrhoeae* • *Chlamydia trachomatis* • *Mycoplasma genitalium* • *Ureaplasma urealyticum* • Genital herpes *Vaginitis* • *Candida spp* • *Trichomonas vaginalis* • Bacterial vaginosis	• Gynecological conditions: Endocervical polyp, fistulae, tumors • Retained tampon • IUCD • Douches

Examination

- ***Character of discharge***: May indicate etiology but not specific.
- ***Vulval skin changes***: Superficial erosions, excoriations, edema or tiny pustules.
- ***Per speculum examination***: To determine origin of discharge—vaginal *vs* cervical. And to note cervical changes.
- ***Per vaginal examination***: For cervical motion tenderness and forniceal tenderness to rule out pelvic inflammatory disease (PID).

Features of Individual Infections

Gonococcal cervicitis

- ***Symptoms:*** Asymptomatic frequently. When symptomatic, mucopurulent vaginal discharge. Dysuria; intermenstrual and post coital bleeding.
- ***P/S examination:*** Mucopurulent discharge from cervical os. Erythema, edema of cervical os. Cervical bleeding.
- ***Vulva:*** Usually normal. In children, vulvitis.

Chlamydial cervicitis

- ***Symptoms:*** Asymptomatic mostly. If symptomatic minimal mucoid discharge. Other symptoms include post coital/intermenstrual bleeding.
- ***P/S examination:*** Minimal mucoid discharge from cervical os. Erythema of os and cervical friability.
- ***Vulva:*** Normal.

[1]**Risk assessment:** For high risk assessment, indicate a high risk of acquiring pathogens causing cervicitis.

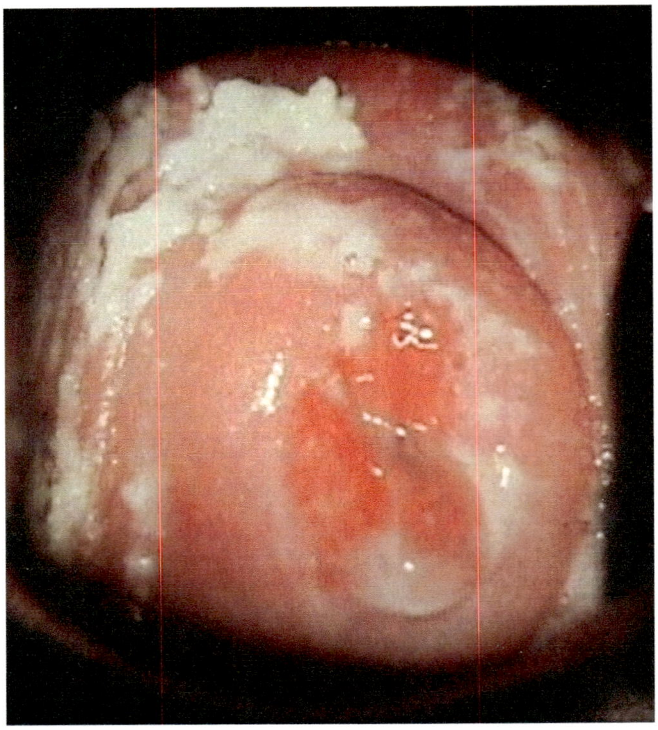

Vaginal discharge due to candida: Curdy white discharge coating the vaginal walls and cervical os.

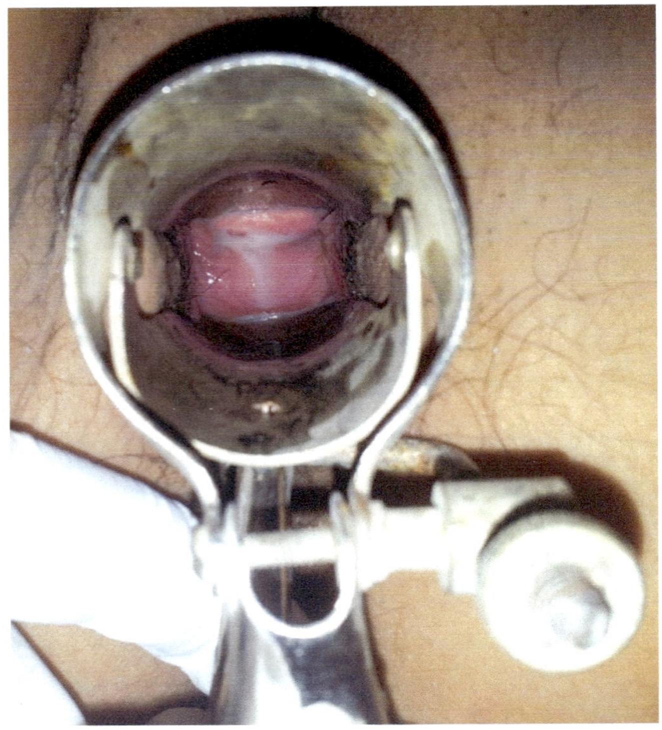

Vaginal discharge due to bacterial vaginosis: Moderate white homogeneous discharge.

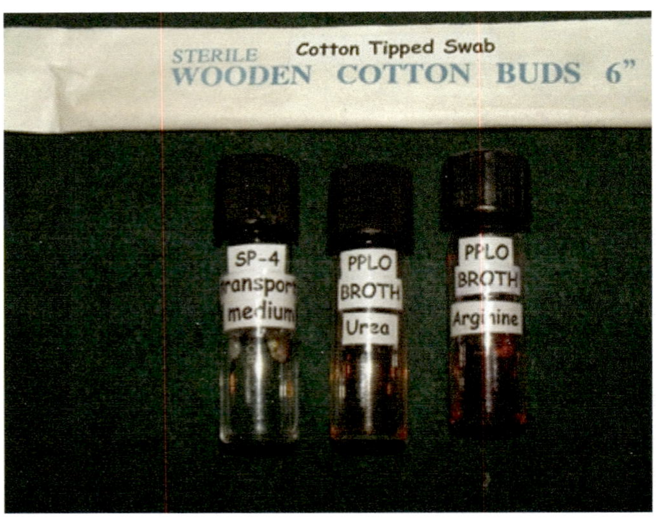

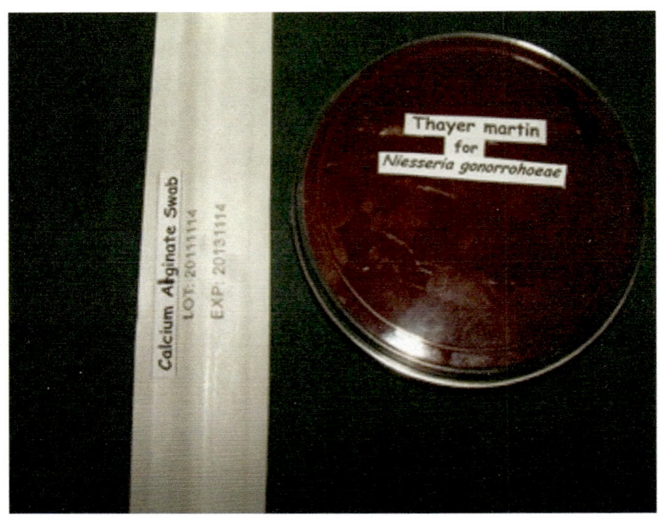

Sample collection in patients with vaginal discharge due to cervicitis: Samples are collected for identification of *C. trachomatis, N. gonorrhoeae, M. genitalium* and *U. urealyticum*. In this case samples are being collected for culture. For *C. trachomatis* the samples are collected using cotton tipped swab (or cytobrush) and transported to lab in transport medium. For *U. urealyticum* and *M. genitalium* samples are collected using a cotton swab and inoculated into PPLO broth with urea and PPLO broth with arginine respectively and for *N. gonorrhoeae* the sample is collected using a calcium alginate swab and plated on Thayer-Martin (modified) medium.

Candidal vulvovaginitis

- ***Symptoms:*** Vulval pruritus. External dysuria. Vaginal discharge-moderate, white, cheesy (curdy), adherent.
- ***P/S examination:*** Discharge (curdy) on vaginal walls.
- ***pH:*** < 4.5.
- ***Vulva:*** Vulvar dermatitis. Erythema, edema, erosions. Sometimes intense.

Trichomonas vaginitis

- ***Symptoms:*** Profuse malodorous white-yellow-green, homogeneous, watery, often frothy discharge. External dysuria and irritation.
- ***P/S examination:*** Discharge on vaginal walls. Cervical os shows pinpoint hemorrhagic spots (strawberry cervix).
- ***pH:*** Usually > 5.0
- ***Vulva:*** Vulvar dermatitis.

Bacterial vaginosis

- ***Symptoms:*** Foul smelling vaginal discharge-moderate to profuse, white or gray homogeneous. Conspicous after sexual intercourse.
- ***P/S examination:*** Discharge uniformly coating vaginal walls. Positive whiff test.
- ***pH:*** Usually > 4.5.
- ***Vulva:*** Usually normal.

HIV AND PATHOGENS OF VAGINITIS

- ***HIV and candidal infection:***
  - *Effect of candidal vaginitis on HIV:* amplified transmission.
  - *Effect of HIV on candidal vaginitis:*
    - Increased prevalence. Also of non-albicans candidal vaginitis.
    - Increased severity and extent.
    - Fluconazole prophylaxis often recommended. Resistance to treatment.
- ***HIV and bacterial vaginosis:***
  - *Effect of bacterial vaginosis on HIV:* amplified transmission of HIV.
  - *Effect of HIV on bacterial vaginosis:* clinical presentation in HIV negative and positive patients probably similar.
- ***HIV and trichomonas vaginitis:***
  - *Effect of trichomonas vaginitis on HIV:* amplified transmission of HIV due to increased HIV shedding as also presence of inflammation and microabrasions.
  - *Effect of HIV on trichomonas vaginitis:* probably no change.

COMPLICATIONS

- ***Pelvic inflammatory disease:*** Chlamydia, gonococcus.
- ***Tubal infertility:*** Chlamydia, gonococcus.
- ***Enhanced transmission of HIV:*** All.
- ***Obstetric complications:*** Preterm birth, low birth weight babies in mother's with bacterial vaginosis.

DIAGNOSIS

Based on Clinical Features

- Based on nature and source of discharge, presumptive diagnosis may be made.
- Both a low sensitivity and specificity.
- Confirmation done by side laboratory procedures and identification of organisms.

Laboratory Investigations (Table 13.2)

For diagnosis of cervicitis

- Unlike urethritis, no clear cut definition.
- Presence of > 30 WBCs/high power field (HPF) on Gram stained cervical smear. Or > 10 WBCs/HPF on Gram stained vaginal smear.

For chlamydial cervicitis

- ***Samples collected:***
  - Endocervical swab, using cotton tipped swabs. Or cytobrush. Self obtained vaginal samples (SOVS). And first void urine (FVU) give similar yield for sensitive tests (PCR).
- ***Direct identification:***
  - *Giemsa staining:* not sensitive. Shows basophilic intracytoplasmic bodies.
  - *Iodine staining:* not sensitive. Shows brown intracytoplasmic bodies.
  - *Direct fluorescent test:* sensitive, specific, but expensive and laborious.
  - *EIA:* sensitive and specific. And simple.
  - *Point of care (rapid) tests:* several available like Chlamydia rapid test.
- ***Nucleic acid-base tests:***
  - *PCR:* very sensitive and specific. Multiplex PCR for *C. trachomatis* and *N. gonorrhoeae* (pathogens commonly causing cervicitis) also available.
  - *Others:* like ligase chain reaction.

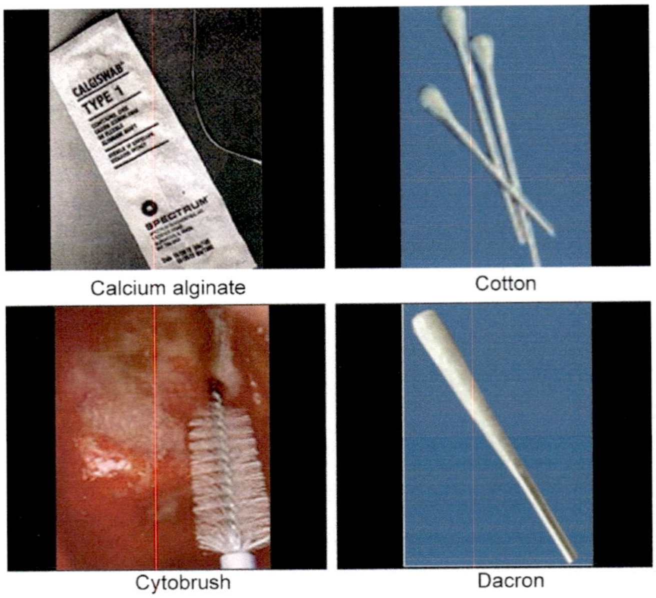

Swabs used to collect specimens from cervical discharge: Calcium alginate and dacron for *N. gonorrhoeae*, cotton tipped swab and cytobrush for *C. trachomatis*, rayon-tipped and cotton-tipped swabs for *M. genitalium* and *U. urealyticum*.

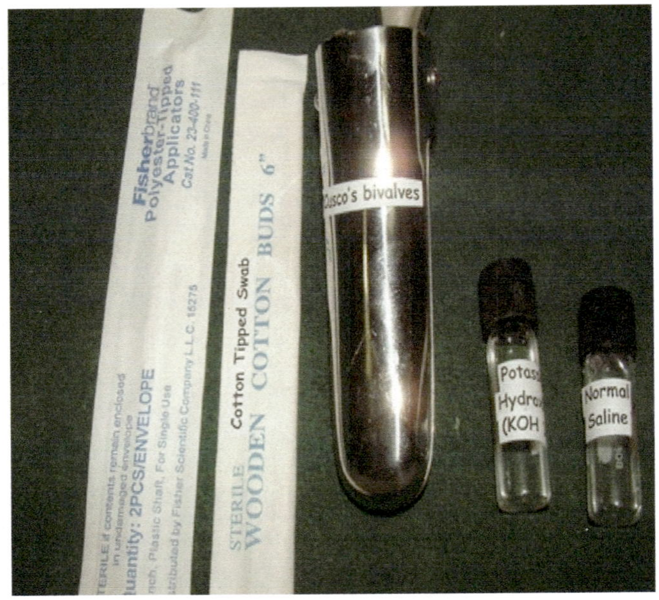

Sample collection in patients with vaginal discharge due to vaginitis: Samples are collected for diagnosis of candidal vaginitis (for a potassium hydroxide mount), trichomonas vaginitis (for a saline mount) and bacterial vaginosis (for a saline mount or Gram stain).

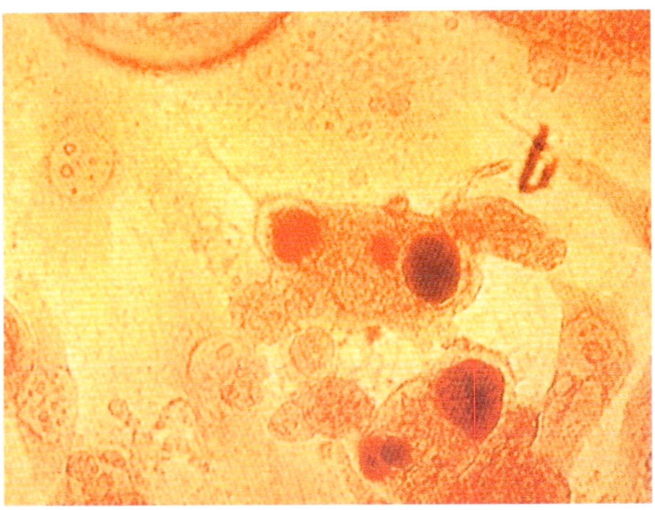

Chlamydial cervicitis: Iodine staining of cervical smear showing brown intracytoplasmic iodine stained chlamydia bodies.

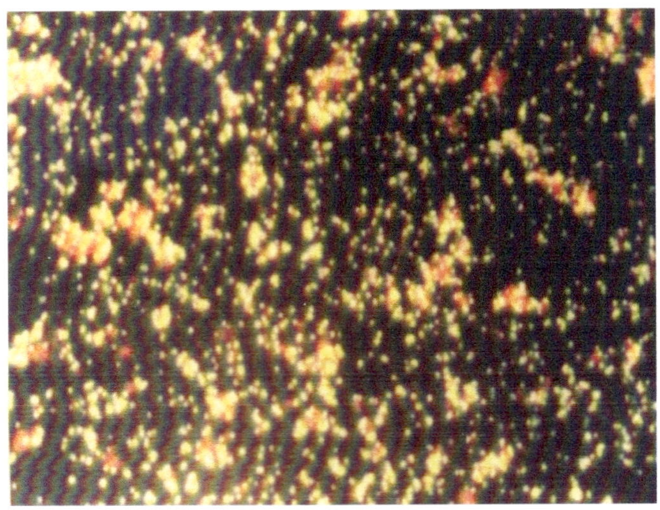

Chlamydial cervicitis: Microimmunofluoroscence to detect chlamydial antigen (seen as greenish refractile particles 100x).

- ***Culture:*** Earlier considered gold standard. On irradiated McCoy cells, Hela-229 and BHK-2. Confirmed by Giemsa/iodine staining or direct fluorescent test.
- ***Serology:*** Not reliable for lower genital infection. May help for upper genital infection in women where isolation not possible.

For gonococcal infections

Chapter 6.

For mycoplasma and ureaplasma

- ***Samples collected:*** As for *C. trachomatis*. Cervical swabs, using rayon/cotton tipped swabs collected.
- ***Culture:*** Using PPLO broth and agar. For *Mycoplasma* in PPLO enriched with arginine and *Ureaplasma* in PPLO with urea. *Mycoplasma* colonies with classical fried egg appearance. *Ureaplasma* colonies pinpoint (difficult to see without magnification). Stain blue with Dienés stain. Colonies further serotyped.
- ***PCR:*** Available both for direct samples. And for identification of colonies on culture.
- ***Serological tests:*** Not standardized.

For T. vaginalis

- ***Samples collected:*** Posterior fornix. For nucleic acid based tests, urine and SOVS also useful.
- ***Wet mount:*** Under 40x. Visible as pear shaped flagellate motile (jerky movements) organisms.
- ***Culture:*** On modified Diamond's media.
- ***Others:*** Latex agglutination—Sensitive and rapid, point of care test. Nucleic acid based tests sensitive.

For candida

- ***Samples collected:*** Posterior fornix, vulva.
- ***Potassium hydroxide(KOH)/saline mount. Or Gram stained smear:*** Budding cells and pseudomycelia.
- ***Culture:*** On Sabouraud's dextrose agar. Or media with chromogenic substrates. Very sensitive but not diagnostic.

For bacterial vaginosis

- ***Samples collected:*** Vaginal discharge from lateral or posterior fornix.
- ***Vaginal pH:*** Of > 4.5. Tested using short range pH paper 3.8-5.4. Color changes from yellow to dark green to deep blue.
- ***Whiff test:*** Add 10% KOH to discharge on blade of speculum. Smell for fishy odor.
- ***KOH mount:*** More than 20% clue cells-squamous epithelial cells studded with coccobacilli and fuzzy borders.
- ***Gram stain:*** Clue cells; paucity of lactobacillus (normal flora) with predominance of Gram negative coccobacilli.

TREATMENT (TABLE 13.3)

- In vaginal discharge, etiology-based treatment often not useful because:
  - Low sensitivity and specificity of clinical diagnosis alone.
  - High incidence of mixed infections.
- Syndrome-based treatment better especially in vaginitis if P/S examination and side lab procedures not available.

Table 13.2: Culture of vaginal discharge

	Swabs for collection of samples	Culture media used
N. gonorrhoeae	Non-cotton swab stick (calcium alginate/ dacron/rayon) with plastic or aluminium shaft	Enriched media (Modified Thayer-Martin, New York City, Chacko-Nair)
C. trachomatis	Cotton tipped swab/cytobrush	McCoy cell line, Hela-229
M. genitalium, U. urealyticum	Rayon/cotton tipped swabs	PPLO broth with urea (for *U. urealyticum*) or arginine (for *M. genitalium*)
Candida spp	Polyester swab	Sabouraud dextrose agar
T. vaginalis	Cotton-tipped swab	Modified Diamond's media

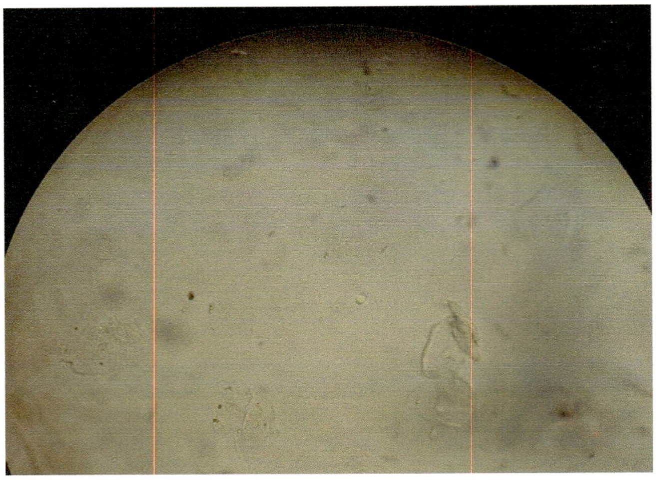

Vaginal discharge due to *T. vaginitis*: Wet mount of discharge showing pear shaped motile organism (40x).

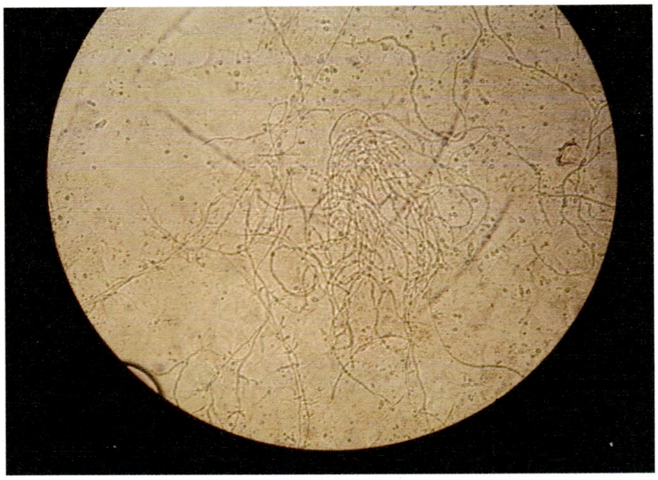

Vaginal discharge due to candida: Potassium hydroxide mount of discharge showing multiple pseudohyphae and budding yeast cells.

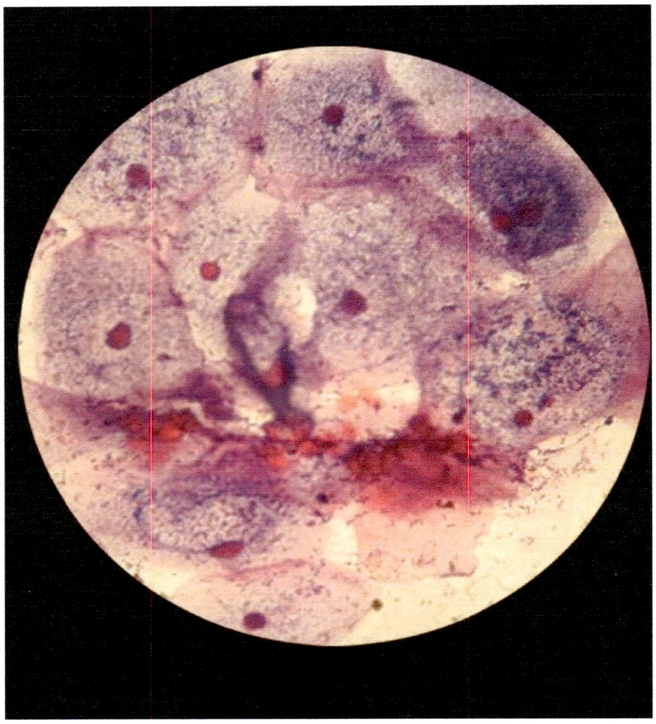

Physiological vaginal discharge: Gram stain showing epithelial squamous cells and multiple Gram-positive coccobacilli (*Lactobacillus spp.*)

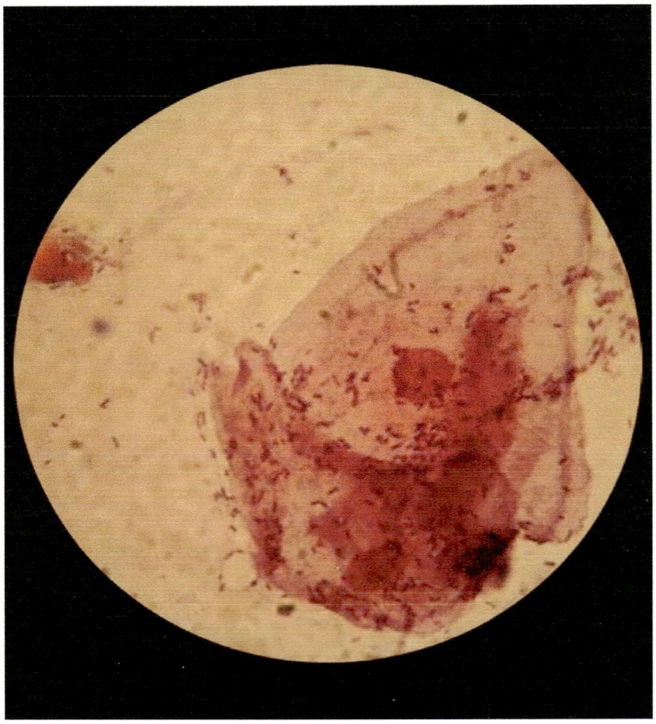

Vaginal discharge: Bacterial vaginosis. Gram stain of vaginal discharge showing clue cells which are squamous epithelial cells studded with Gram negative coccobacilli. Bacterial vaginosis is due to alteration of bacterial flora with over growth of Gardnerella vaginalis, Mobiluncus, Bacteroides and Mycoplasma.

Management of Sex Partners

- ***Of patients with bacterial vaginosis:*** Routinely, treatment not necessary.
- ***Of patients with trichomonas vaginitis:*** Treated with tinidazole/metronidazole.

Table 13.3: Treatment guidelines for vaginal discharge

Organism	CDC 2010	WHO 2003	NACO 2007
N. gonorrhoeae	• Ceftriaxone 250 mg IM stat **OR** • Cefixime 400 mg SOD*	• Ciprofloxacin 500 mg SOD* **OR** • Ceftriaxone 125 mg IM stat **OR** • Cefixime 400 mg SOD* **OR** • Spectinomycin 2 g IM stat	• Cefixime 400 mg SOD*
C. trachomatis	• Azithromycin 1 gm SOD* **OR** • Doxycycline 100 mg bid × 7 days	• Azithromycin 1 gm SOD* **OR** • Doxycycline 100 mg bid × 7 days	• Azithromycin 1 gm SOD*
Bacterial vaginosis	• Metronidazole 500 mg bid × 7 days **OR** • Metronidazole gel, 0.75% one applicator (5 g) intravaginally, od × 5 days **OR** • Clindamycin cream, 2% one full applicator (5 g) intravaginally at bedtime × 7 days	• Metronidazole 500 mg bid × 7 days	• Secnidazole 2 gm SOD* **OR** • Tinidazole 500 mg bid × 5 days
Candida spp	• Clotrimazole 1% intravaginally × 7-14 days **OR** • Fluconazole 150 mg SOD*	• Miconazole or clotrimazole 200 mg intravaginally od × 3 days **OR** • Clotrimazole 500 mg intravaginally, stat **OR** • Fluconazole 150 mg SOD*	• Fluconazole 150 mg SOD* **OR** • Clotrimazole 500 mg stat intravaginally
T. vaginalis	• Metronidazole/tinidazole 2 gm SOD*	• Metronidazole/tinidazole 2 gm SOD*	• Secnidazole 2 gm SOD* **OR** • Tinidazole 500 mg bid × 5 days

*SOD : Single oral dose

Chapter 14

Sexually Transmitted Infestations

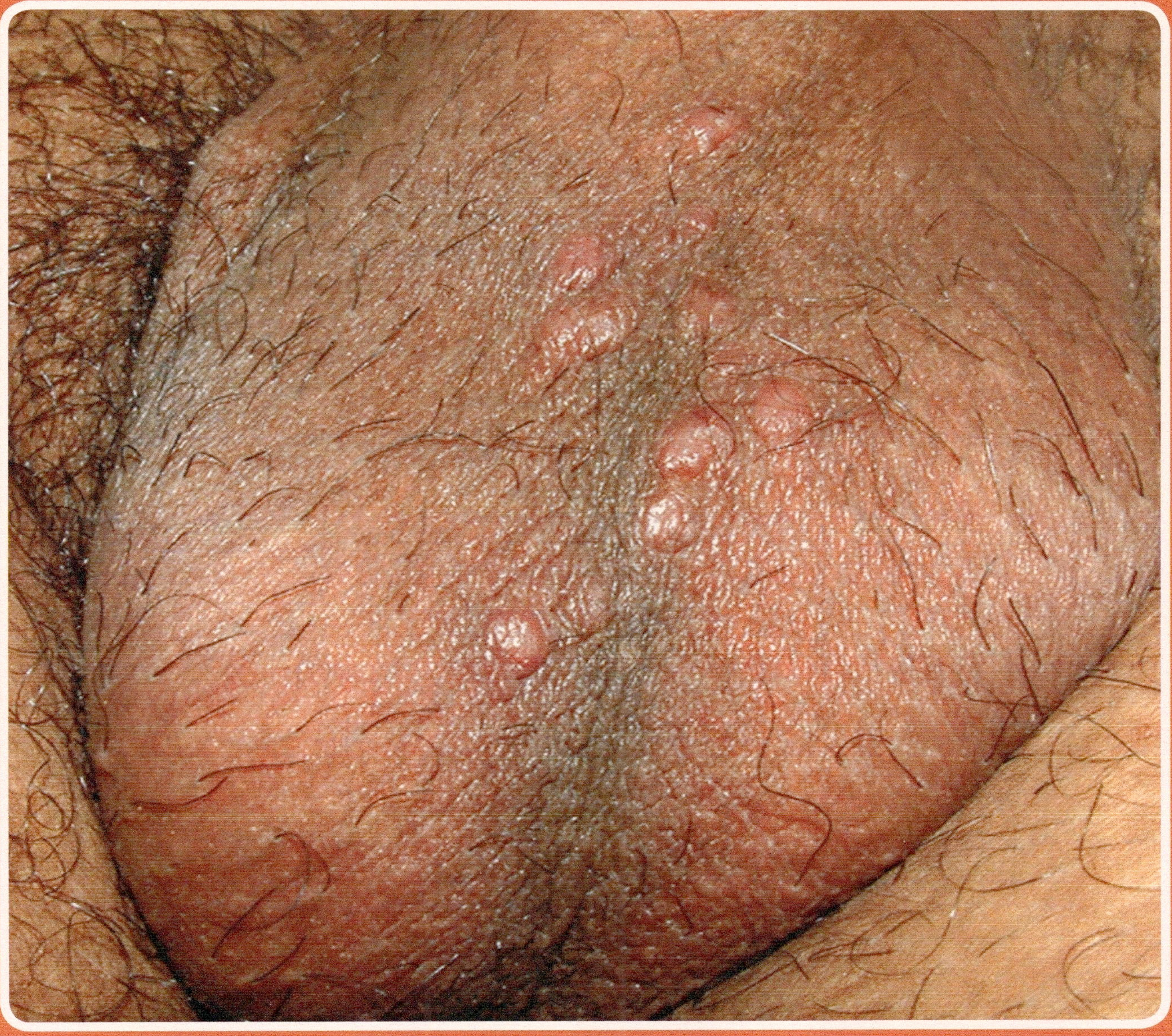

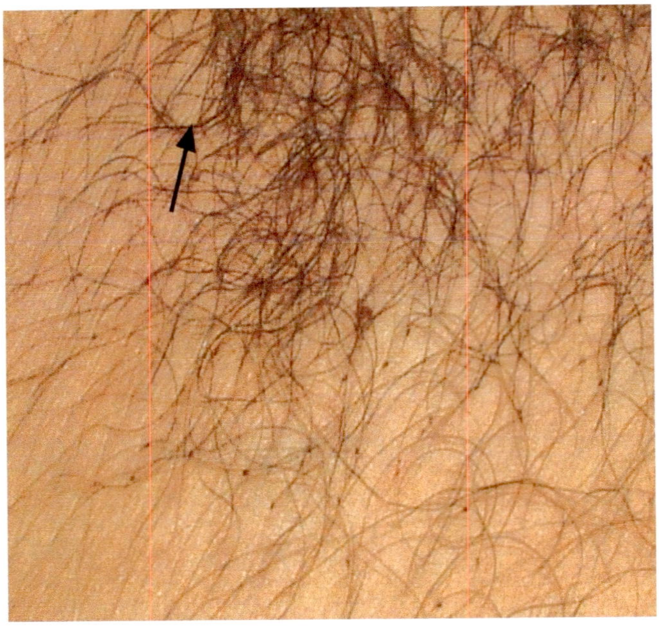

Pediculosis pubis: Crab louse eggs (nits) attached to pubic hair.

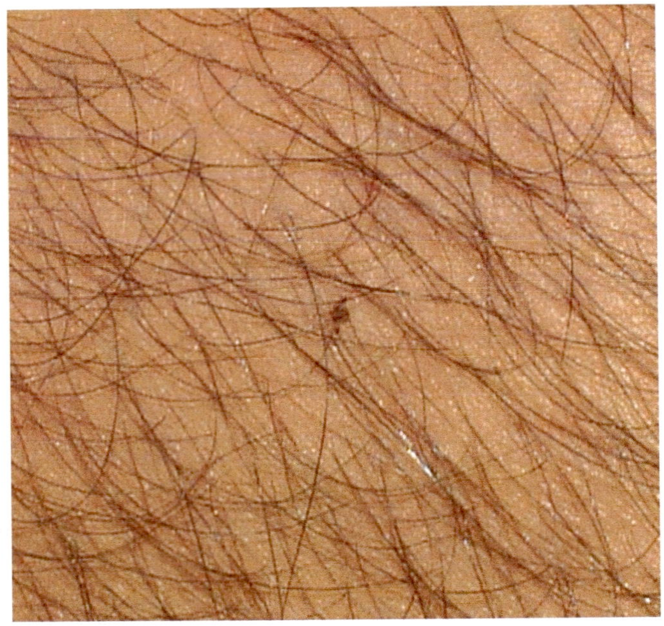

Pediculosis pubis: Crab louse clinging to root of abdominal hair.

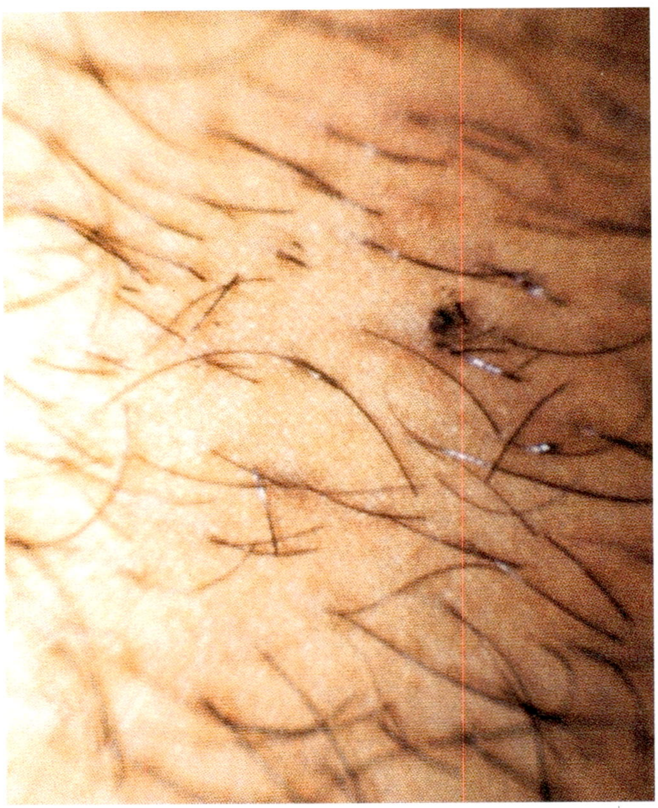

Pediculosis pubis: Maculae ceruleae are blue-gray macules seen on the abdomen. Precise mechanism unknown, but probably due to bite of arthropod.

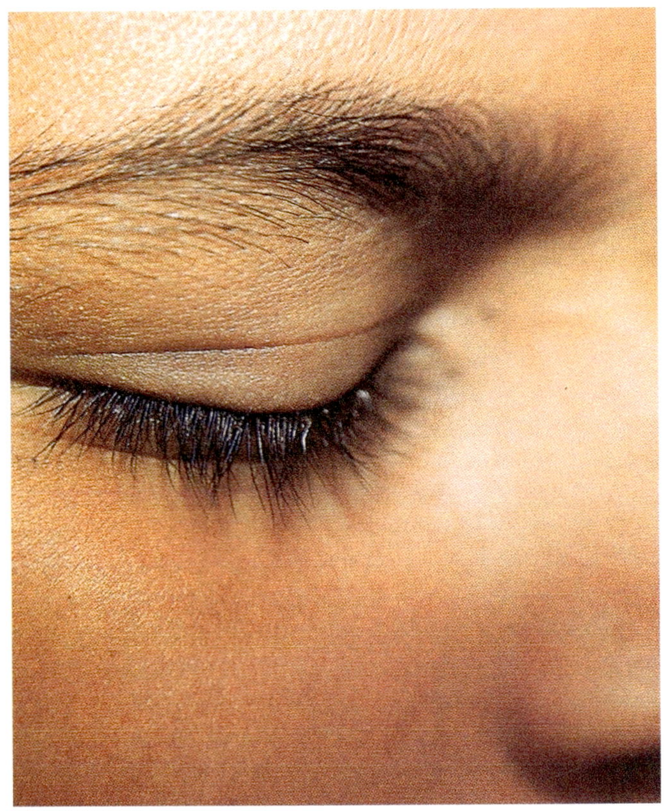

Pediculosis pubis: Crab louse nits on the lashes. When pediculosis pubis is suspected, other body parts should be examined as louse may infest other parts of body with short hairs.

PEDICULOSIS PUBIS

Epidemiology

Also known as pthiriasis pubis.

Geographic distribution

- Worldwide prevalence of 2-10%. Decreasing prevalence due to attributable to waxing of pubic hair.
- Outbreaks in military men, hostels and areas with overcrowding.

Demographic distribution

- In sexually active people. Commonly found as co-infection with other STIs.
- Especially in homeless, unkempt and those not taking regular bath.

Etiology

Etiological agent

- Pubic louse or *Pthirus pubis* or crab lice.
- Small (1 mm).
- Attaches to hair shaft using serrated edges on claws.
- Survives for 2 weeks on human host. And only 36 hours off it.

Transmission

- Sexual transmission.
- Fomites (sharing of towels, underclothes, bedding).

Clinical Features

Manifestations

- Severe itching.
- Lice and eggs (nits) visible. Louse faeces visible as brown specks on body or underclothings.
- Maculae ceruleae (sky-blue macules) seen commonly on thighs or trunk.
- Infests pubic hair, hair on inner aspect of thighs and perianal area. Other hair bearing areas (body hair, axillae, eyelashes, beard) may be infested.

Complications

- Involvement of eyelashes. May manifest as conjunctivitis.
- Secondary impetiginization.

Diagnosis

Based on clinical features

Itching on pubic area with visible lice and nits.

Laboratory Investigations

Saline mount of organism.

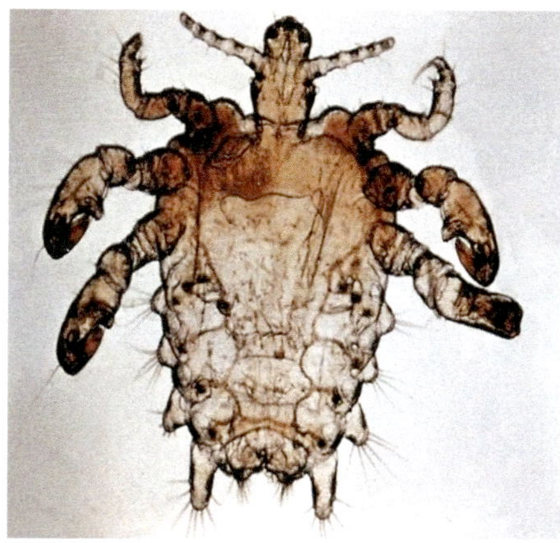

Pthirus pubis: Squat arthropod with 1st claw with serrated edges and 2nd and 3rd pincer like claws. Help to grip hair.

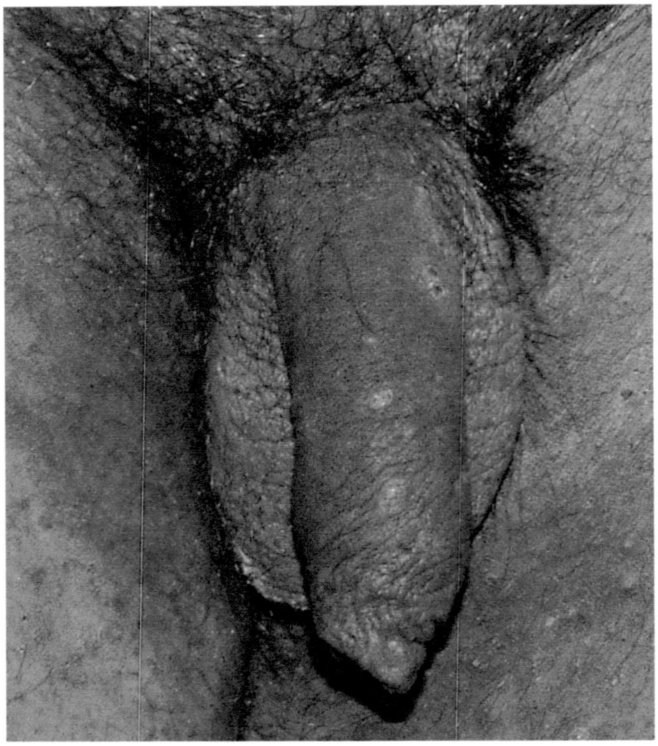

Genital scabies: Multiple excoriated papules on penis and scrotum.

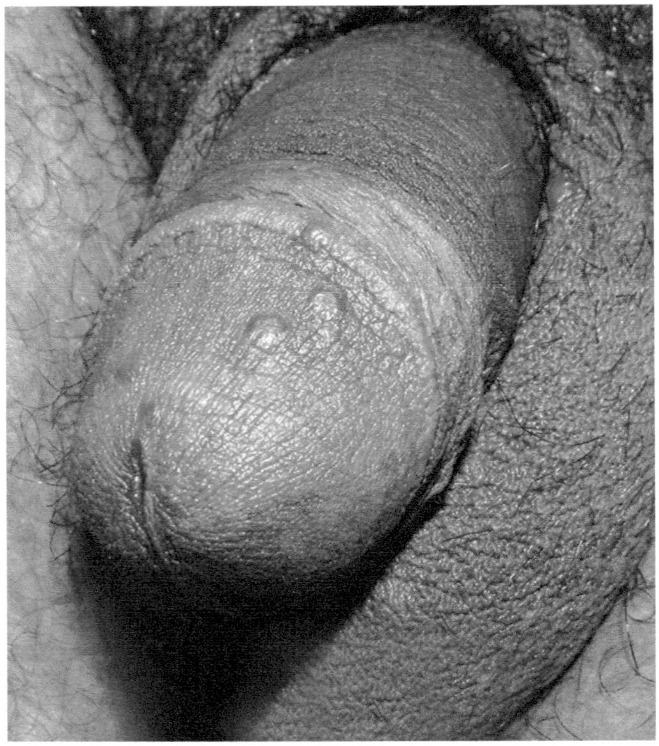

Pubic lice: Multiple excoriated papules on glans.

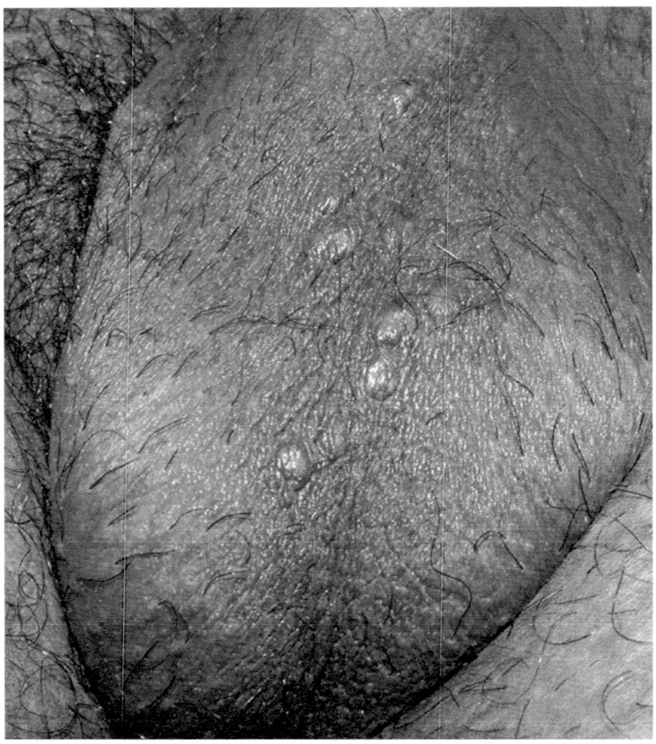

Genital scabies: Erythematous nodules on scrotum in a patient with generalized pruritus.

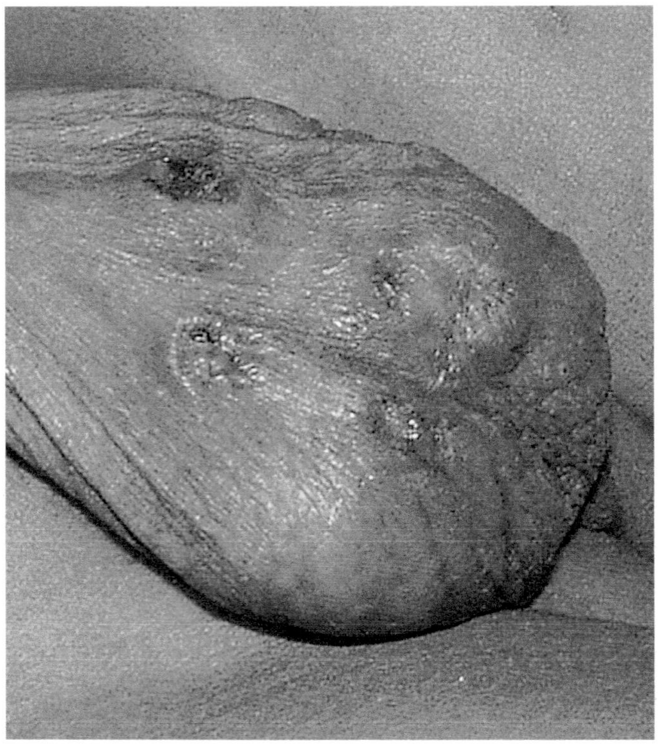

Nodular scabies: Scrotum showing excoriated well defined nodules with crusting indicating secondary infection.

Treatment

- Permethrin, 5%. Whole body overnight application. Repeated 1 week later.
- All sexual contacts to be treated irrespective of symptoms.
- Other drugs like benzyl benzoate, malathion, gamma benzene hexachloride may be used.

SCABIES

Epidemiology

Geographic distribution

- Affects 0.5-3% of STD clinic attendees.

Demographic distribution

- Genital scabies commoner in males.
- Sexually transmitted scabies in age group 15-45 years.
- HIV-positive patients have more severe form of disease (Norwegian scabies).

Etiology

Etiological agent

- *Sarcoptes scabiei var hominis*.
- ***Structure:*** Ovoid body, flattened dorsoventrally with 4 pairs of short legs. Females larger than males.
- ***Life cycle:*** Lifespan of 4–6 weeks. Female lays 40–50 eggs; from these 6 legged larvae emerge after 3–4 days. Larvae transform into nymphs which moults to develop into adult males and females.
- Mites show preference for certain sites to burrow, avoiding areas with high density of pilosebaceous follicles.

Transmission

- Mostly non-sexual. But sexual transmission also occurs.
- Also through fomites (sharing of clothes, bedsheets, towels).

Clinical Features

Incubation period

3-4 weeks between contact and eruption of lesions.

History

- Pruritus, especially nocturnal.
- Family history positive.

Morphology

- 'Burrows' characteristic lesions; seen as serpiginous tracts in skin; due to residence of mite.
- Excoriated papules, vesicles, pustules; due to hypersensitivity.
- Nodules on genitalia (scrotum and shaft of penis).

Sites of lesions

Even when sexually transmitted, distribution similar to non-sexually transmitted infection. Webspaces, flexors of wrist, ulnar aspects of forearms, axillae, breasts and periareolar area, umbilicus, pubic area and inner aspect of thighs medial malleoli (Circle of Hebra).

Variants

- Nodular scabies on genitalia.
- Norwegian scabies in HIV-positive individuals.

Complications

Secondary infection; may ocassionally trigger post-streptococcal glomerulonephritis.

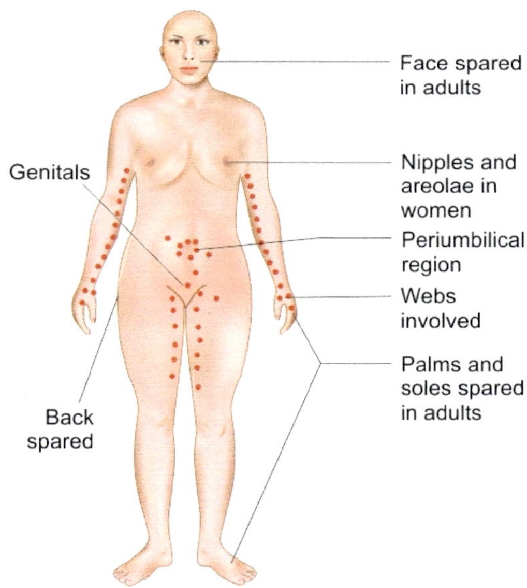

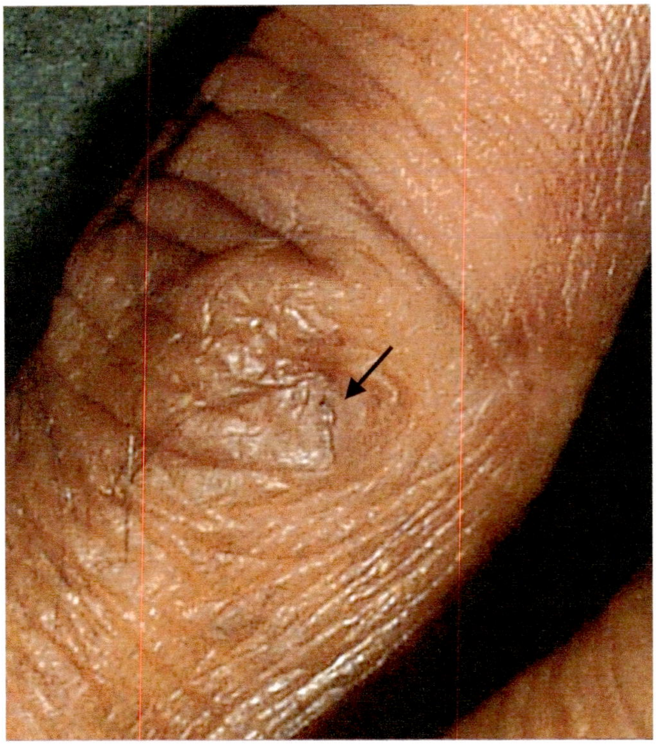

Scabies: Patients with sexually acquired scabies should be examined and treated as for non sexually acquired scabies. Note burrow.

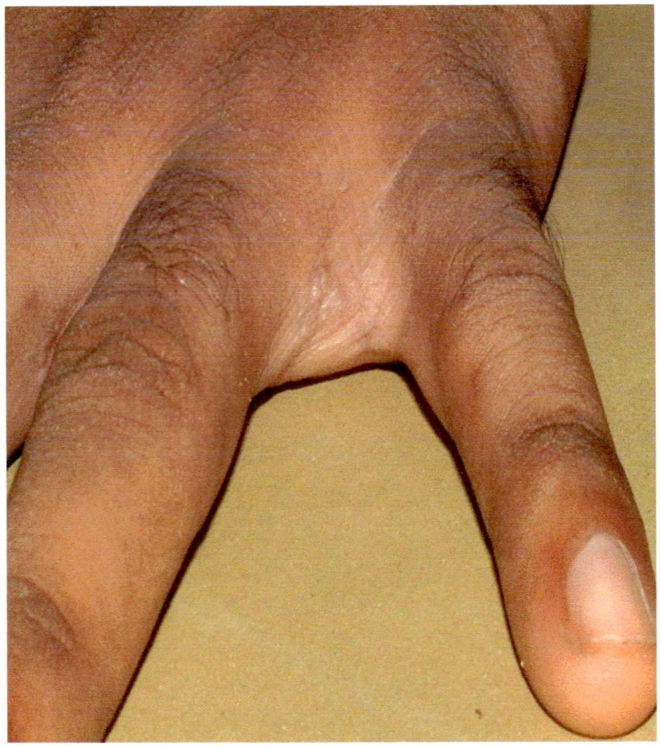

Scabies: Web space (classical site) showing burrow.

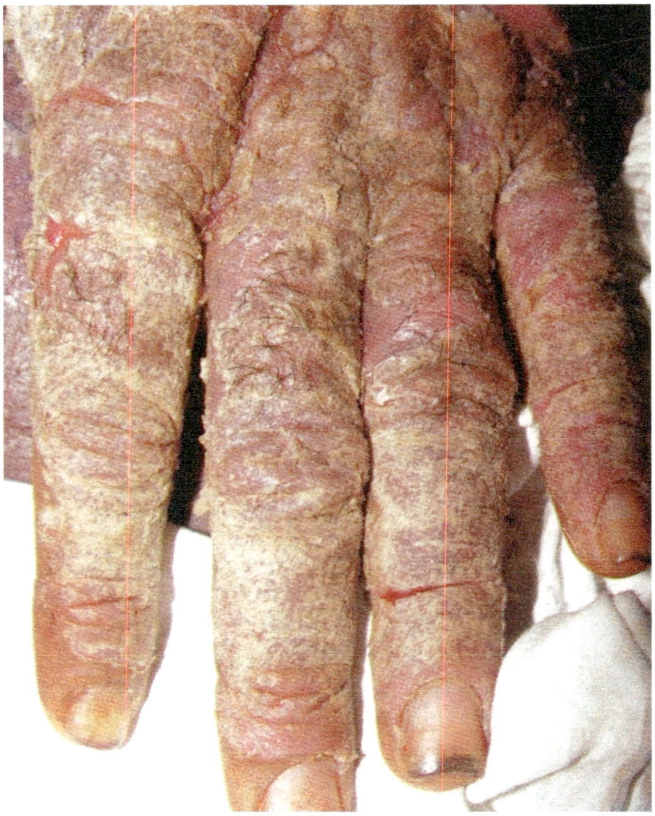

Norwegian scabies: Hyperkeratotic lesions on the dorsa of hand.

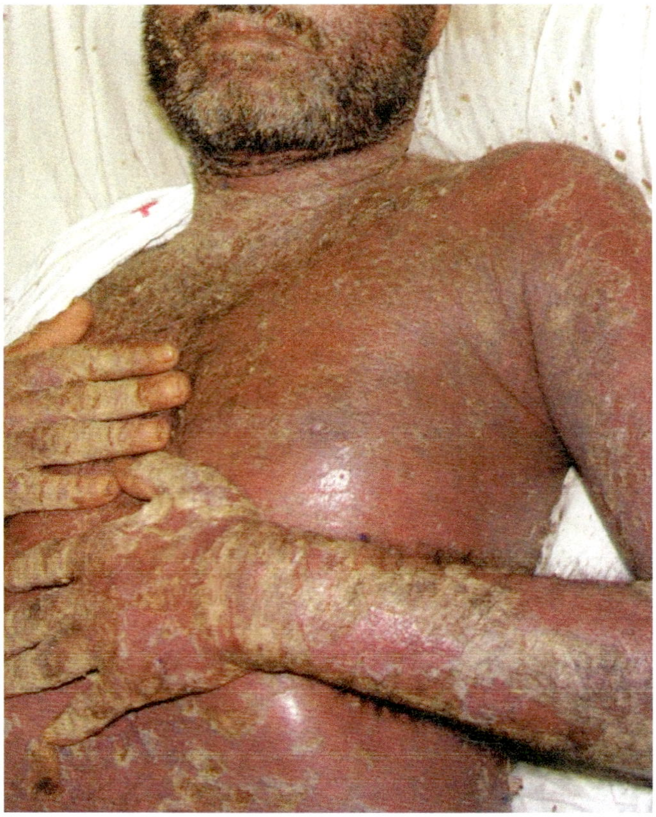

Norwegian scabies: Presenting as exfoliative dermatitis.

Scabies and HIV

- ***Norwegian scabies***
  - Hyperkeratotic crusted lesions on hands and feet. Erythematous plaques to erythroderma on trunk. Highly contagious.
  - Often diagnosed on biopsy.

Diagnosis

Based on clinical features

- Severe pruritus with nocturnal exacerbations.
- Family history of itching similar rash.
- Excoriated papules or burrows at characteristic sites.

Laboratory investigations

- KOH mount of scraping from burrow reveals mite or eggs under low power.
- Methylene blue stain used to highlight burrows.
- ***Biopsy:*** Norwegian scabies—many acari seen.

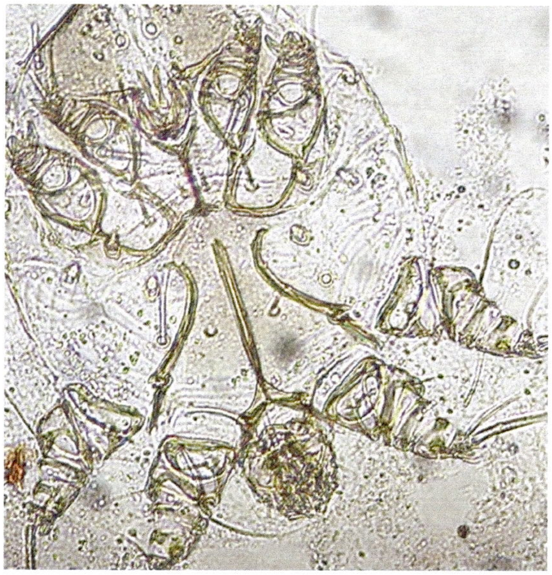

Sarcoptes scabiei: Dorsoventrally flattened organism with four pairs of legs.

Treatment (Table 14.1)

Antiscabicidal drugs

Mostly topicals ivermectin, orally probably less effective. Use limited to mass treatment in orphanages, and mentally challenged patients. Or if compliance in doubt.

Applications

Even if lesions restricted to genitalia, whole body treatment recommended.

OTHER MEASURES

- Entire family/close contacts to be treated.
- Antihistamines important.
- Antibiotics (topical or systemic), if secondary infection.
- Topical steroids (sometimes intralesional) for genital nodules.

Table 14.1: Treatment of scabies

Drug	Method of application
Topical	
Permethrin, 5%	Drug of choice. Whole body application at bedtime. Bathe in morning. Repeat application after a week. Safe in pregnancy and infants.
Malathion, 0.5%	Whole body application for 24 hours. Repeat after a week. Not safe in pregnancy or infants.
Benzoyl benzoate, 25%	Whole body, 2-3 applications in 24 hours. Not safe in pregnancy. Dilute (2-3 times) in infants and children.
Gamma benzene hexachloride, 1%	Whole body, single application for 6-24 hours. Not safe in pregnancy or infants.
Precipitated sulphur, 10%	Whole body, single application for 6-24 hours. Safe in pregnancy and infants.
Oral	
Ivermectin	200 µg/kg single dose. Repeat after 2 weeks. ?similar efficacy to topical permethrin 5%. Useful for mass treatment.

Chapter 15

Non-venereal Genital Conditions

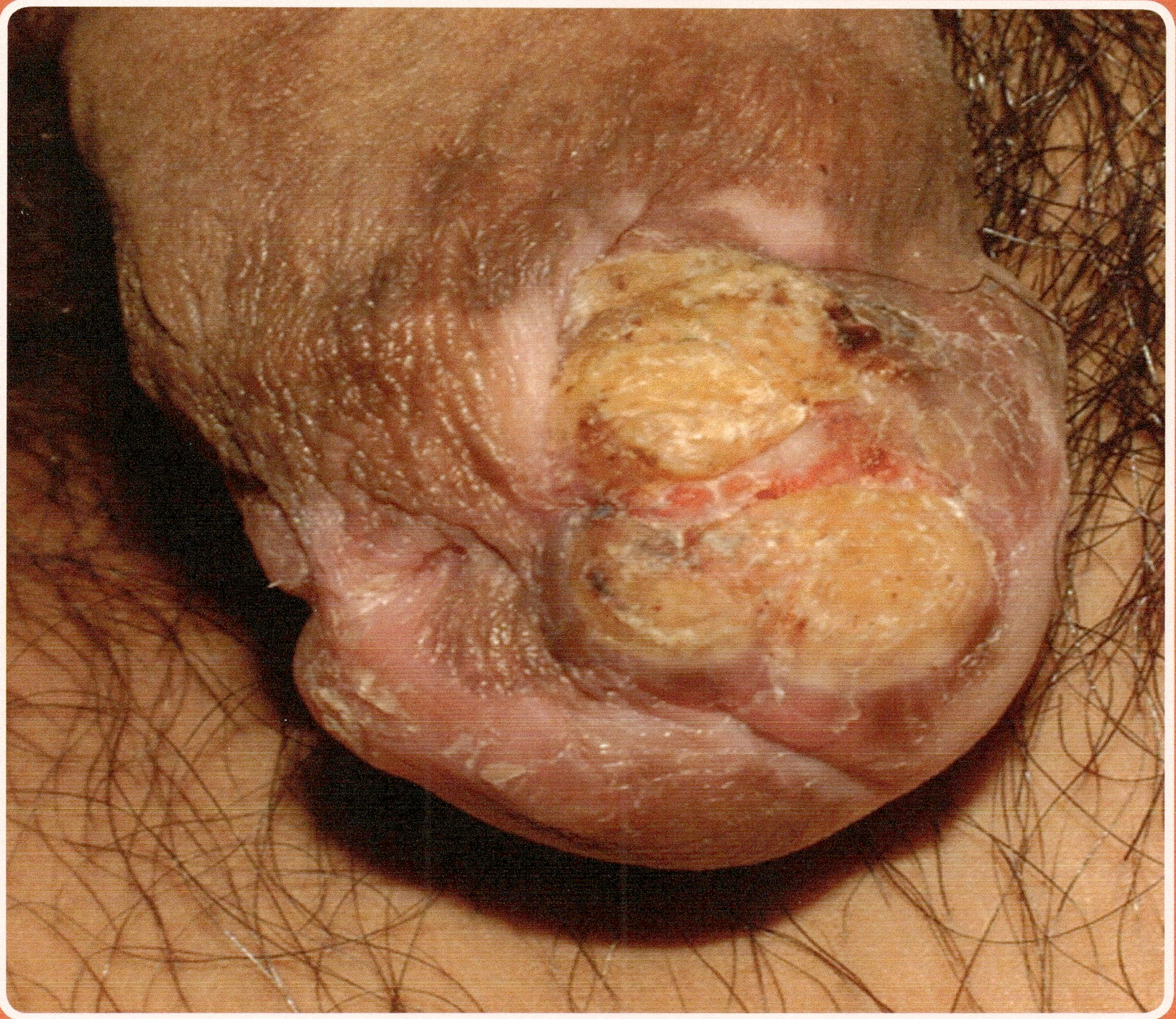

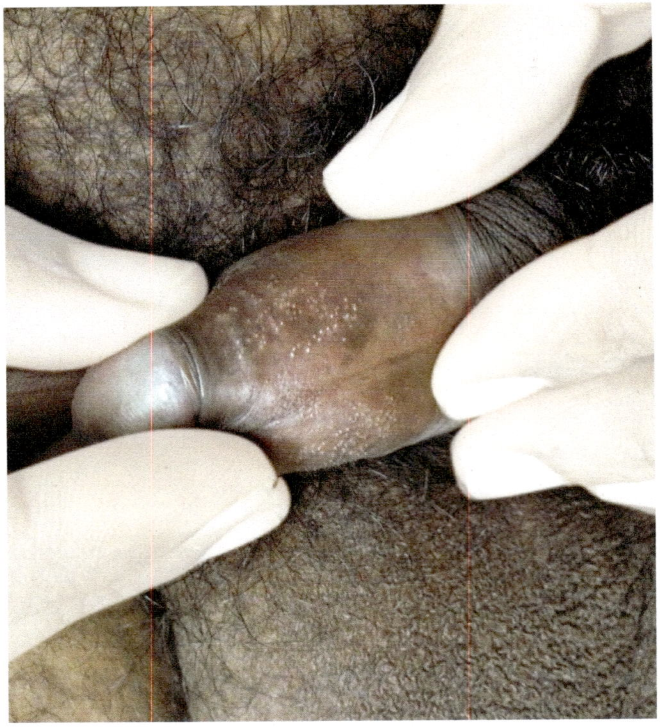

Fordyce spots: Pale skin colored or yellowish papules on the penile shaft.

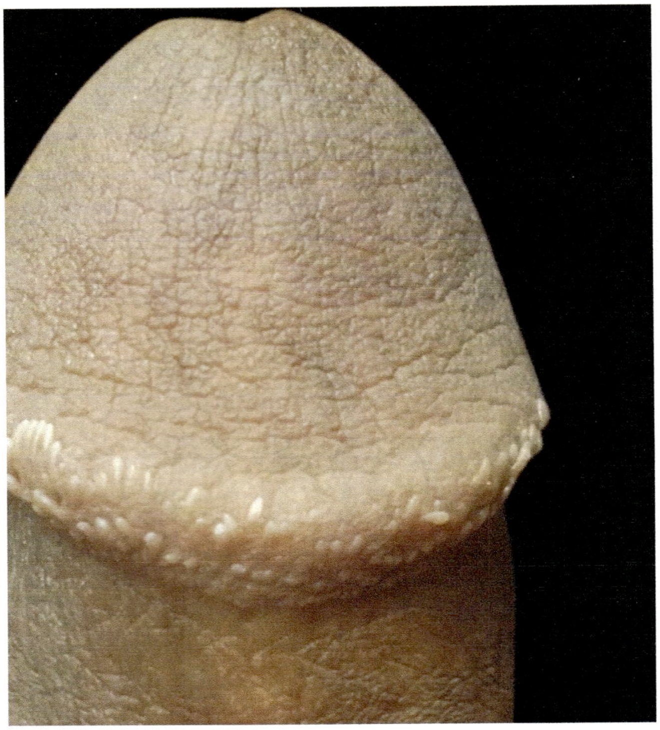

Pearly penile papules: Asymptomatic pink, rounded to acuminate papules on coronal sulcus.

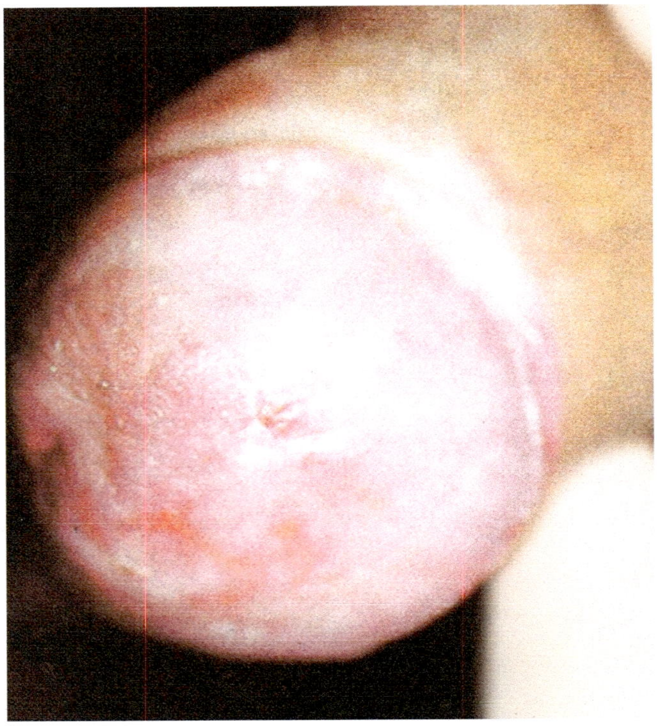

Lichen sclerosus: Ivory white, atrophic plaque on glans obliterating the urinary meatus.

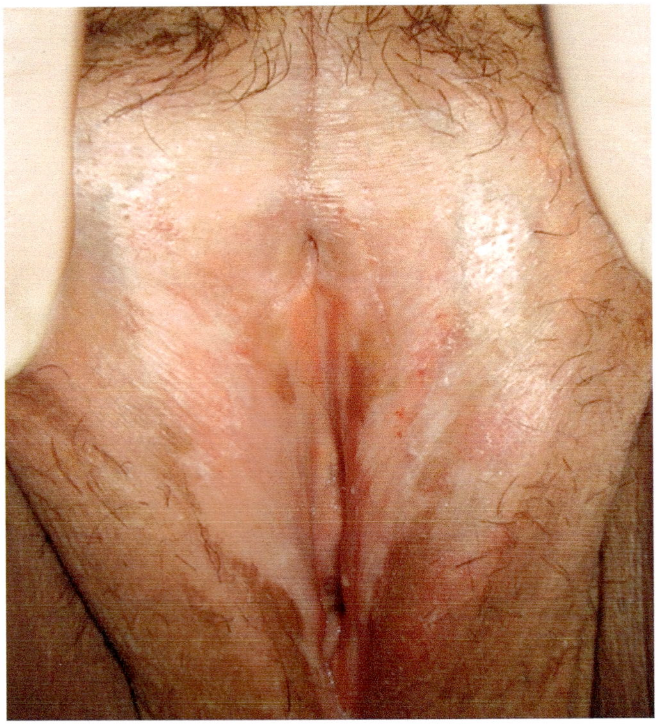

Lichen sclerosus: Ivory white, shiny, atrophic plaque on inner aspect of labia majora, showing follicular plugging at edge.

ECTOPIC SEBACEOUS GLANDS

Known as Fordycés spots.

Etiology

Ectopic sebaceous gland. Normally, sebaceous glands found only in association with a hair follicle.

Clinical Features

Morphology

- May appear at birth, during puberty or adulthood.
- Asymptomatic small, painless, well-defined, skin colored-yellowish papules, 1 to 3 mm in diameter.
- Often misdiagnosed as anogenital warts (AGW).

Sites

- ***Genital:*** Scrotum, shaft of the penis in males. Labia in females.
- ***Extragenital:*** Inner surface of buccal mucosa and vermilion border of the lips.

Treatment

- ***Counselling:*** Reassure—normal, not an STI (AGW).
- ***Specific treatment:*** Offered if patient distressed. Therapies include destruction of glands by radiofrequency or CO_2 laser ablation.

PEARLY PENILE PAPULES

- Common, seen in upto 50% of males.
- Normal. Histologically angiofibroma.

Clinical Features

Morphology

- Asymptomatic.
- Flesh colored-pink, smooth, rounded/acuminate 1–3 mm papules.
- Often misdiagnosed as AGW.

Sites

Coronal sulcus.

Treatment

- ***Counselling:*** Reassure—normal, not an STI (AGW).
- ***Specific treatment:*** Offered if patient distressed. Therapies include destruction of glands by radiofrequency or CO_2 laser ablation.

LICHEN SCLEROSUS (LS)

Epidemiology

- Common in adults with peak in 4th decade. Can affect prepubertal children also.
- Females affected more than males.
- Anogenital involvement more frequent (85-98%) than extragenital involvement (15-20%).

Etiology

?Autoimmune.

Clinical Features

Symptoms

- ***In males:*** Uncircumcised male complains of itching, incomplete erection, phimosis.
- ***In females:*** Dyspareunia, anogenital itching, burning sensation.

Morphology

- Erythematous, ivory white to white plaques on genitals with atrophy (manifesting as wrinkling) and sclerosis of skin.
- Erosions, fissures and ulcers may develop.
- Follicular lesions observed in periphery of plaque in hair bearing area.
- Needs differentiation from genital vitiligo (Table 15.1).

Table 15.1: Differences between LS and genital vitiligo

LS	Genital vitiligo
Hypopigmented to depigmented plaque	Hypopigmented to depigmented macule
Atrophy and sclerosis present	Absent
Fissuring present	Absent
Pruritus and burning sensation present	Absent
Lesions of LSA may be present at other sites	Lesions of vitiligo present at other sites

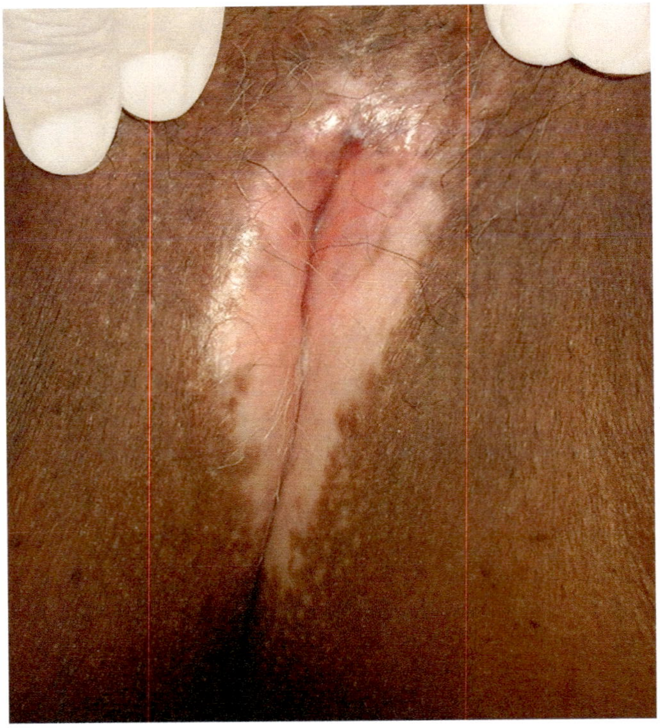

Lichen sclerosus: Vulvar lesion showing narrowing of introitus.

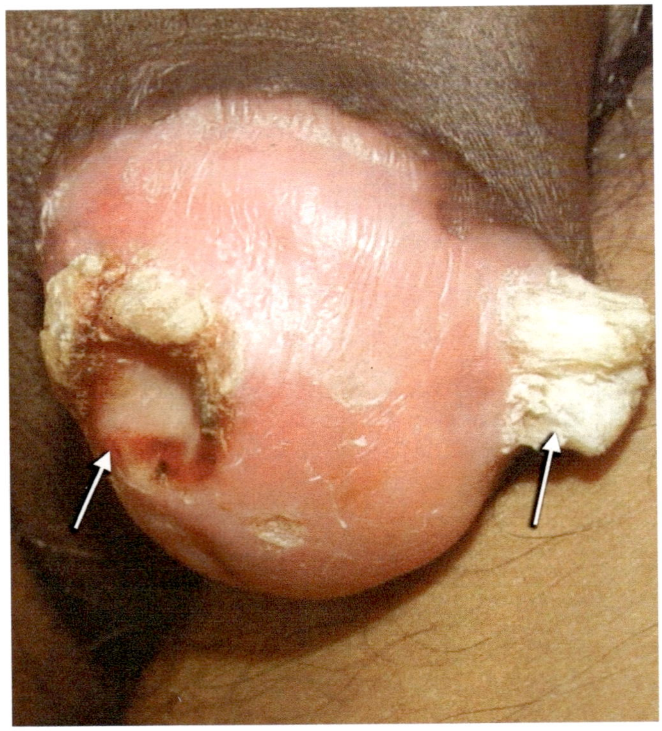

Lichen sclerosus with complications: Lesion of LS has developed (A) Squamous cell carcinoma and (B) cutaneous horn.

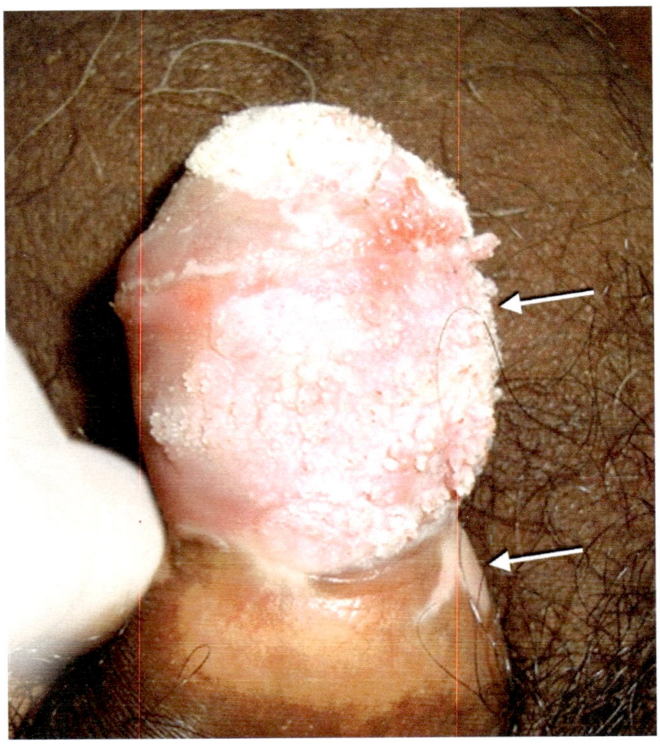

Lichen sclerosus with complications: Penile lesion with constriction (waisting) and squamous cell carcinoma.

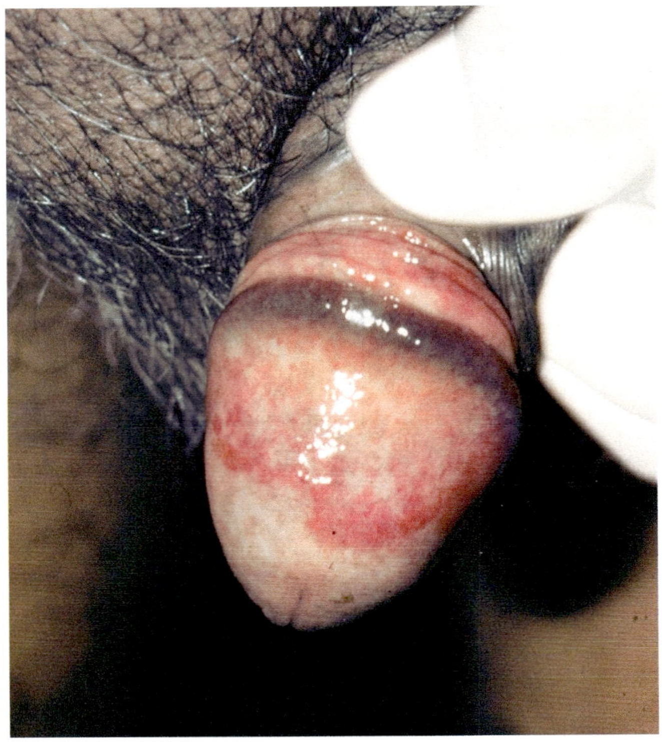

Zoon's balanitis: Well-defined erythematous plaque on glans with prominent erythematous stippling at the periphery.

Sites of lesions

- *Males:* Urinary meatus, prepuce, glans penis, penile shaft.
- *Females:* Vulva, inner aspect of labia majora, labia minora, vaginal introitus. Perianal area involvement gives figure of 8 appearance.

Complications

- ***Sexual dysfunction:*** In males, due to erectile compromise; in females due to dyspareunia (reduced size of introitus due to vulvar sclerosis).
- ***Malignant transformation:*** 1% in females and 5-30% in males with genital LS. Look for induration, friable area and ulceration. Biopsy suspicious lesions.

Diagnosis

Based on clinical features

Hypopigmented to depigmented plaque on genitals with atrophy and sclerosis.

Laboratory investigations

Skin biopsy

- Lichenoid tissue reaction. Orthokeratotic hyperkeratosis, hydropic degeneration of basal cells, edema of upper dermis. And homogenization of collagen associated with lymphocytic inflammatory infiltrate.

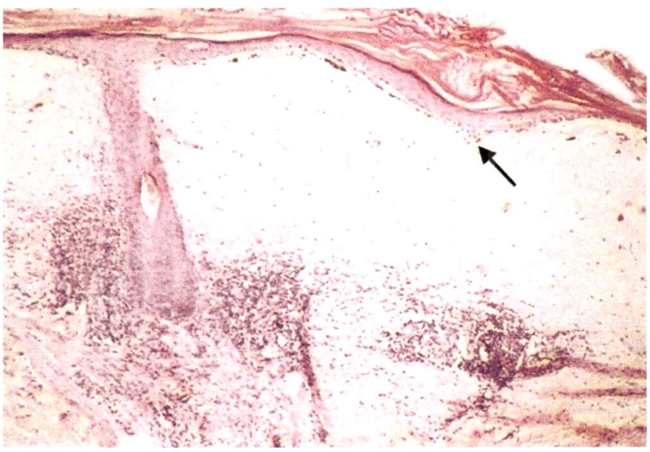

Lichen sclerosus *et* atrophicus: Epidermal atrophy, keratotic plugs, edema and hyalinized upper dermis with inflammatory infiltrate in mid dermis.

- Biopsy from representative area, to document diagnosis. Or from suspicious area, to rule out malignancy.

Treatment

Treatment necessary for symptomatic relief. And to reduce risk of malignant transformation.

Topical therapy

- Ultrapotent steroid like clobetasol propionate.
- Topical immunomodulators like tacrolimus and pimecrolimus (as effective as topical corticosteroids).
- Calcineurin inhibitors; variable efficacy.
- Topical androgens and progesterone not effective.

Physical modalities

- Light therapy. Monochromatic excimer light. Laser division of adhesions.
- ***Surgery:***
  - *In males:* Circumcision, resurfacing of glans, meatotomy, urethroplasty.
  - *In females:* Fenton's procedure (median perineotomy).

ZOON'S BALANITIS

- Reactive (to irritants) balanitis.
- Indolent but asymptomatic.
- Well demarcated, moist erythematous lesion with cayenne pepper stippling.
- Histopathology typical.
- Topical steroids, tacrolimus. And physical modalities.

PAPULONECROTIC TUBERCULIDE OF GENITALIA

Nongenital locations common sites of occurrence of tuberculide. Glans and vulva uncommon localized sites of involvement.

Epidemiology

- Mostly reported from Africa, Asian subcontinent and Japan.
- Affects young to middle aged males (less frequently females).

Pathogenesis

Tuberculide-a delayed hypersensitivity reaction to *M. tuberculosis*.

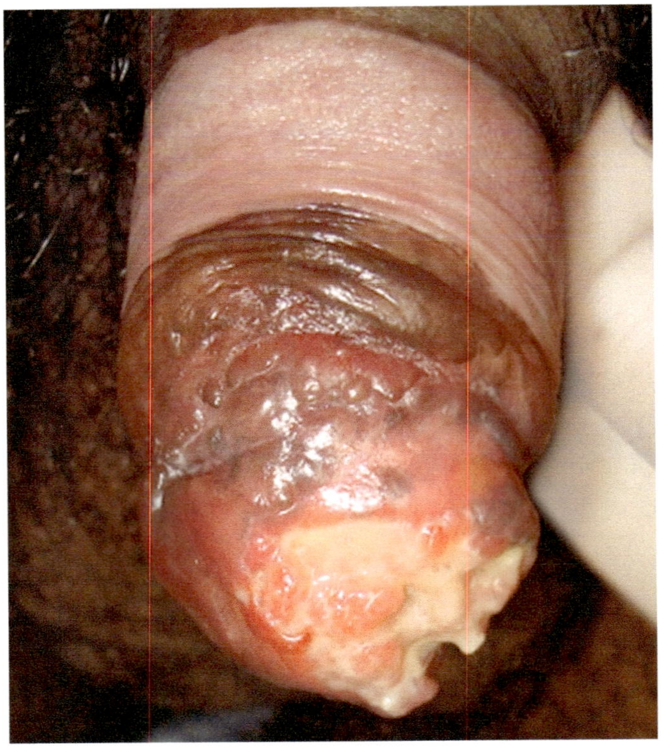

Papulonecrotic tuberculid of glans: Recurrent episodes of necrotic ulcer. Note healed punched out and bridging scars (worm eaten appearance).

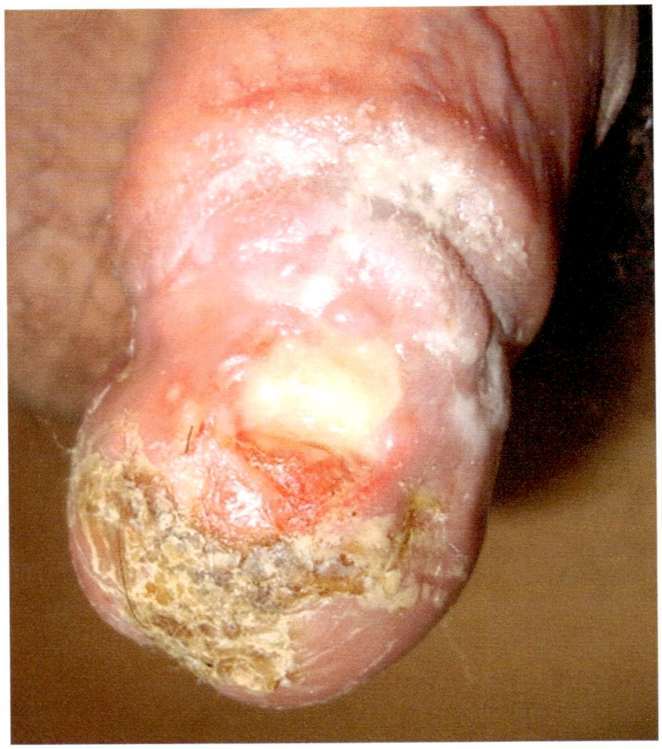

Papulonecrotic tuberculid: Papules, crusted and punched out ulcers with scars causing mutilation of glans penis.

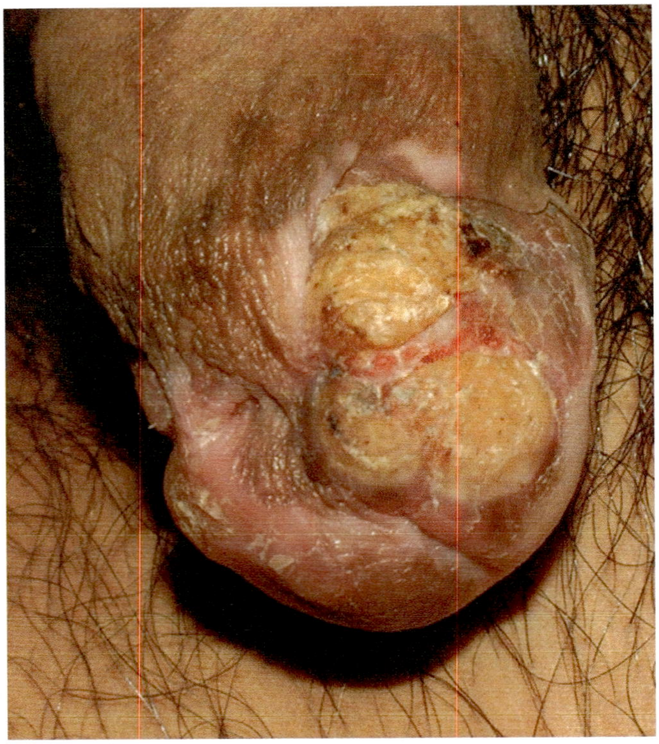

Pseudoepitheliomatous keratotic and micaceous balanitis: Early stage. Crusted plaque showing adherant mica like scales.

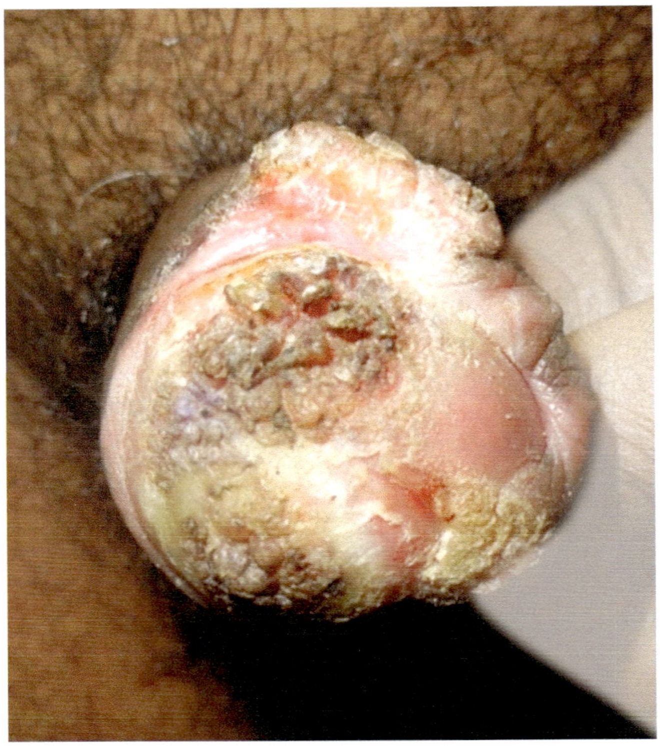

Pseudoepitheliomatous keratotic and micaceous balanitis: Indurated plaque with verrucosity and thick adherant scaling.

Clinical Features

Morphology

- Cyclical episodes of variable duration. Papules which ulcerate in center. And self-heal to leave punched out and bridging or varioliform scars giving a 'worm-eaten appearance'.
- Tuberculosis of another organ/system present historically or concurrently. Sometimes not.

Diagnosis

Diagnostic criteria

- Strongly positive Mantoux test.
- Chronic recurrent papular eruption occurring in crops, with necrosis, ulceration, and scarring.
- Tuberculoid histology with endarteritis and thrombosis of dermal vessels.
- Absence of tubercle bacilli in lesion.
- Response to antituberculous treatment.

Treatment

- Antituberculous therapy.

PSEUDOEPITHELIOMATOUS KERATOTIC AND MICACEOUS BALANITIS

Morphological diagnosis. Histologically ranges from benign to locally invasive verrucous carcinoma to invasive squamous cell carcinoma (SCC).

Epidemiology

- Elderly males.
- Rarely middle aged males.

Etiology

?Infection by human papilloma virus.

Clinical Features

- Progresses in 4 stages:
    - *Plaque stage:* Thin plaque with silvery white scaling.
    - *Tumor stage:* Slow-growing. Thick, non tender, plaque with hyperkeratotic mica-like scales and crusts. Can form cutaneous horn.
    - *Verrucous carcinoma*
    - *Squamous cell carcinoma:* Locally invasive verrucous tumor with low grade atypia. May evolve into SCC.
- Lymphadenopathy absent in early stages. Suspect SCC, if present.

Histopathology

- Initially, pseudoepitheliomatous hyperplasia without atypia. And band-like dermal inflammatory infiltrate.
- Later, low-grade atypia with no local invasion seen.
- Ocassionally frank changes of invasive SCC.

Treatment

- Surgery with wide excision, treatment of choice.
- Resistant to medical therapy such as 5-fluorouracil, cryotherapy or partial surgical excision.

PSORIASIS

Morphology

- Genital lesions not uncommon in psoriasis vulgaris. Isolated genital lesions also seen.
- In uncircumcised males, present as solitary distinctive well defined, brightly erythematous plaque but bereft of classical scales.
- In circumcised males and in females, with typical lesions of psoriasis.
    - If corroborative lesions elsewhere absent, diagnostic biopsy necessary.

Sites

On glans. And vulva. Also pubic region and natal cleft.

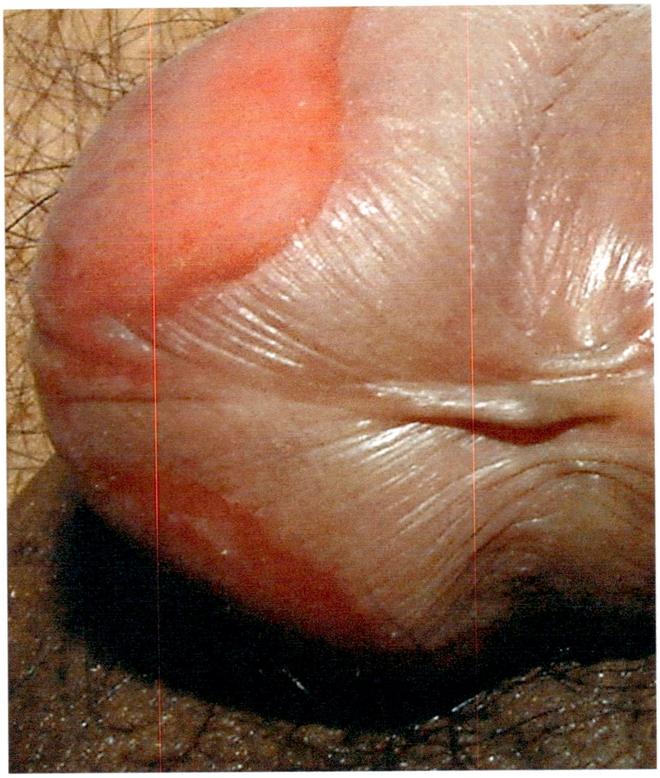

Psoriasis in uncircumcised male: Well defined erythematous plaque with minimal scaling.

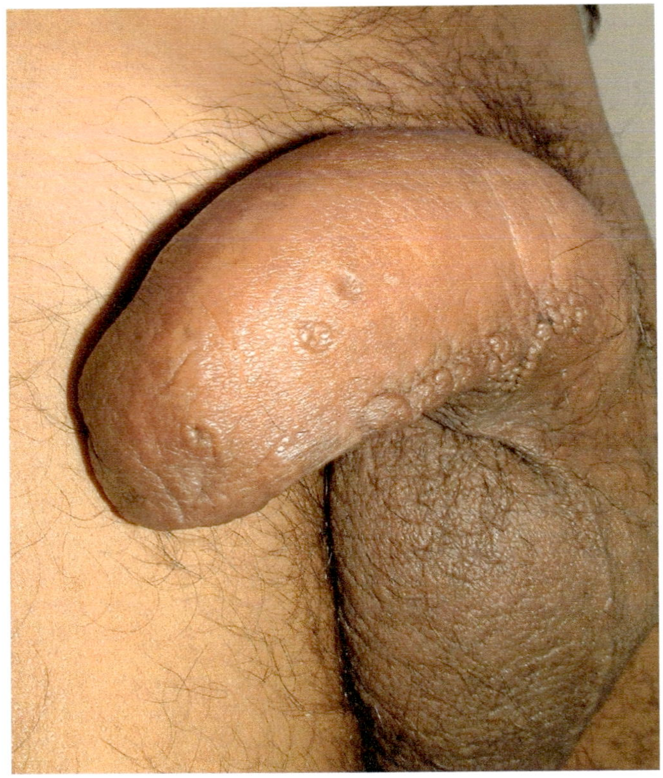

Lichen planus: Annular violaceous lesions on shaft of penis.

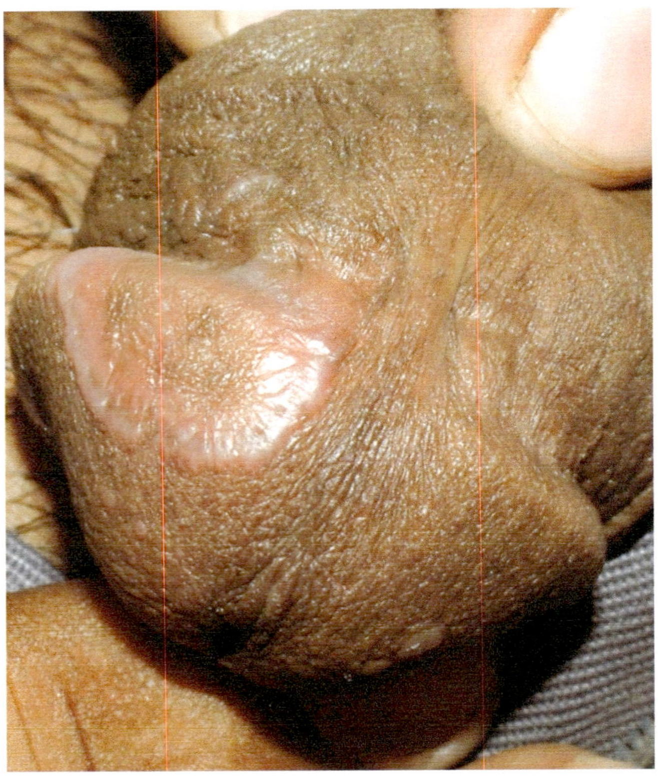

Lichen planus: Annular violaceous lesion on the glans.

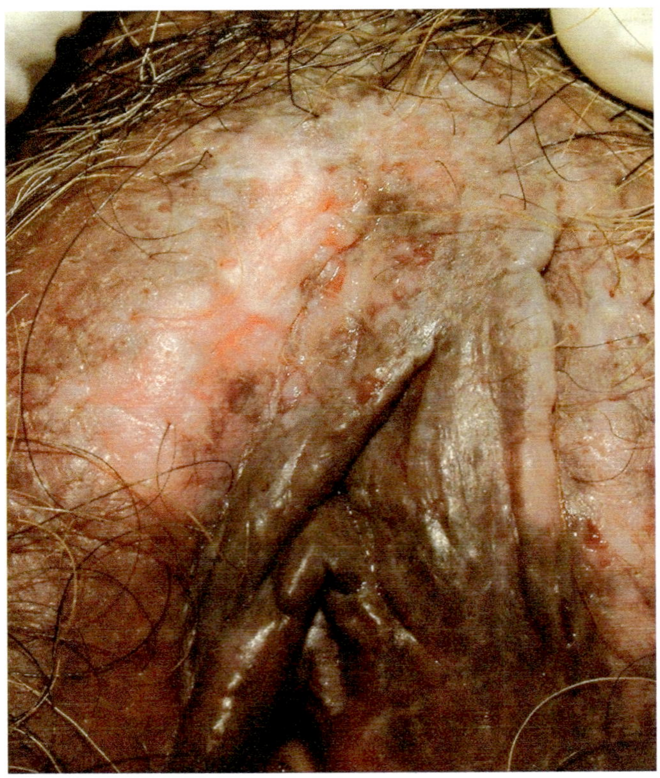

Lichen planus: Violaceous papules and erosions on the vulva. Patient presented with itching, dyspareunia and dysuria.

Treatment

- ***For localized lesions:*** Topical corticosteroids. Or topical tacrolimus/pimecrolimus.
- ***For extensive disease:*** As warranted by extent of disease.

LICHEN PLANUS

Morphology

- ***In men:*** Lesions sometimes restricted to genitalia. Or be part of widespread involvement. Lesions typical; often annular and usually not ulcerative.
- ***In females:*** Lesions on female genitalia fairly common. Occur alone. Or be part of widespread involvement. Or combined with lesions in buccal mucosa (erosive lesions in vulva and gingiva termed vulvovaginal–gingival syndrome). Variable clinical presentation -- fine, reticulate papules (complaints of itching) to severe erosive disease (accompanied by dyspareunia).

Sites

- ***In men:*** Penile shaft, glans penis, prepuce or scrotum.
- ***In females:*** Mainly vulva

Treatment

- ***For localized lesions:*** Topical corticosteroids. Or topical tacrolimus/pimecrolimus.
- ***For extensive disease:*** As warranted by extent of disease.

CHAPTER 16

Premalignant and Malignant Lesions of Genitals

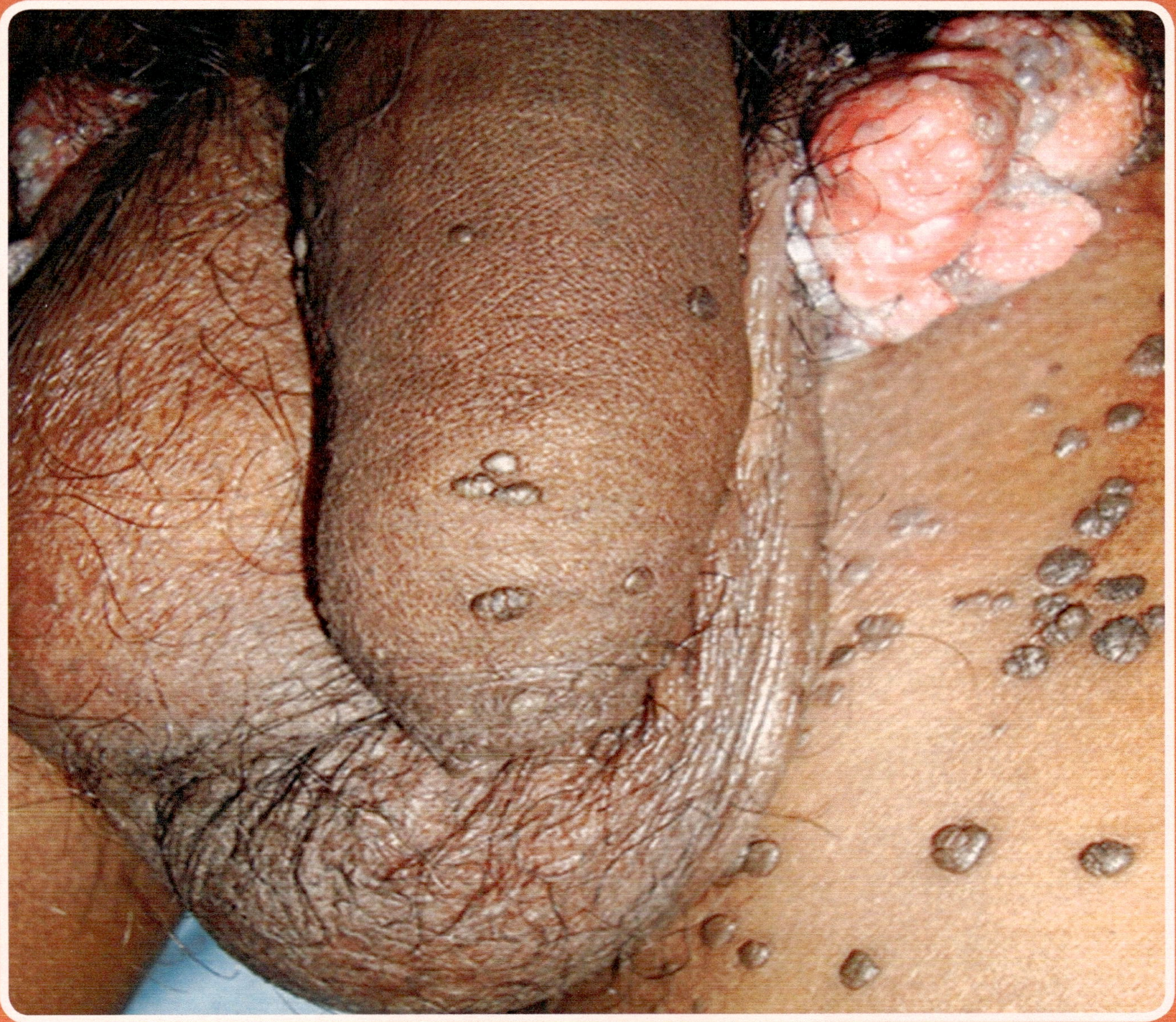

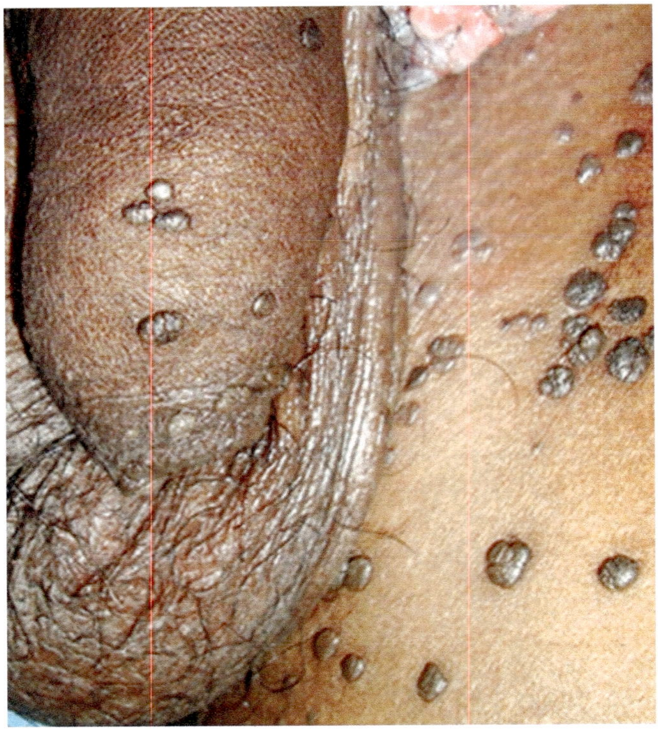

Bowenoid papulosis: Multiple hyperpigmented papules with mildly velvety surface. Caused by human papilloma virus (most commonly 16, 18).

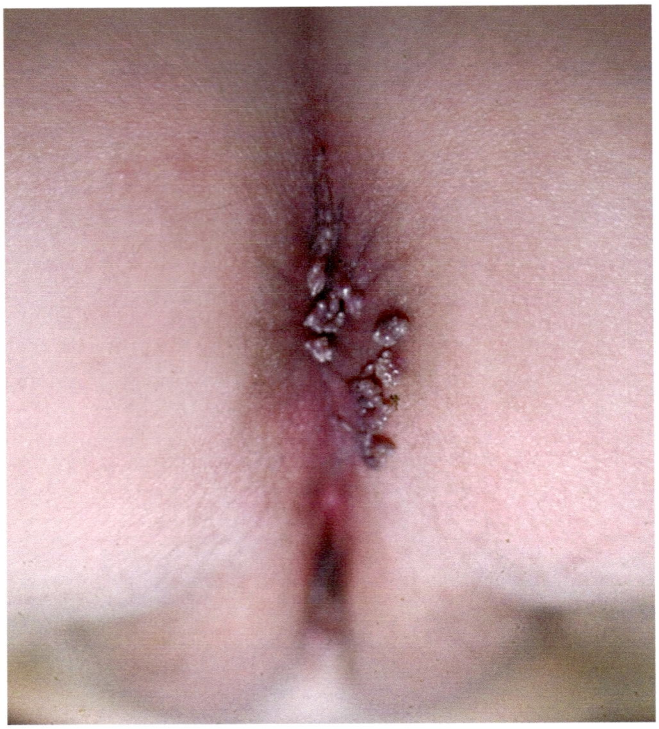

Bowenoid papulosis: Multiple 2-3 mm hyperpigmented papules, discrete, firm with velvety surface. Most frequently due to HPV 16. May sometimes regress spontaneously.

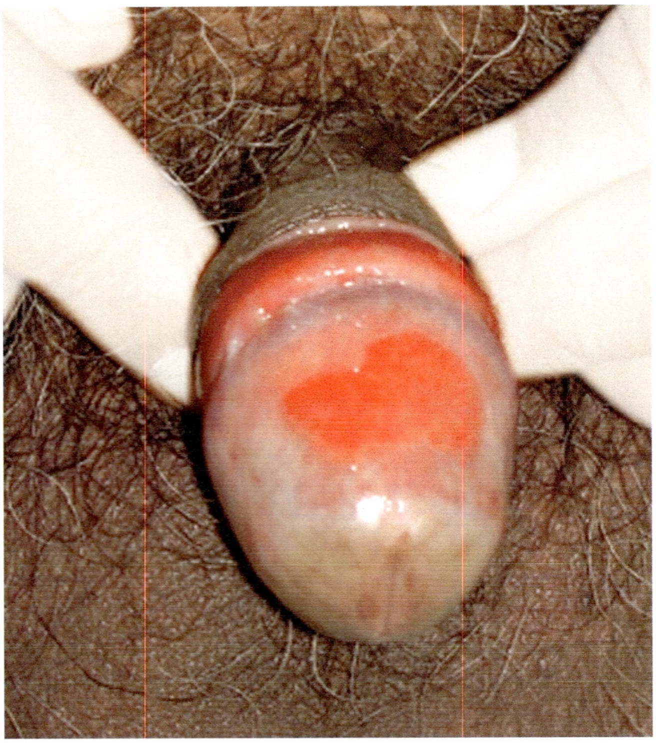

Erythroplasia of Queyrat: Well defined persistent, shiny erythematous plaque on glans. Should be biopsied to confirm diagnosis and differentiate from Zoon's balanitis.

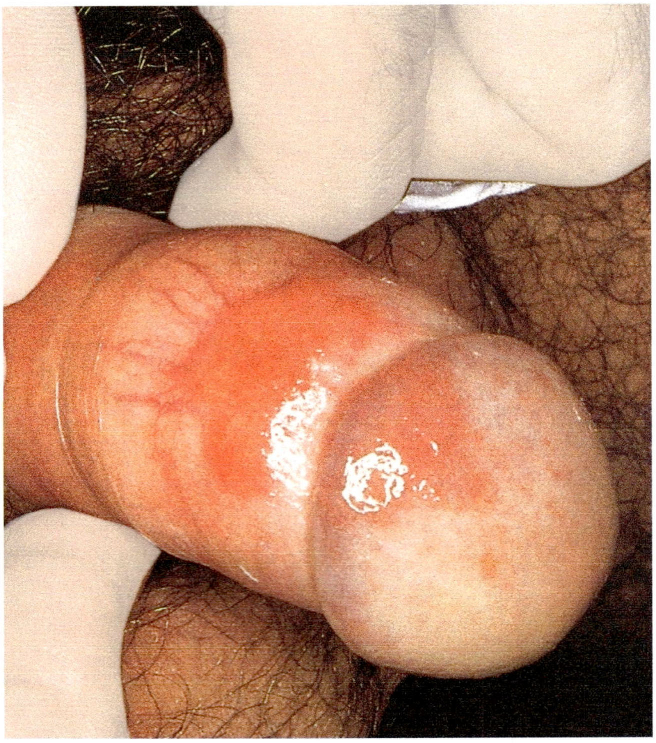

Erythroplasia of Queyrat: Well defined persistent, glazed erythematous plaque on glans.

SQUAMOUS CELL CARCINOMA *IN SITU*

Nomenclature

- Squamous cell carcinoma *in situ* characterized by atypical cells (hyperplasia of a typical keratinocytes, nuclear atypia, and mitotic activity) restricted to epidermis/epithelium.
- ***In males:*** Known as penile intraepithelial neoplasia (PIN). Histologically, PIN classified based on degree of differentiation (differentiated and undifferentiated types). Or on vertical level of atypia (PIN I, II, III). PIN I being mild atypia limited to upper-third of epidermis/epithelium, PIN II being atypia limited to upper 2/3 and PIN III being full thickness atypia, but without breaching basement membrane.
- ***In females:*** On vulva known as vulvar intraepithelial neoplasia (VIN), and on cervix as cervical intraepithelial neoplasia (CIN). VIN classified based on vertical extent of atypia into VIN I, II, III, as for PIN. Recent classification of VIN changed to include usual type of VIN (uVIN) and differentiated VIN (dVIN).
- Bowenoid papulosis (BP) erythroplasia of Queyrat (EQ), and Bowen's disease (BD) premalignant subtypes of PIN and VIN. All clinically distinct but, histopathologically similar with features of squamous cell carcinoma *in situ*. BP conforms to PIN II/VINII, and EQ and BD to PIN III/VIN III. Though terms VIN and PIN now preferred, older terms still widely used.

Epidemiology

- EQ and BD in elderly; BP in young adults.
- Females less frequently affected.
- BP more common in HIV positive patients.

Etiology

Predisposing factors include

- ***Infections.***
  - *HPV infection:* HPV-16 and 18 most implicated. HPV DNA detected in a quarter. Presence of HPV-associated CIN in female partners predisposes.
  - *HIV infection.*
- ***Poor hygiene:*** Most patients uncircumcised. Probably associated poor hygiene/smegma predisposes.
- ***Pre-existing disease:*** Lichen sclerosus *et* atrophicus, lichen planus, pseudoepitheliomatous and micaceous balanitis.

Clinical Features

Three conditions conventionally included.

Bowenoid papulosis

Morphology

- Multiple, hyperpigmented papules, small nodules or plaques with velvety surface.
- Often regresses spontaneously. And in HIV-positive patients, on institution of antiretroviral therapy.

Sites of lesions

- Penile shaft, external genitalia, vulva (keratinized skin).

Erythroplasia of Queyrat

Morphology

- Well-defined, shiny, erythematous, non-scaly velvety red plaque.
- Usually solitary, rarely can be multiple.
- Induration, ulceration and nodularity absent. If present, rule out of malignant transformation (to SCC).

Sites of lesions

- Glans, coronal sulcus, prepuce.

Bowen's disease

Morphology

- Erythematous well-defined plaque with indented (reniform) margins and silvery white scales.
- Usually single. Sometimes multiple.

Sites of lesions

- Follicle bearing skin of genitalia.

Complications

Malignant transformation

- ***In males:*** Occurs in a third of patients. Higher in BD or EQ, least for BP.
- ***In females:*** In 80% of untreated VIN transform to malignancy.
- ***Predisposing factors:*** For malignant transformation include smoking, immunosuppression, high risk HPV-types.

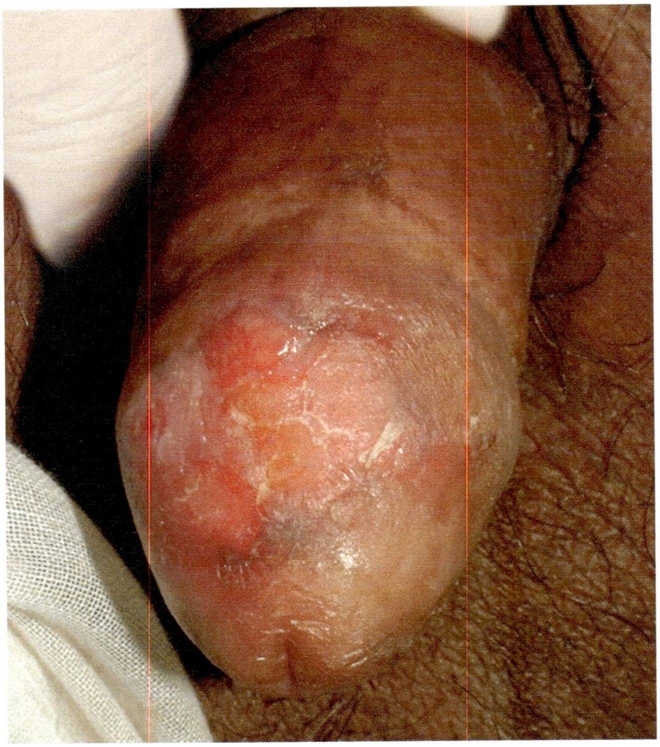

Bowen's disease: Well defined, irregular (indented) erythematous, scaly, mildly indurated plaque on glans.

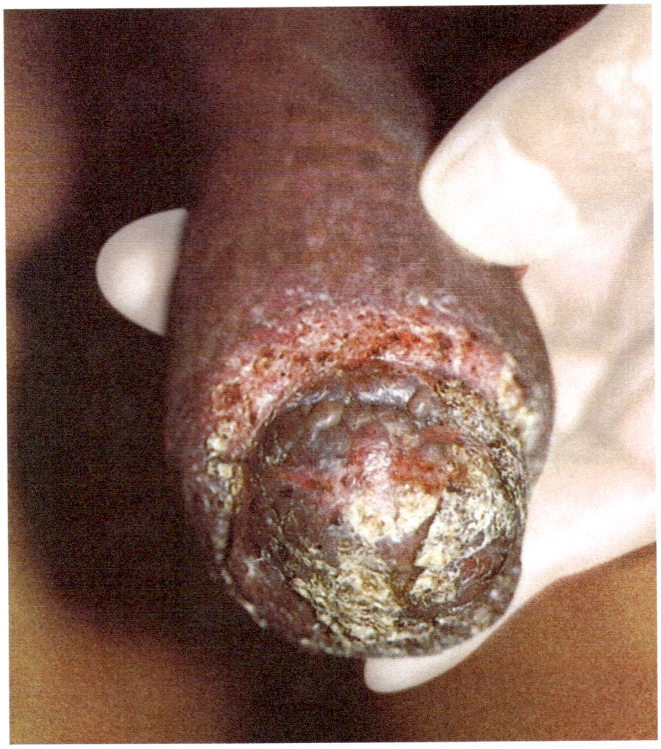

Squamous cell carcinoma: Erythematous exophytic growth with an indurated base.

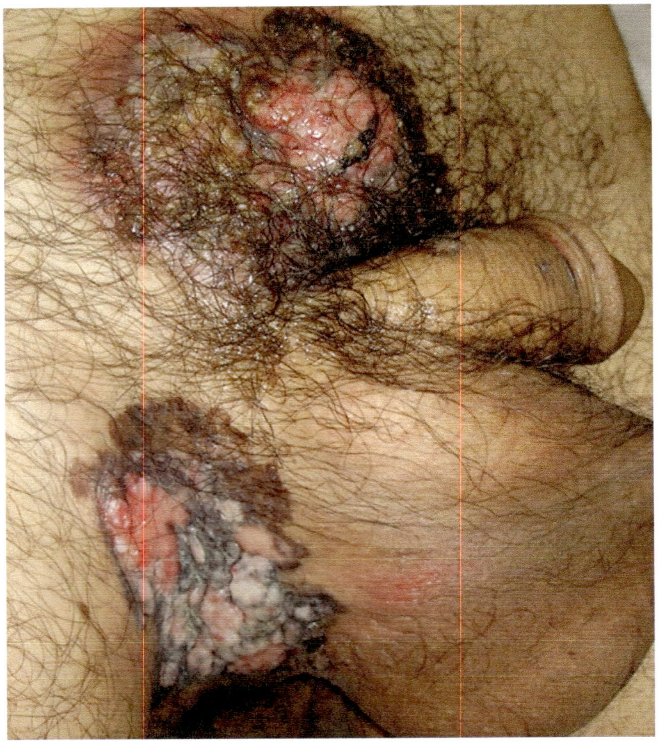

Squamous cell carcinoma: Well defined indurated plaques on pubic area and inguinal area with crusting, maceration and foul-smelling discharge.

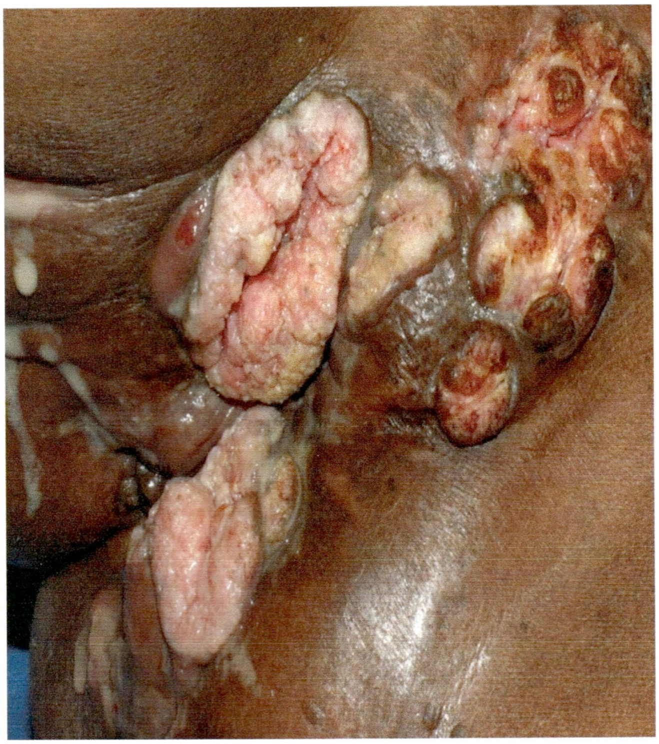

Squamous cell carcinoma: Fungating verrucous growth with induration and foul smelling discharge.

- ***Progress to:*** Basaloid or warty type of SCC.

Diagnosis

Histopathology

Squamous intraepithelial neoplasias on histopathology diagnosed on presence of atypical keratinocytes, nuclear atypia and mitotic activity not breaching epithelium.

- ***PIN I/VIN I:*** Mild atypia limited to upper one-third of epidermis. Seen only in condyloma acuminata, hence not considered malignant now and so removed from classification.
- ***PIN II/VIN II:*** Atypia limited to upper two-thirds of epidermis. Clinically correlates with BP.
- ***PIN III/VIN III:*** Full-thickness atypia of the epidermis but no breach in basement membrane. Clinically correlates with BD and EQ.

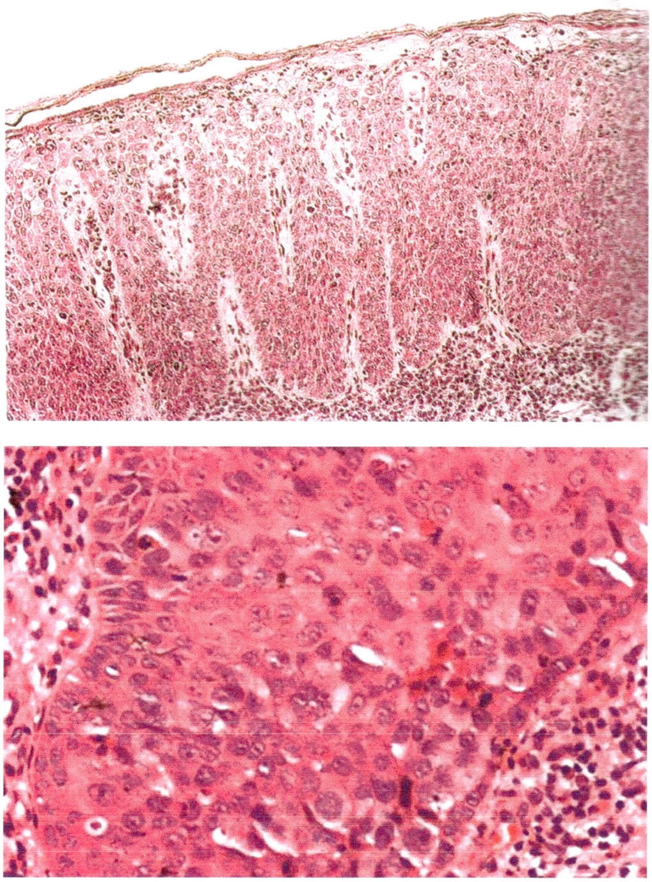

Bowen's disease: Disorganized acanthotic epidermis with atypical cells (Bowenoid cells).

Courtesy: Prof. M. Ramam, Department of Dermatology, AIIMS, New Delhi.

Treatment

- ***Topical applications:*** 5 fluorouracil and imiquimod.
- ***Physical modilities:*** Cryotherapy, Moh's micrographic surgery, total glans resurfacing, laser excision or ablation.

SQUAMOUS CELL CARCINOMA

Squamous cell carcinoma (SCC) commonest penile and vulvar malignancy.

Epidemiology

Penile and vulvar carcinoma commoner in developing countries. Commoner in poor socioeconomic strata. Commoner in older patients.

Etiology

Several risk factors for development of SCC:

- ***Human papilloma virus (HPV) infection:*** HPV 16 and 18. HPV demonstrable in half of penile and vulvar carcinoma. Differentiated tumors HPV-negative.
- ***Poor hygiene:*** Neonatal circumcision highly protective. Phimosis, predisposes. Probably related to local hygiene.
- ***Pre-existing skin lesions:*** Lichen sclerosus, erosive—lichen planus and pseudoepitheliomatous keratotic and micaceous balanitis. And premalignant lesions like PIN and VIN (bowenoid papulosis, erythroplasia of Queyrat, Bowen's disease).
- ***Sexual history:*** Peno-oral sex. Lifetime number of sexual partners. And lifetime number of intercourse.
- ***Immunosuppression:*** As in HIV infection.
- ***Miscellaneous factors:*** Older age (> 50 years), smoking and use of smokeless tobacco predisposes.

Clinical features

Morphology

Several morphological presentations:

- ***Nodular lesions:*** Most common presentation. Erythematous, exophytic growth with an indurated base. And areas of ulceration with foul-smelling discharge. Several histological variants-verrucous carcinoma, warty carcinoma and papillary carcinoma. Less aggresive course.
- ***Ulcerative lesions:*** Excavated irregular, non-healing ulcer with indurated base. Floor covered with

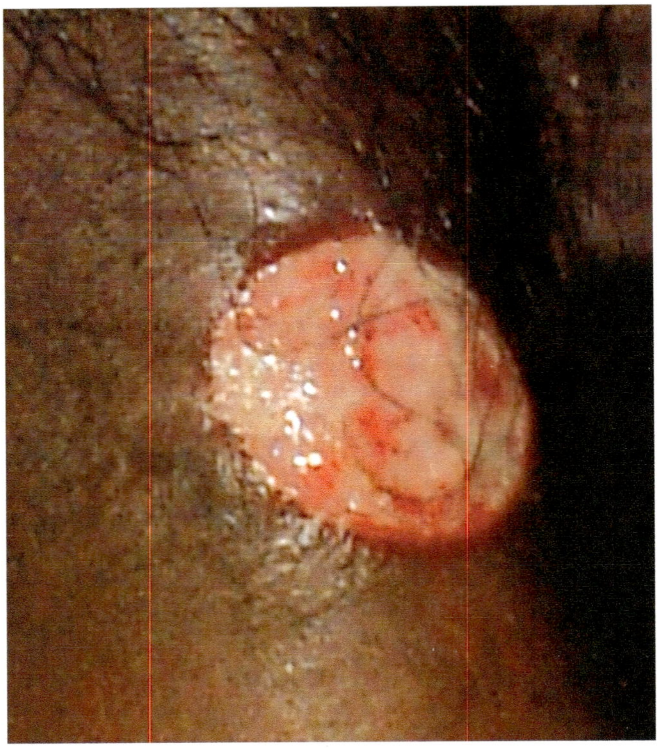

Squamous cell carcinoma: Irregular non healing ulcer with an indurated base.

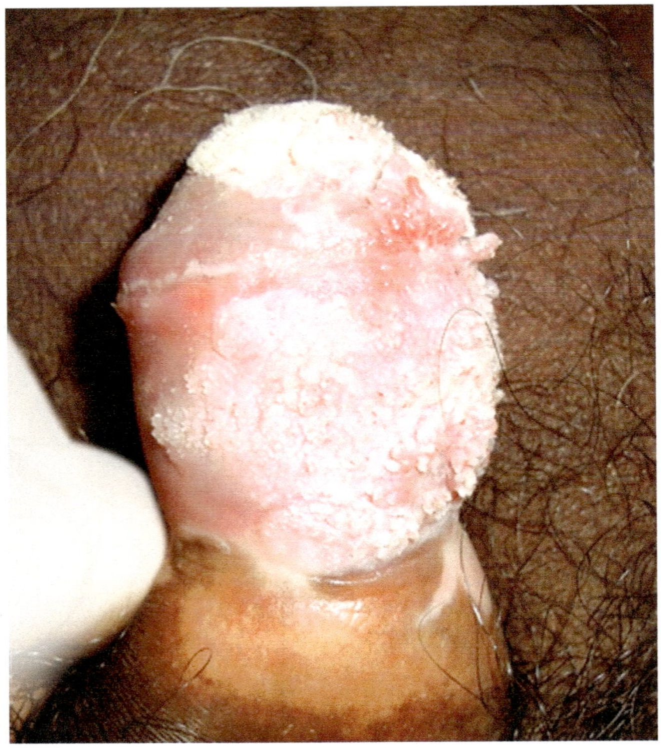

Lichen sclerosus with squamous cell carcinoma: Note constriction visible on penis due to lichen sclerosus (waisting).

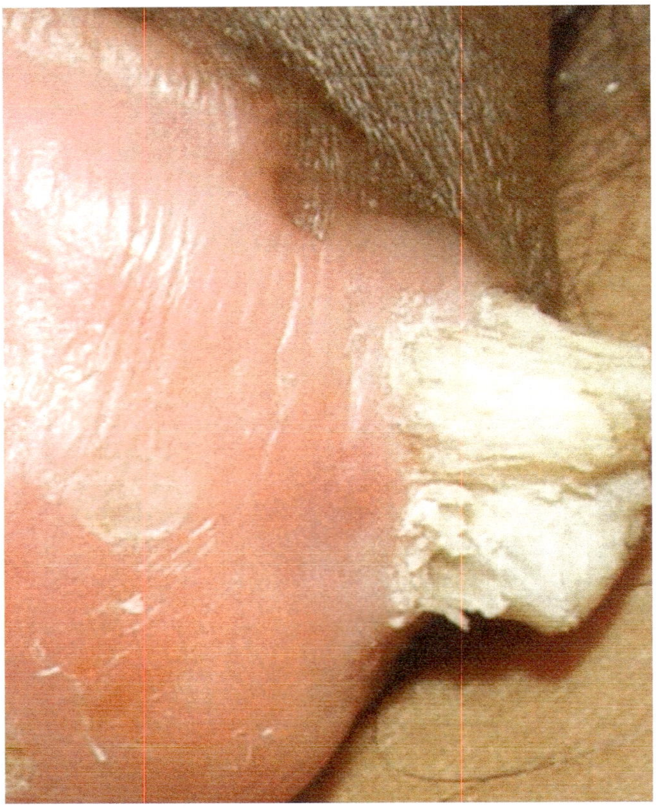

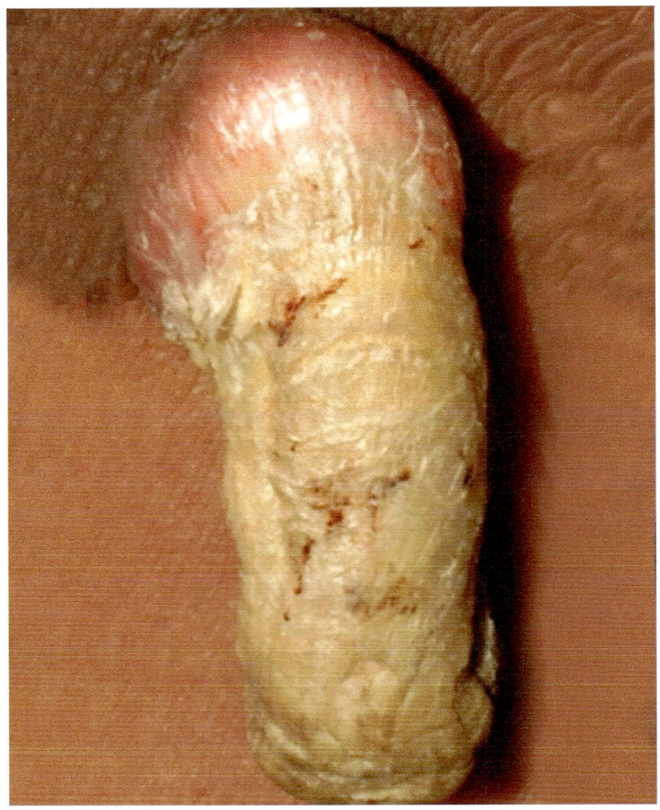

Cutaneous horn: With underlying induration. On histopathology shows a squamous cell carcinoma.

necrotic, foul-smelling slough. Several histological variants-basaloid, sarcomatoid or adenosquamous carcinoma. Highly aggressive with high metastatic potential.

- ***Other variants:***
  - *Plaque:* erythematous indurated lesion.
  - *Phimosis:* incidental finding during circumcision.
  - *Cutaneous horn:* when diagnosed on histopathology.

Sites of lesions

- ***In males:*** Glans penis, prepuce and shaft.
- ***In females:*** Vulva, labia majora, labia minora, fourchette.

Complications

- ***Local invasion:*** Into urethra.
- ***Metastasis:***
  - *To lymph nodes:* may lead to lymphedema, lymphangiectasis.
  - *To internal organs.*

Diagnosis

Histopathology

Depending on grade of differentiation, penile carcinoma classified into grade 1 (well-differentiated), grade 2 (moderately differentiated) and grade 3 (poorly differentiated). Well-differentiated types include keratinizing and verrucous carcinoma. Undifferentiated types include warty, basaloid and warty-basaloid types. Keratinizing being the most common type and basaloid and warty carcinomas being HPV associated.

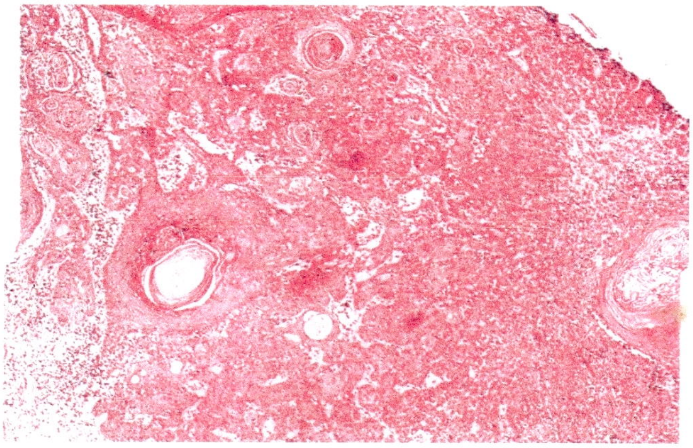

Squamous cell carcinoma: Well differentiated squamous cell carcinoma showing horn cysts.

Treatment

- Management includes assessment of depth of involvement and metastasis. Specific treatment depends on stage of the disease.
- Best managed by surgeons/oncosurgeons.

Chapter 17

Sexually Transmitted Infections in Pregnancy

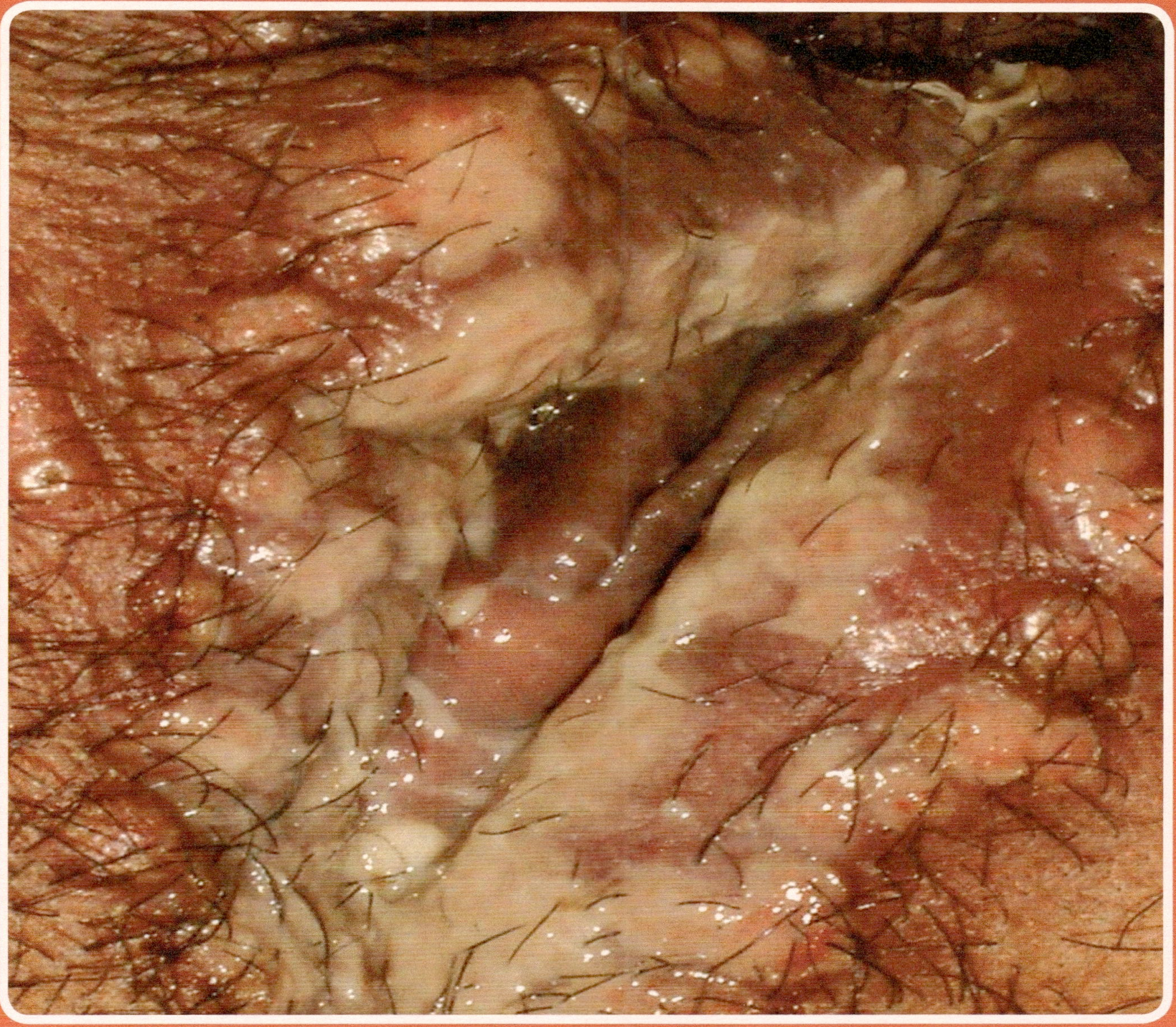

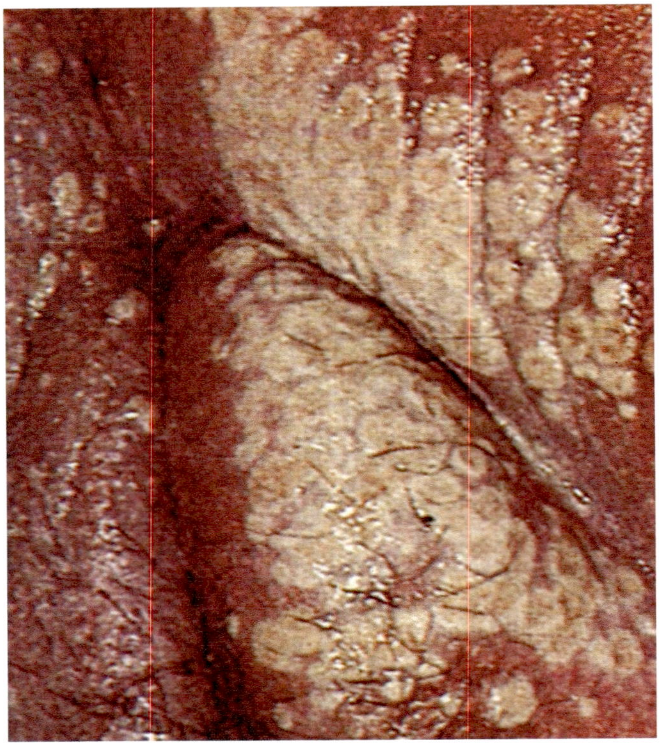

Genital herpes in pregnancy: Primary episodes more severe. Presence of such lesions near delivery warrants caesarian section.

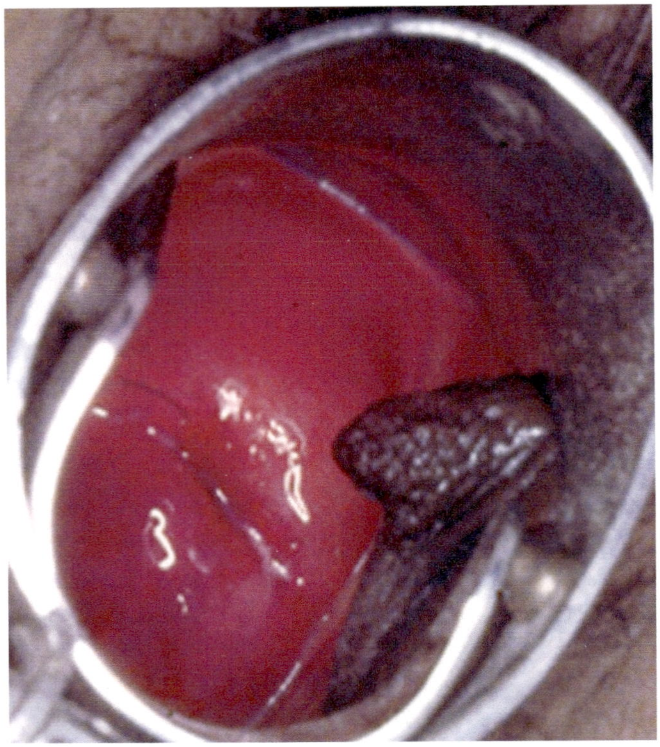

Genital herpes in pregnancy: Cervical lesions more frequent.

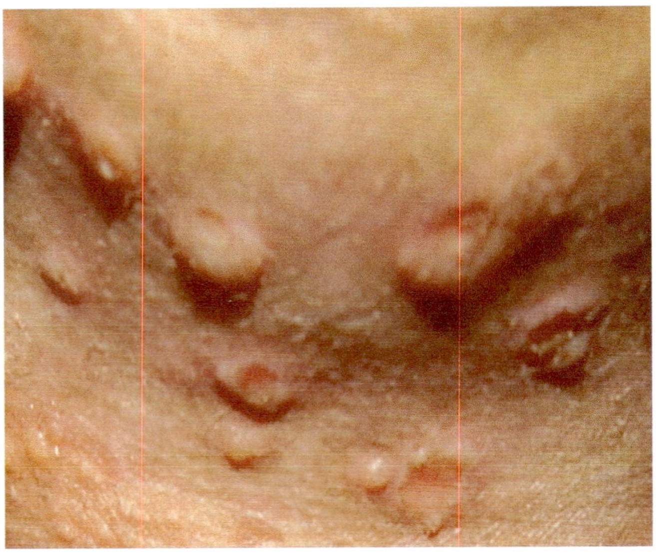

Neonatal herpes: Grouped vesicles on the neck.

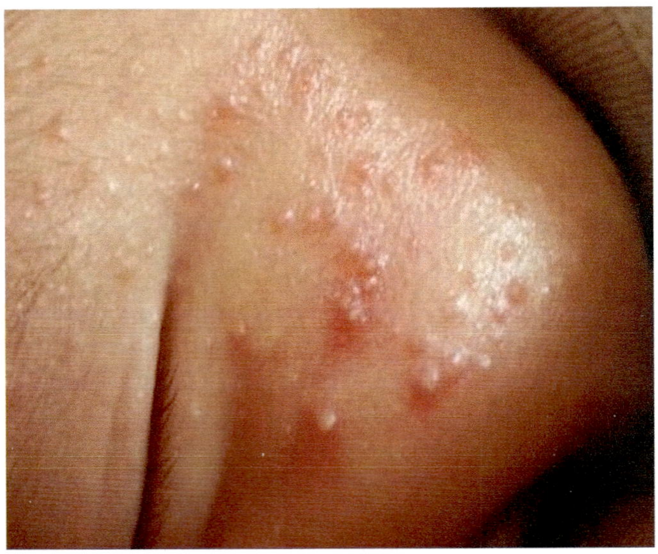

Neonatal herpes: Cutaneous manifestations include grouped vesicles around eyes, mouth.

GENITAL HERPES (GH)

Interaction of GH and Pregnancy

Effect of GH on Pregnancy

- Neonatal HSV infection due to *in utero* transplacental transmission (5%). Or during delivery (85%), due to asymptomatic shedding from cervix or lower genital tract during delivery. Or after delivery (10%).
- Highest risk of transmission if mother has primary GH in late pregnancy. GH early in antenatal period leads to development of protective IgG antibodies which are transmitted to the fetus preventing neonatal HSV infection.
- ***Neonatal infection***
  - *Antenatal infection:* microcephaly, intrauterine growth retardation, hepatosplenomegaly and intrauterine fetal death.
  - *Intrapartum infection:* neonatal herpes.
- ***Neonatal herpes***
  - Most neonatal infections acquired from asymptomatic mothers.
  - *Factors affecting acquisition of neonatal infection:*
    - Higher with primary 1st episode infection acquired in 3rd trimester (30-50%) than recurrent GH (< 1%).
    - Higher with HSV-1 than HSV-2.
  - *Manifestations:* 3 types recognized:
    - Localized form: Vesicles, bullae occurring around eyes, mouth or localized area of skin.
    - Disseminated form: Dissemination to internal organs. Serious condition.
    - Central nervous system: Encephalitis. Serious condition, with poor prognosis.

Effect of Pregnancy on GH

- Primary episode more severe. Frequency of cervical lesions increased.
- Asymptomatic shedding increased.
- Frequency of recurrences probably same.
- Risk of dissemination higher (hepatitis, encephalitis, pneumonia).

Treatment

- ***Primary episode:*** Acyclovir 400 mg tid × 7 days.
- ***Recurrent episode:*** Acyclovir 400 mg tid × 5 days.
- ***Suppressive therapy:*** In antenatal period not protective against neonatal HSV infection.

ANOGENITAL WARTS (AGW)

Interaction of AGW and Pregnancy

Effect of AGW on Pregnancy

- Large condyloma acuminata cause obstruction during delivery. Episiotomy needed. Sometimes even caesarian section.
- Transmission during labor leading to laryngeal papillomatosis in newborn.

Effect of pregnancy on AGW

Condyloma acuminata larger in size, more numerous, fleshy and vascular in pregnancy.

Treatment

Some treatments (podophyllin/podophyllo toxin) not safe in pregnancy. Some of doubtful safety (imiquimod). So both avoided. Safe treatments include—trichloroacetic acid, cryotherapy, radiofrequency ablation.

SYPHILIS

Interaction of Syphilis and Pregnancy

Syphilis detected in pregnancy either clinically (presence of lesions of primary, secondary or tertiary syphilis). Or more frequently serologically. Routine serological screening for syphilis (VDRL or RPR, sometimes TPHA) mandatory on first antenatal visit globally. Repeated in populations with high prevalence of syphilis, at 28-32 weeks and at delivery.

Effect of syphilis on pregnancy

- Syphilis acquired *in utero* through transplacental transmission from a syphilitic mother.
- Early syphilitic mother more infective. And infection rare before 16 weeks of gestation.
- About a third of pregnancies escape infection, another third abort or are stillborn and a third get congenital syphilis.
- Two stages of congenital syphilis recognized:
  - *Early congenital syphilis:* similar to secondary stage of acquired syphilis–cutaneous lesions (all types including vesicobullous lesions) and mucosal; lymphadenopathy, hepatosplenomegaly, and bone (osteochondritis. Or periostitis) involvement.
  - *Late congenital syphilis:* similar to late stage of acquired syphilis, but cardiovascular involvement rare. Triad of ocular involvement (interstitial

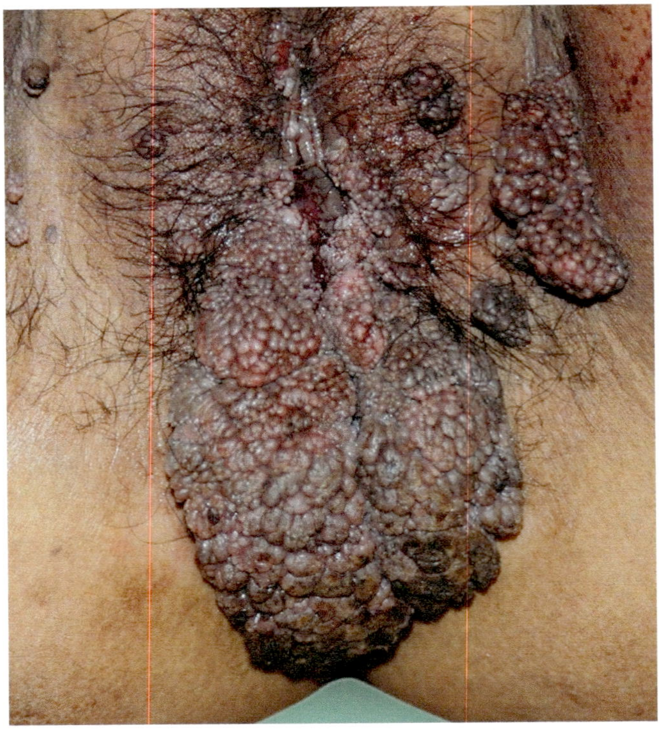

Anogenital warts in pregnancy: AGWs become exuberant in pregnancy.

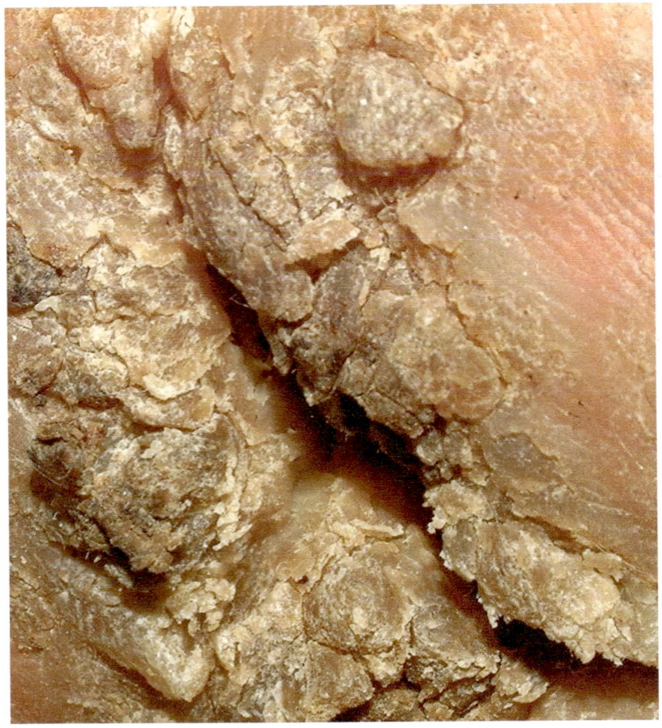

Anogenital warts in pregnancy: Exuberant lesions obstructing birth canal.

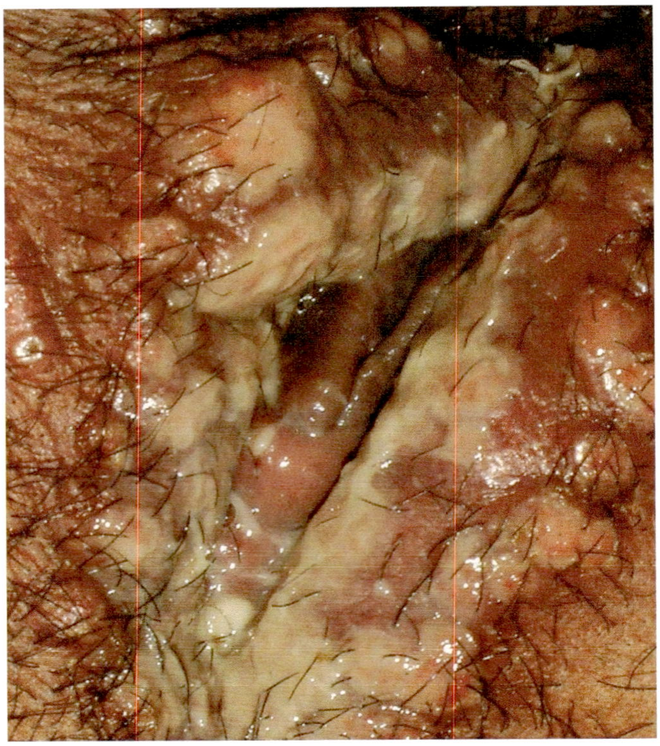

Condyloma lata in a pregnant women: Course of syphilis does not change in pregnancy but syphilis has a deleterious effect on the child.

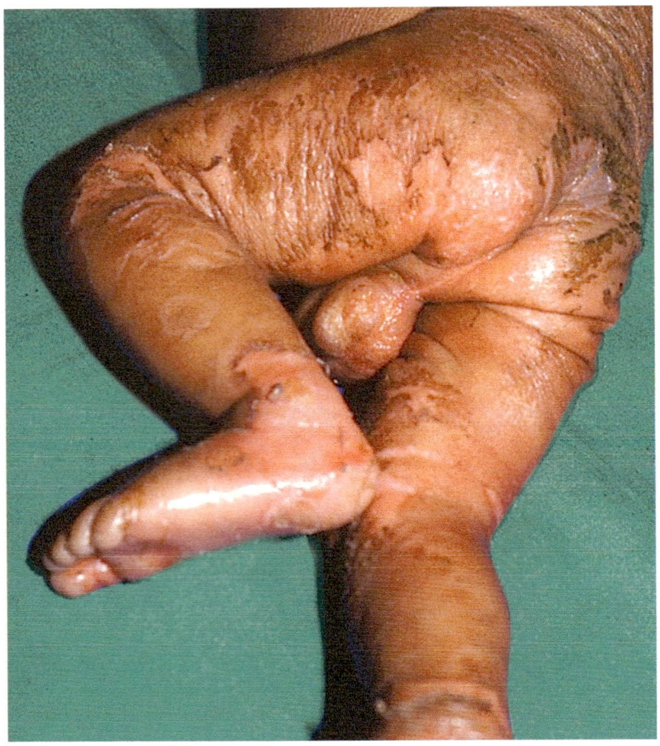

Congenital syphilis: Child born with erythematous scaly plaques. Erosions due to preceding bullae.

keratitis), eighth nerve deafness and abnormalities of permanent dentition (notched incisors and mulberry molars) comprise Hutchinson's triad. Palatal or nasal septal perforation, collapse of nose, periosteitis with laying down of new bone clinically appearing as anterior bowing of tibia—sabre tibia. But cutaneous and mucosal lesions rare.

Effect of pregnancy on syphilis

- Probably no change in clinical picture.
- Biological false positive with VDRL/RPR high, so need confirmation with TPHA.

Treatment

Seropositive pregnant women considered infected unless clear documentation of adequate treatment with declining sequential antibody titers. Serofast low antibody titers do not warrant treatment but persistent higher titer antibody tests require treatment.

Of pregnant women

- ***1st line of therapy:*** Penicillin effective for preventing maternal-fetal transmission. And also for treating fetal infection. Optimal penicillin regimens not defined but regimen appropriate for stage of syphilis recommended.
- ***In penicillin-sensitive women:*** Desensitize (as no proven alternative to penicillin available for maternal syphilis).
- ***In penicillin sensitive pregnant women, who cannot be desensitized:*** Erythromycin stearate (never estolate) 2 g daily (in 4 doses) × 14 days (early syphilis)–28 days (late syphilis). However erythromycin not ideal, as does not reliably cure infected fetus. So treat such neonate at birth.
- ***Other management considerations***
  - *In early syphilis:* 2nd dose of benzathine penicillin 2.4 million units, 1 week after 1st dose sometimes recommended.
  - *In 2nd half of pregnancy:* management facilitated by sonographic evaluation of fetus (for hepatomegaly, ascites, hydrops) and placenta (for thickening). Women treated for syphilis in 2nd half of pregnancy at risk for premature labor and/or fetal distress, due to Jarisch-Herxheimer reaction, so careful monitoring for uterine contractions or decreased fetal movements. Stillbirth a rare complication of treatment.
  - *Missed doses:* not acceptable in pregnant patients. If any dose missed, repeat full course.

Of newborn

Treatment decision based on:

- Presence of syphilis in mother.
- Inadequacy of maternal treatment.
- Presence of clinical/laboratory/radiographic evidence of syphilis in infant.

CHANCROID

Interaction of Chancroid and Pregnancy

Effect of chancroid on pregnancy

Adverse outcomes not reported.

Effect of pregnancy on chancroid

Presentation and clinical features of chancroid similar to non-pregnant women.

Treatment

- Azithromycin 1 gm single oral dose. Or ceftriaxone 250 mg intramuscular stat (same as non-pregnant women).
- Ciprofloxacin (as also other fluoroquinolones) contraindicated.

DONOVANOSIS

Interaction of Donovanosis and Pregnancy

Effect of donovanosis on pregnancy

Adverse events not common.

Effect of pregnancy on donovanosis

- Number of lesions and size of lesions increased.
- More aggressive course. Risk of hematogenous dissemination higher. Recurrences frequent.
- Response to treatment slow.

Treatment

- Erythromycin 500 mg four times daily for 3 weeks. Or azithromycin 1 gm weekly for 3 weeks.
- Doxycycline and ciprofloxacin contraindicated.

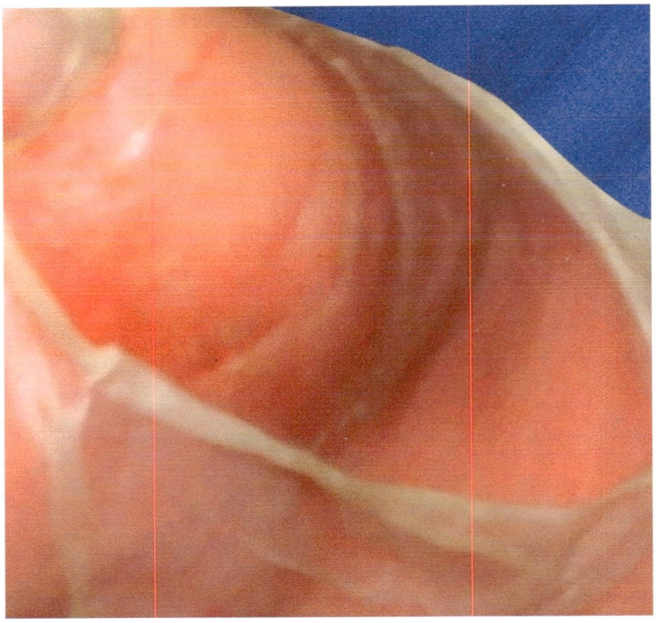

Syphilis: Congenital syphilis. Bullous lesions (usually on normal skin) presenting at birth or soon thereafter (pemphigus syphiliticus).

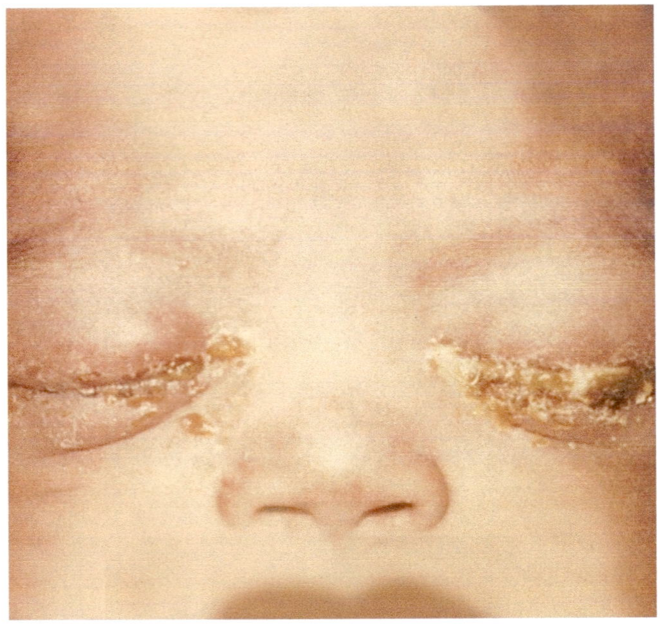

Ophthalmia neonatorum: Infection of birth passage with *N. gonorrhoeae* and *C. trachomatis* may lead to conjunctivitis in neonate.

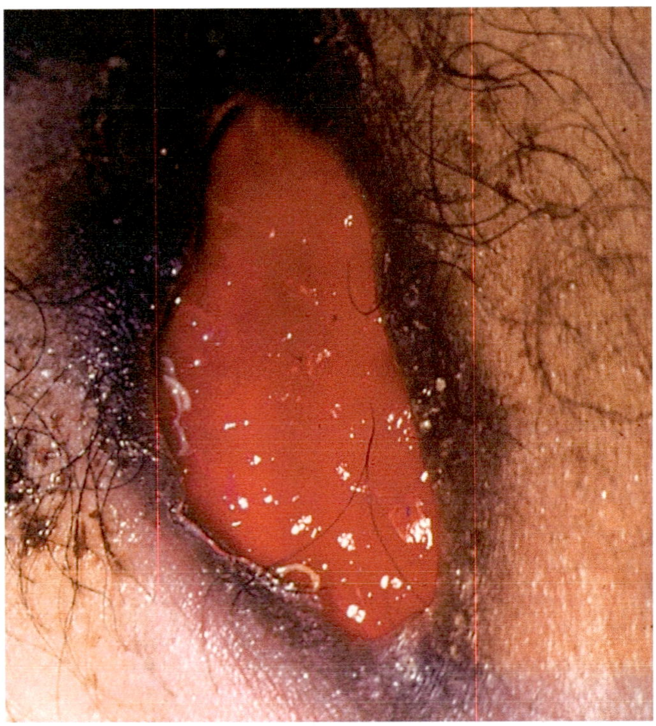

Donovanosis: Lesions often larger and more numerous.

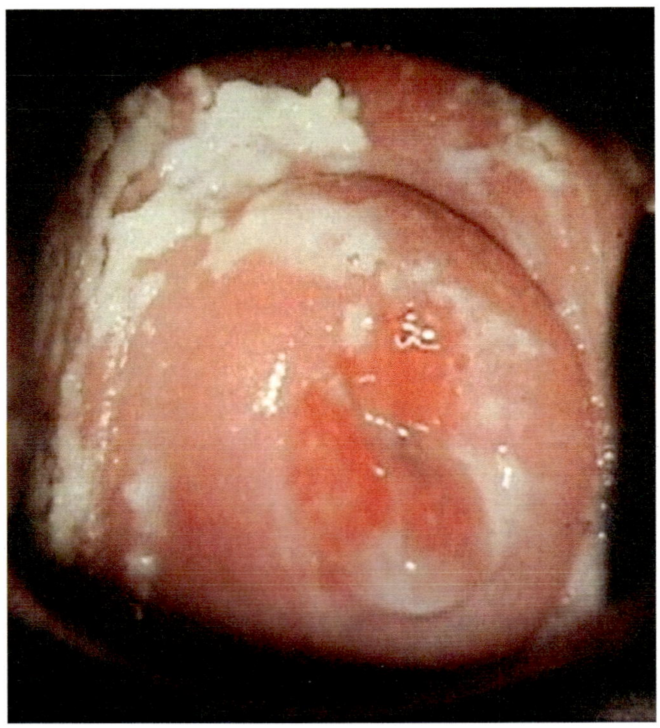

Candidal vulvovaginitis in pregnancy: More frequent and recurrent.

LYMPHOGRANULOMA VENEREUM (LGV)

Interaction of LGV and Pregnancy

Effect of LGV on pregnancy

Adverse outcomes not reported.

Effect of pregnancy on LGV

Complications (genital hypertrophy, rectal strictures) commoner.

Treatment

- Erythromycin 500 mg qid × 3 weeks.
- Doxycycline contraindicated.

GONORRHOEA

Interaction of Gonorrhoea and Pregnancy

Effect of gonorrhoea on pregnancy

- ***Effect on fetus:*** Preterm delivery, premature rupture of membranes, small for date baby chorioamnionitis.
- ***Effect on neonate:*** Transmission during contact with vaginal discharge during delivery. *In utero* transmission does not occur. Ophthalmia neonatorum, pharyngitis, proctitis, scalp abscess, vaginal, joint and disseminated infection.
- ***Effect on mother:*** Postpartum sepsis, endometritis, salpingitis, pelvic inflammatory disease more common.

Effect of pregnancy on gonorrhoea

- Mainly asymptomatic.
- Disseminated gonococcal infection, oropharyngeal infection more common.

Treatment

- Azithromycin, 2 gm single oral dose. Or cefixime, 400 mg single oral dose.

UREAPLASMA AND MYCOPLASMA

Effect of Ureaplasma and Mycoplasma on Pregnancy

- ***In fetus:*** Spontaneous abortion, chorioamnionitis, preterm birth.
- ***In neonate:*** Congenital pneumonia, chronic neonatal lung disease.
- *Mycoplasma genitalium* infection not associated with adverse fetal outcomes.

BACTERIAL VAGINOSIS (BV)

Interaction of BV and Pregnancy

Effect of BV on pregnancy

- ***Fetus:*** Spontaneous abortion, premature rupture of membranes, preterm labor and birth, intra-amniotic infection.
- ***Mother:*** Postpartum endometritis, pelvic inflammatory disease.

Effect of pregnancy on BV

Presentation similar to non-pregnant women.

Treatment

Metronidazole, 500 mg bid × 7 days. Or 250 mg tid × 7 days.

TRICHOMONIASIS

Interaction of Trichomoniasis and Pregnancy

Effect of trichomoniasis on pregnancy

Can lead to premature rupture of membranes, preterm delivery and low birth weight babies.

Effect of pregnancy on trichomoniasis

Similar presentation as non-pregnant women.

Treatment

Metronidazole, 2 gm single oral dose.

VULVOVAGINAL CANDIDIASIS (VVC)

Interaction of VVC and Pregnancy

Effect of VVC on Pregnancy

- No adverse fetal outcome.

Effect of Pregnancy on VVC

- Frequency markedly increased.

Treatment

Clotrimazole 1% intravaginally for 7 days.

Recommended screening tests for pregnant women

- HIV, VDRL, HBsAg in all pregnant women at first antenatal visit.
- Routine screening for *C. trachomatis* and hepatitis C recommended by CDC at first antenatal visit.
- Routine screening for trichomoniasis or HSV infections not recommended.

Chapter 18

Sexually Transmitted Infections in Adolescents

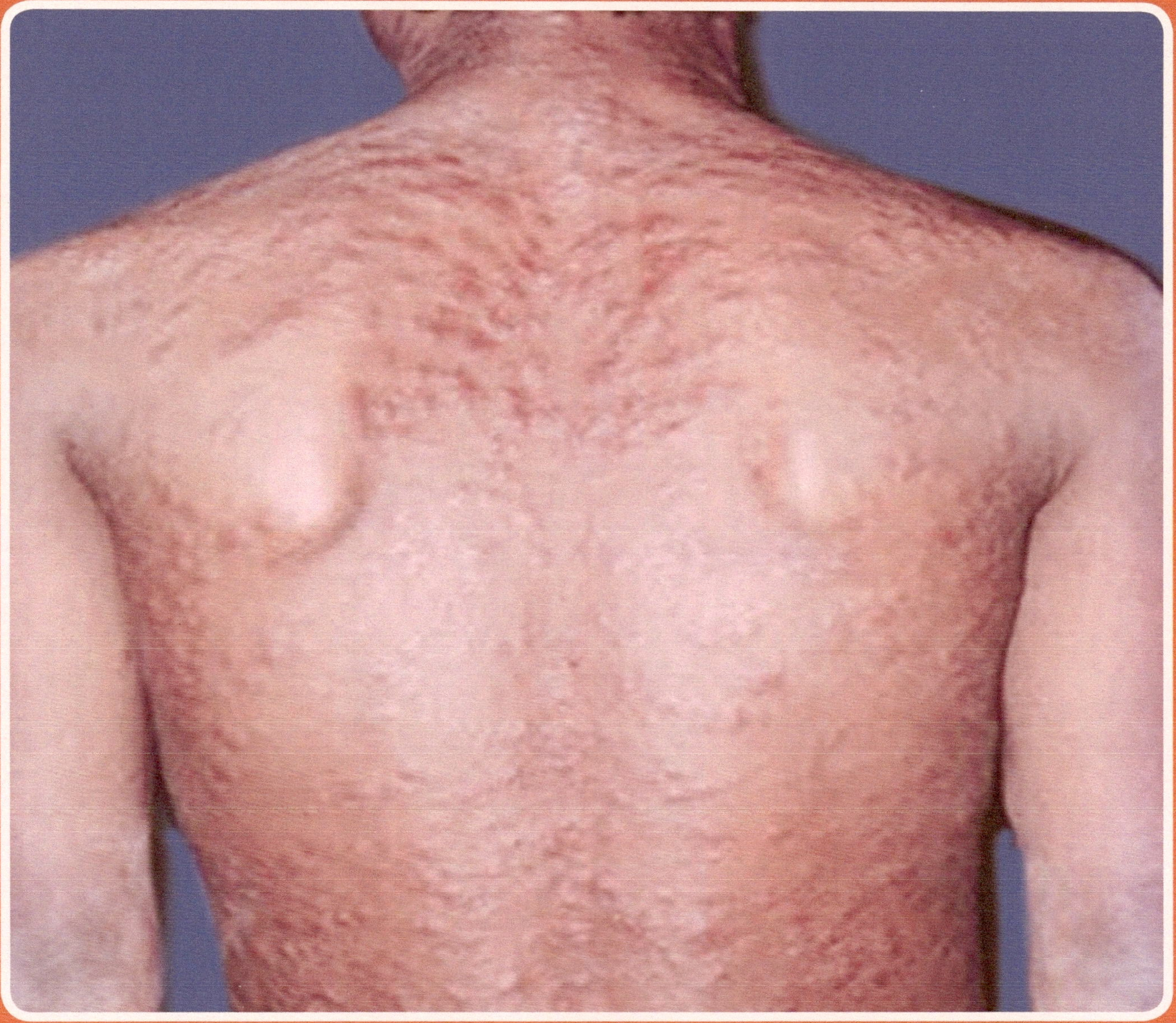

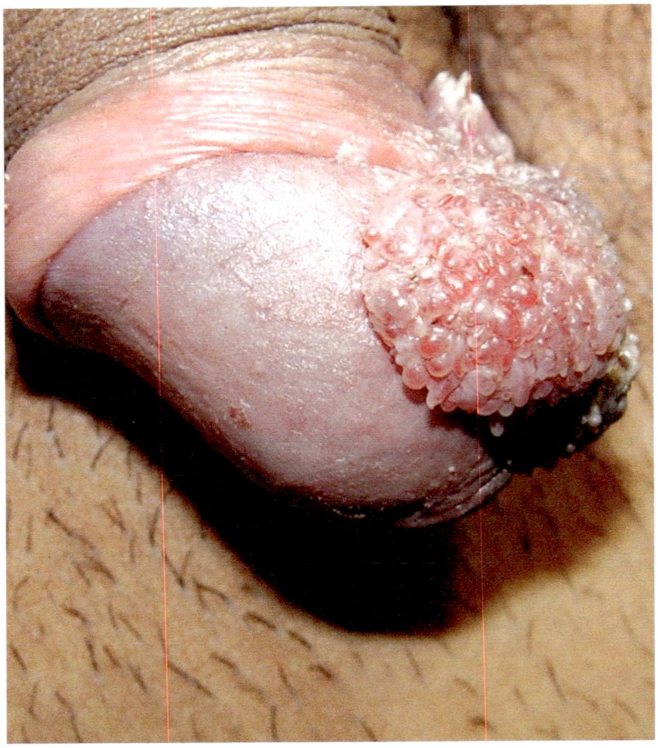

Anogenital warts: Frequent due to unprotected sex with multiple partners, including anogenital sex.

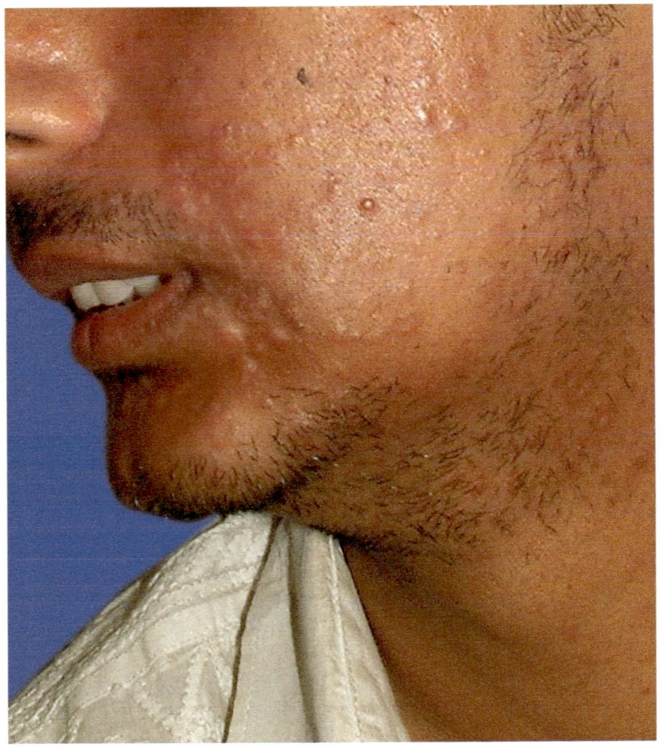

Secondary syphilis in adolescent: Adolescence is a period of high risk behavior and prominently.

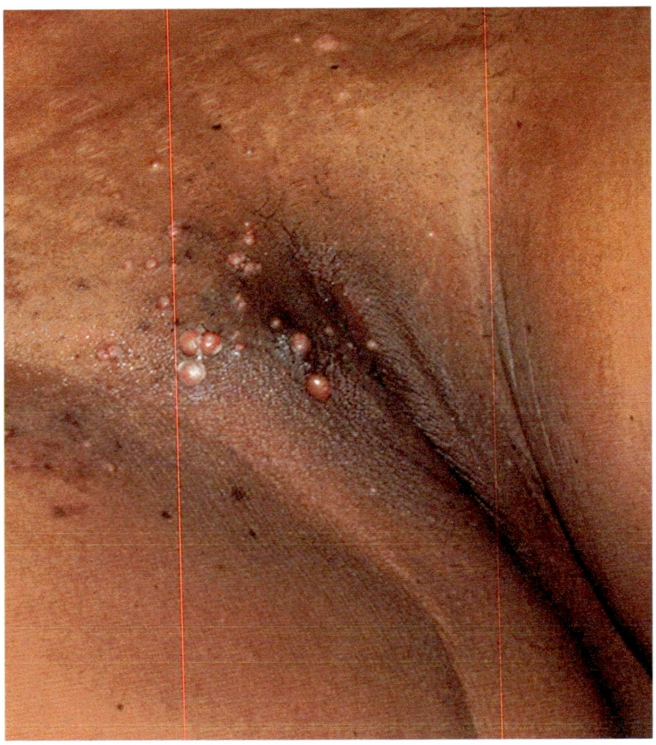

Molluscum contagiosum: Another common sexually transmitted infection.

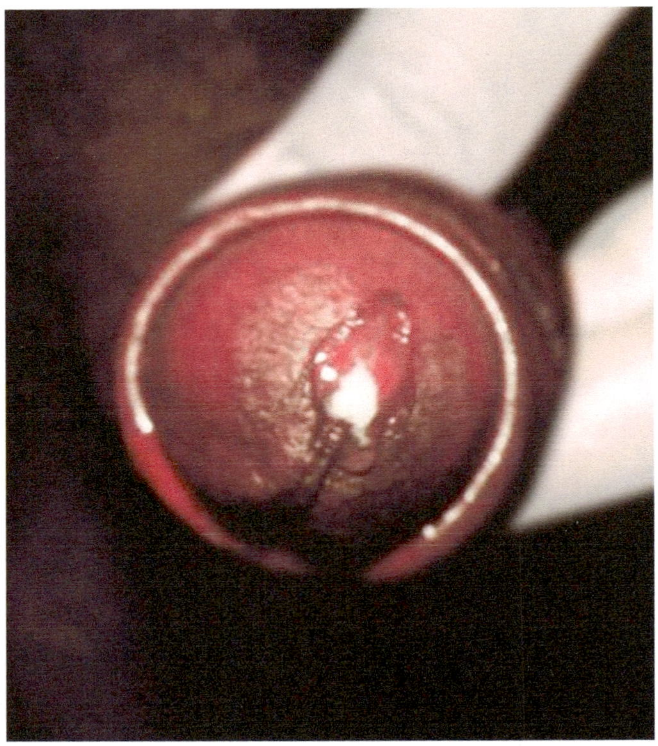

Urethral discharge: Prevalence of gonococcus and chlamydial infection higher in adolescence.

EPIDEMIOLOGY

Prevalence

Prevalence of sexually transmitted pathogens such as gonococcus and chlamydia already very high in adolescents in developed countries. Similar trend In developing countries—due to wider exposure through media, increased networking through internet and easy access to money, travel (for education and work). And liberalization of economy and culture.

Predisposing Factors

Adolescence a period of change and curiosity. And high risk behavior (Table 18.1). Sexually transmitted infections (STIs) in adolescents (aged 15-19 years) either due to promiscuous behavior. Or sexual abuse.

Table 18.1: High risk factors for STIs
• Early age of intercourse
• Multiple partners
• Unprotected sex
• Experimental sex
• Homosexuality
• Drug abuse
• Persons living in detention centers, orphanages
• Lack of access to health care facility

MANAGEMENT OF STIs IN ADOLESCENCE

Issues related to management of STIs in adolescence include taboo (though less now) associated with premarital sex and obstacles/delay in seeking treatment (and consequent spread to partners). So compassionate attitude, gentle probing, maintenance of confidentiality and high index of suspicion paramount.

PREVENTION

Efforts to reduce STIs in adolescents at all levels–individual, family, school, college, society. And importantly government. Measures likely to help:

- IEC activities
- Vaccines

IEC activities

- Providing information regarding safe sexual practices (including barrier protection, avoiding casual sex) at level of primary education.
- Spreading awareness on HIV and STIs *via* media, holding group discussions, forums, blogs.
- Encouraging treatment seeking behavior if any suspicion of STIs. Seeking treatment at traditional health care centers preferred over treatment on internet.

Vaccines

- ***Hepatitis B vaccine:*** For all.
- ***HPV vaccine:***
  - Two HPV vaccines available.
    - Bivalent protects against high risk HPV (type 16 and 18) which cause 80% of cervical cancers.
    - Quadrivalent protects against both high risk HPV (type 16 and 18) and low risk HPV (6 and 11) which cause most of anogenital warts.
  - Vaccines most effective when all doses administered before sexual contact.
    - In females: Either vaccine given at 11-12 years of age, but can be given upto 13-26 years.
    - In males: Quadrivalent vaccine given at 9-26 years of age.

GUIDELINES FOR SCREENING

Guidelines regarding screening and treatment not well-defined. And vary from country to country. Certain recommendations regarding screening in adolescence (CDC 2010):

- ***Routine screening recommended:***
  - Yearly screening for *Chlamydia trachomatis* for all sexually active females < 25 years.
  - Yearly screening for gonorrhoea for all sexually active women at high risk.[1]
  - Routine screening for HIV for all sexually active persons and those involved in injectable drug abuse.
  - Pap smear for sexually active women > 21 years.
- ***Routine screening not recommended:*** For syphilis, trichomoniasis, bacterial vaginosis, herpes simplex, hepatitis B virus in asymptomatic persons.

[1] **High risk:** < 25 years of age, previous history of gonococcal infection, presence of other STIs, new or multiple sex partners, inconsistent condom use, drug abuse and commercial sex work.

5 SECTION

ANNEXURES

ANNEXURE 1

Relevant Anatomy of Male Genital Tract

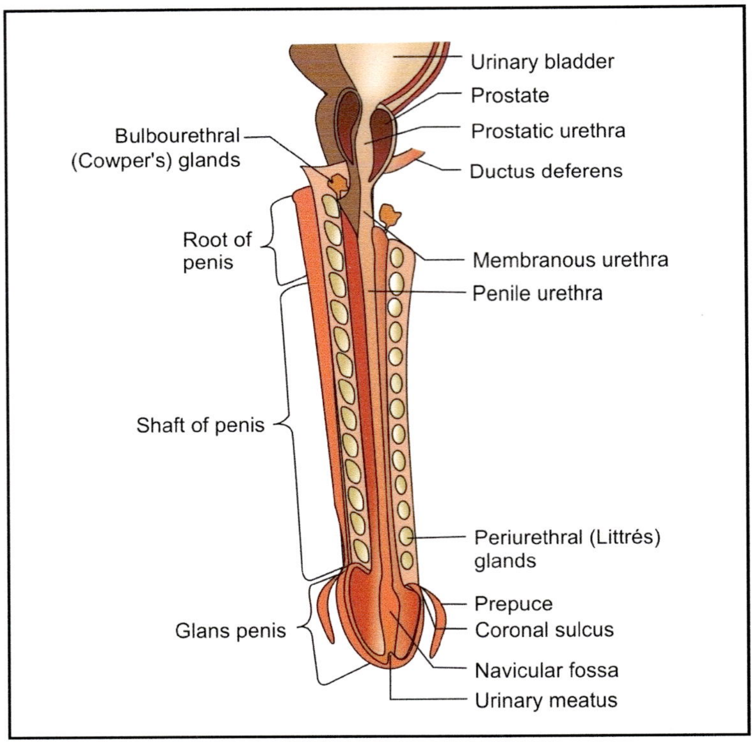

Sagittal section of penile shaft

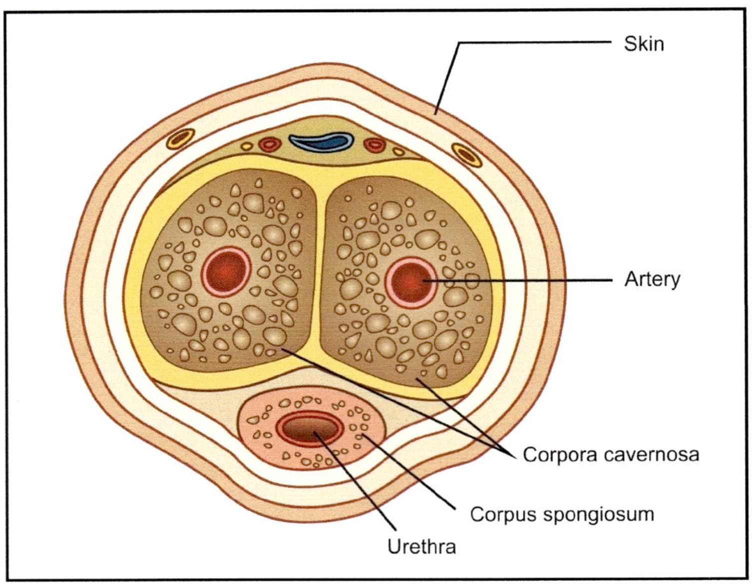

Cross-section of penile shaft

PENIS

- ***Function:*** Male organ of sexual activity. Also contains penile urethra which transports urine and semen.
- ***Composed of:***
  - *Glans:* most distal part. In uncircumcised, covered by prepuce (foreskin). Prepuce normally retractable (unless patient phimosed) except at frenulum (fibrous band attaching prepuce to glans ventrally). Retraction or surgical removal of prepuce (circumcision) exposes underlying glans. Junction between glans and penile shaft–corona. Urethra opens on tip of glans at urethral meatus.
  - *Shaft:* cylindrical organ with upper surface known as dorsal surface and lower as ventral surface. Covered by (outside inwards) skin (lacks hair follicles), Dartos layer, (smooth, discontinuous muscle layer), penile fascia (loose connective tissue with blood vessels, dorsal veins, nerve bundles and adipocytes) and tunica albuginea, (dense fibrous membrance). Composed of corpora cavernosa (2 in number) and corpus spongiosum which contains urethra.
  - *Root.*

URETHRA

- ***Length:*** About 20 cm.
- ***Consists of 3 parts:***
  - *Prostatic urethra:* proximal part, starts from bladder. And surrounded by prostate. Lined by pseudostratified columnar epithelium.
  - *Membranous urethra:* extends from lower pole of prostate to bulb of corpus spongiosum. Lined by stratified columnar epithelium.
  - *Penile/distal urethra:* passes through corpus spongiosum. Ends distally at urethral meatus. Terminal part dilated (fossa navicularis) before opening at urethral meatus. This part lined with stratified (non-keratinized) squamous epithelium.

SCROTUM AND CONTENTS

Scrotum

- Sac of skin to hold testes and epididymis.
- Located directly behind the penis and in front of anus.
- Covered by thin layer of rugosed (thrown into folds) skin. Skin more hairy, more pigmented with more sebaceous and sweat glands.
- Maintains temperature lower than human body to optimize spermatogenesis.

Testes

- Organ both of reproductive and endocrine system.
- Covered by fibrous capsule called tunica albuginea.
- Divided by fibrous tissue partitions into 200 to 400 wedge shaped sections or lobes.
- Each lobe, has 3 to 10 coiled tubules, called seminiferous tubules, to produce sperm cells. Testis contains 2 important cell types—Sertoli cells which assist in spermatogenesis. And Leydig cells which produce testosterone.

Epididymis

- Comma shaped structure located on posterior border of testis. Three parts (head—caput, body—corpora and tail—cauda).
- Composed of single long (6 m) fine highly coiled tubular structure which tapers distally to form ductus deferens (vas deferens).
- Helps in maturation and storage of sperms.

GLANDS

Several glands associated with male genital tract.

- ***Seminal vesicles:*** Paired glands. Located on posterior surface of urinary bladder, immediately inferior and lateral to ductus deferens. Constrict to form short ducts which join ductus deferens to form ejaculatory ducts. And ejaculatory ducts enter prostate.
- ***Prostate:*** Lies below bladder and surrounds prostatic urethra. Is composed of two parts-glandular portion and fibromuscular portion. May be involved in gonococcal and chlamydial infection (prostatitis).
- ***Bulbourethral (Cowper's) glands:*** Paired glands. Open into membranous urethra. May be involved in gonococcal and chlamydial infections (Cowperitis).
- ***Periurethral (Littre's) glands:*** Innumerable. Present along entire length of penile urethra. May be involved in gonococcal and chlamydial infections (Litteritis).

LYMPHATIC DRAINAGE

Table 1: Lymphatic drainage of male genital tract

Organ	Draining lymph node
Penile skin, prepuce, scrotum, perineum	Superficial inguinal lymph nodes
Glans, penile urethra	Deep inguinal nodes. Occasionally external iliac nodes
Vas deferens, ejaculatory duct, prostate	External and internal iliac lymph nodes
Seminal vesicles	Internal iliac lymph nodes
Testis, epididymis	Pre- and para-aortic group

ANNEXURE 2

Relevant Anatomy of Female Genital Tract

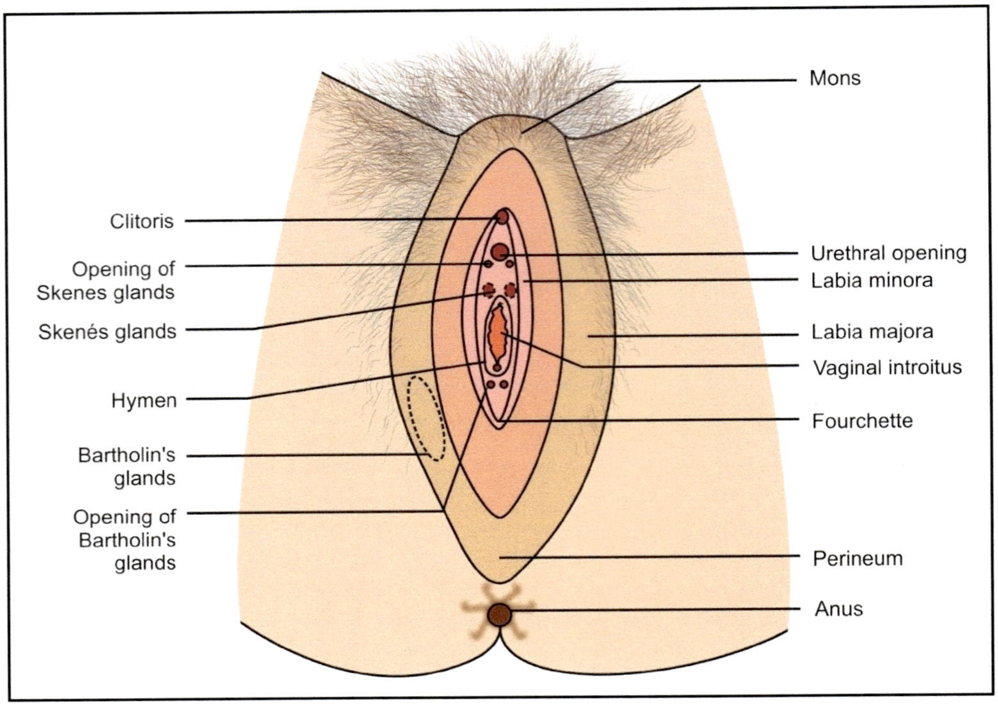

Structure of vulva and related structures

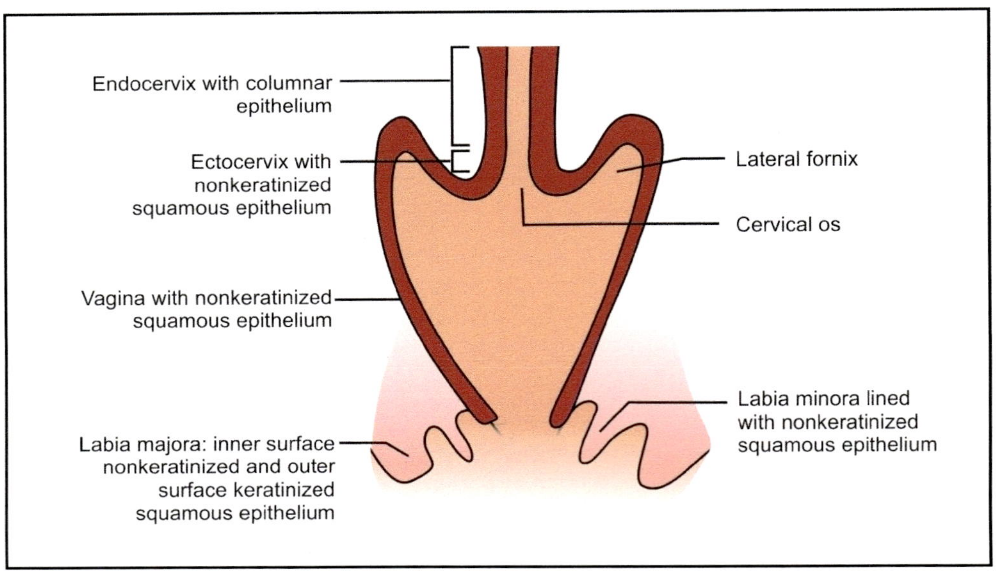

Section of female genitalia

VULVA

Vulva (female external genitalia) consists of pubis, labia majora and labia minora and structures enclosed within.

- ***Mons pubis:*** Small mound raised by underlying pad of fat. Is covered with pubic hair.
- ***Labia majora:*** 2 folds of skin and subcutaneous fat having internal mucosal and outer cutaneous lining. Appear as large lips starting from mons pubis superiorly (anteriorly) and join perineum inferiorly (posteriorly).
- ***Labia minora:*** Smaller folds of mucosa within labia majora, enclosing vestibule. Upper end of labia minora join around clitoris (female penis) to form small prepuce. And posteriorly meet at fourchette.
- ***Vestibule:*** Almond shaped area enclosed by labia minora. Extend superiorly (anteriorly) from clitoris to fourchette inferiorly (posteriorly). Contains vaginal and urethral openings. And openings of greater vestibular (Bartholin's) glands.
  - *Urethral orifice:* present below clitoris and above vaginal introitus. Lesser vestibular (Skene's) glands open on either side of urethral orifice.
  - *Vaginal opening (introitus):* is covered by thin membrane (hymen). Ducts of greater vestibular (Bartholin's) glands open on either side of vaginal introitus.
- ***Perineum:*** Area between vaginal introitus and anal opening. Consists of muscle for supporting pelvic area.

INTERNAL STRUCTURES

Vagina

- Is a fibromuscular organ.
- Consists of 4 walls (anterior, posterior and two lateral walls) and roof.
- Roof (vault) contains cervical opening or cervical os which juts into vagina to form fornices.
- Lined by stratified squamous epithelium, so resistant to infection by gonococcus.

Cervix

- Connection between uterus and vagina.
- Consists of ectocervix (distal part) and endocervix (proximal part).
- Ectocervix lined by nonkeratinized squamous epithelium while the endocervix lined by columnar epithelium. Former resistant to gonococcus, latter susceptible.

GLANDS

- ***Greater vestibular (Bartholin's) glands:*** Mucus secreting, paired pea sized glands. Lie in posterior part of labia majora. And open in vestibule. May be involved in gonococcal and chlamydial infections. However, more frequently infection not sexually transmitted.
- ***Lesser vestibular (Skene's) glands:*** Paraurethral mucus secreting glands. Open into urethra or periurethral area.

Table 1: Lymphatic drainage of female genital tract

Organ	Draining lymph node
Vulva	Superficial inguinal and femoral lymph nodes
Vagina	Upper-third: external iliac nodes Middle-third: internal iliac nodes Lower-third: superficial iliac nodes
Cervix	External and internal iliac and sacral nodes
Uterus	Para-aortic, external iliac, superficial inguinal nodes
Fallopian tubes	Para-aortic nodes
Ovaries	Pre- and para-aortic nodes

ANNEXURE 3

STI Syndromes

Syndrome of urethral discharge

RTIs/STIs: Gonorrhoea, Chlamydial infection, Trichomoniasis

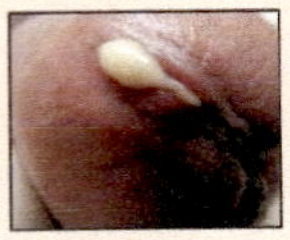

Causative organisms
- *Neisseria gonorrhoeae*
- *Chlamydia trachomatis*
- *Trichomonas vaginalis*

History of:
- Urethral discharge (UD)
- Pain/burning while passing urine, increased frequency of urination
- Sexual exposure of either partner to a high risk behaviour including orogenital sex

→

Examination:
- Examine urethral meatus for redness and swelling
- If UD absent, gently massage urethra from base of penis towards meatus. Look for thick, creamy greenish-yellow or mucoid discharge

↓

Laboratory Investigations: If available
- Gram stain of urethral smear: ≥ 5 neutrophils/oil immersion field (OIF)
  - ➢ In gonococcal urethritis: Gram-negative intracellular diplococci
  - ➢ In non-gonococcal urethritis: No organisms seen
- Gram stain of sediment of 1st void urine: ≥ 10 neutrophils/OIF

Treatment:

1st visit:

As dual infections common, treatment of UD to cover both gonococcal and chlamydial infections.
- Recommended regimen for uncomplicated* UD:
  - –Cefixime 400 mg SOD**
  - **PLUS**
  - –Azithromycin 1 g SOD**

  } under supervision
- If patient allergic to azithromycin: Erythromycin 500 mg qid x 7 days.

2nd visit: after 7 days
- If symptoms subside: Counsel and send.
- If symptoms (discharge/dysuria) persist:
  - –Check for compliance. And for reinfection
  - –Treat for *Trichomonas vaginalis*: Secnidazole 2 gm SOD*

3rd visit: If the symptoms still persist
- Refer to higher centre as early as possible

* Disease limited to lower anogenital tract (anterior urethritis and proctitis)

** Single oral dose

Syndrome specific guidelines for partner management:
- Treat all recent partners:
  - –Female partners: as above after ruling out pregnancy and history of allergies.
  - –Male partners: as above after ruling out allergies
- Advise sexual abstinence during course of treatment
- Provide condoms, educate about correct and consistent use
- Refer for counselling and voluntary testing for HIV, syphilis and Hepatitis B
- Schedule return visit after 7 days

Management of pregnant partner:

Pregnant partners of patients with UD should be examined (P/S and P/V examination) and treated for both gonococcal and chlamydial infections:
- Gonococcal infection: Cefixime 400 mg SOD*. Or Ceftriaxone 125 mg single intramuscular injection

PLUS
- Chlamydial infection: Erythromycin 500 mg qid x 7 days. Or Amoxicillin 500 mg tid x 7 days

Quinolones (like ofloxacin, ciprofloxacin) and doxycycline contraindicated in pregnancy

*Single oral dose

Syndrome of scrotal swelling

RTIs/STIs: Gonorrhoea, Chlamydial infection

Causative organisms
- *Neisseria gonorrhoeae*
- *Chlamydia trachomatis*

History of:
- Swelling and pain in scrotum
- Pain or burning while passing urine
- Systemic symptoms like malaise, fever
- Sexual exposure of either partner to high risk practices including orogenital sex

Examination:
- Scrotal swelling
- Redness and edema of overlying skin
- Tenderness of epididymis and vas deferens
- Associated urethral discharge/genital ulcer/inguinal lymph nodes and if present refer to respective flowchart
- A transillumination test to rule out hydrocele

Laboratory Investigations: If available
- Gram stain of urethral smear: ≥ 5 neutrophils/OIF
- In gonococcal urethritis: Gram-negative intracellular diplococci
- In non-gonococcal urethritis: No organisms seen
- Gram stain of sediment of 1st void urine: ≥ 10 neutrophils/OIF

Differential diagnosis (non RTIs/STIs):

Infections causing scrotal swelling: Tuberculosis, filariasis, coliforms, pseudomonas, mumps virus infection

Non infectious causes: Trauma, hernia, hydrocele, testicular torsion, and testicular tumors

Treatment
- Treat for both gonococccal and chlamydial infections
  - –Cefixime 400 mg orally bid × 7 days

  PLUS

  - –Doxycycline 100 mg orally, bid × 14 days
  - –And refer to higher center as early as possible since complicated infections need parenteral and longer duration of treatment
- Supportive therapy. To reduce pain (bed rest, scrotal elevation with T-bandage and analgesics)

Note: Delay in therapy may result in damage and scarring of testes leading to subfertility

Syndrome specific guidelines for partner management:

Partner needs to be treated depending on the clinical findings

Management protocol in case pregnant partner:
- Depending on the clinical findings in pregnant partner (whether vaginal discharge or endocervical discharge or PID is present) appropriate drug regimens used.
- Drugs safe: Erythromycin base/erythromycin estolate/amoxicillin
- Drugs contraindicated: Doxycycline, erythromycin estolate

Syndrome of vaginal discharge

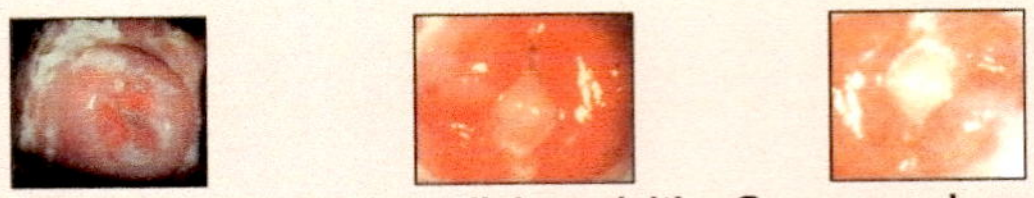

Vaginits   Chalamydial cervicitis   Gonococcal cervicitis

Causative organisms of vaginitis
- *Trichomonas vaginalis (TV)*
- *Candida albicans*
- *Gardnerella vaginalis*
- *Mycoplasma*

Causative organisms of cervicitis
- *Neisseria gonorrhoeae*
- *Chlamydia trachomatis*
- *Trichomonas vaginalis*
- *Herpes simplex virus*

History of:
- Menstrual history to rule out pregnancy
- Nature and type of discharge (amount, smell, consistency)
- Genital itching
- Burning while passing urine increased frequency
- Presence of any ulcer, swelling on vulval or inguinal region
- Genital complaints in sexual partners
- Low backache

→

Examination:
- Per speculum examination to differentiate between vaginitis and cervicitis
- **Vaginitis:**
  - *Trichomoniasis:* greenish frothy discharge
  - *Candidiasis:* curdy white discharge
  - *Bacterial vaginosis:* adherent discharge
  - *Mixed infections:* atypical discharge
- **Cervicitis:**
  - Cervical erosion/cervical ulcer/ mucopurulent cervical discharge
  - Bimanual pelvic examination to rule out pelvic inflammatory disease
  - If speculum examination is not possible or client is hesitant, treat both for vaginitis and cervicitis

→

Laboratory investigations:
- *Wet mount microscopy:* for *Trichomonas vaginalis* and clue cells
- *10% KOH preparation:* for *Candida albicans*
- *Gram stain of vaginal smear:* for clue cells seen in bacterial vaginosis
- *Gram stain of endocervical smear:* to detect gonococci

↓

Treatment

Treatment of vaginitis (TV+BV+ Candida)
- ***To cover trichomonoasis and bacterial vaginosis:***
  - Secnidazole 2 gm orally, stat

    OR
  - Tinidazole 500 mg orally, bid × for 5 days
  - Metoclopropramide taken 30 minutes before secnidazole, to prevent gastric intolerenace
- ***To cover candidiasis***
  - Fluconazole 150 mg stat

    OR
  - Clotrimazole 500 mg vaginal pessaries stat

Treatment of cervicitis (chlamydia and gonorrhoea)
- *To cover gonorrhoea:* Cefixime 400 mg orally stat

  PLUS
- *To cover chlamydia:* Azithromycin 1 g, 1 hour before lunch
- If vaginitis and cervicitis are present treat for both
- Instruct client to avoid douching
- Pregnancy, diabetes, HIV to be ruled out in recurrent infections
- Follow-up after one week

↓

Syndrome specific guidelines for partner management
- Treat current partner only if no improvement after initial treatment
- If partner symptomatic, treat client and partner using above protocols
- Advise sexual abstinence during the course of treatment
- Provide condoms, educate about correct and consistent use
- Schedule return visit after 7 days

↓

Management of pregnant patient

Per speculum examination should be done to rule out pregnancy complications like abortion, premature rupture of membranes

Treatment for vaginitis (TV+BV+ Candida)
- In first trimester of pregnancy
  - Local treatment with clotrimazole vaginal pessary/cream only for candidiasis. Oral flucanozole contraindicated in pregnancy
  - Metronidazole pessaries or cream intravaginally if trichomoniasis or BV is suspected.
- In second and third trimester oral metronidazole can be given
  - Secnidazole 2 gm orally stat

    OR

    Tinidazole 500 mg orally bid × 5 days
  - With metodopropramide taken 30 minutes before Metronidazole, to prevent gastric intolerance

Syndrome of genital ulcer disease

RTIs/STIs: Genital herpes, Syphilis and Chancroid

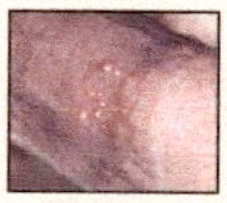

Genital herpes

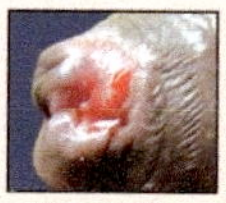

Syphilis

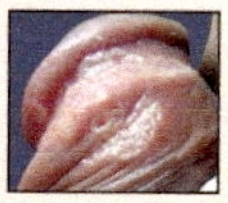

Chancroid

Causative organisms:
- ***Common:***
  - *Genital herpes: Herpes simplex virus*
  - *Syphilis: Treponema pallidum*
  - *Chancroid: Haemophilus ducreyi*
- ***Infrequent:***
  - *Granulomas inguinale: Klebsiella granulomatis*
  - *Lymphogranuloma venereum: Chlamydia trachomatis*

History of:
- Genital ulcer/vesicles
- Sexual exposure of either partner to high risk practices including orogenital sex

→

Examination:
- Presence of vesicles/ulcer
- Look for inguinal lymph node swelling and if present refer to respective flowchart

→

Laboratory investigations:
- RPR test for syphilis
- For further investigations refer to higher center

Treatment
- ***If vesicles or multiple painful ulcers present. Or recurrences***: Treat as herpes genitalis: Acyclovir 400 mg orally, tid x 7 days
- **If only ulcers seen. *And no recurrences***: Treat for syphilis and chancroid:
  - ***To cover syphilis:***
    - ➢ Benzathine penicillin 2.4 million IU IM after test dose half dose in each buttock (with emergency tray ready)

      OR
    - ➢ In individuals allergic or intolerant to penicillin, Doxycycline 100 mg orally, bid x 14 days.

    PLUS
  - ***To cover chancroid:***
    - ➢ Azithromycin 1 g SOD

      OR
    - ➢ Ciprofloxacin 500 mg orally bid x 3 days

Refer to higher center
- If not responding to treatment
- Genital ulcers co-existent with HIV
- Recurrent lesions

Treatment should be extended beyond 7 days if ulcers have not epithelialized (not formed a new layer of skin over the sore)

Syndrome specific guidelines for partner management:
- Treat all partners of previous 3 months for syphilis and chancroid
- Advise sexual abstinence during course of treatment
- Provide condoms and educate about correct and consistent use
- Refer for voluntary counseling and testing for HIV, Syphilis and Hepatitis B
- Schedule return visit after 7 days

Management of pregnant partner:
- All RPR-positive pregnant women considered infected unless documentation of adequate treatment and decreasing sequential serologic antibody titers.
  - Benzathine penicillin, 2.4 million IU IM after test dose (vide supra) (with emergency tray ready) Second similar dose of benzathine penicillin, 2.4 million units IM administered 1 week after initial dose in women with early (primary, secondary, or early latent) syphilis
  - Quinolones (like ofloxacin, ciprofloxacin), doxycycline, sulphonamides contraindicated in pregnancy
  - Pregnant women allergic to penicillin treated with erythromycin (base or ethylsuccinate, never stearate) 500 mg orally qid x 15 days. And neonate treated for syphilis after delivery
- All pregnant women asked for history of genital herpes and examined for herpetic lesions:
  - Women without signs and symptoms of genital herpes or its prodrome deliver vaginally
  - Women with genital herpetic lesions at the onset of labor→ delivered by Caesarean section (to prevent neonatal herpes)
  - Acyclovir may be administered orally to pregnant women with 1st episode genital herpes or severe recurrent herpes

Syndrome of inguinal bubo

RTIs/STIs: LGV, Chancroid

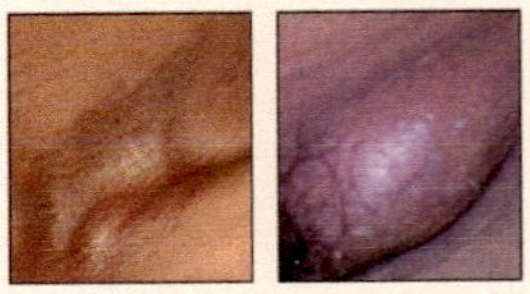

Causative Organisms

- *Bubo of LGV: Chlamydia trachomatis* serovars L1,L2,L3
- *Bubo of chancroid: Haemophilus ducreyi*

History of:

- Swelling in inguinal region which may be painful
- Preceding history of genital ulcer ±
- Sexual exposure of either partner to high risk practices including orogenital sex
- Systemic symptoms like malaise, fever

Examination:

- Localized enlargement of lymph nodes in groin which may be tender and fluctuant
- Inflammation of skin over swelling
- Presence of multiple sinuses
- Edema of genitals and lower limbs
- If genital ulcer present, refer to respective flow chart

Laboratory Investigations:

Diagnosis is on clinical grounds

Differential diagnosis (non RTIs/STIs):

- Tuberculosis, filariasis
- Any acute infection of skin of pubic area, genitals, buttocks, anus and lower limbs can also cause inguinal swelling. If malignancy or tuberculosis suspected, refer to higher center for biopsy.

Treatment

- *To cover LGV:* Doxycycline 100 mg orally bid × 21 days

PLUS

- *To cover chancroid:*
  –Azithromycin 1 g stat

  OR

  –Ciprofloxacin 500 mg bid × 3 days
- Refer to higher center as early as possible.

Note:

- Bubo never to be incised and drained at primary health center, even if it is fluctuant, due to high risk of fistula formation and chronicity. If bubo fluctuant always refer for aspiration to higher center
- Severe cases with vulval edema in females, referred to higher center forsurgical intervention

Syndrome specific guidelines for partner management:

- Treat all partners who are in contact with client in last 3 months
- Partners should be treated for chancroid and LGV
- Azithromycin 1 g orally single dose to cover chancroid + Doxycycline 100 mg orally bid × 21 days to cover LGV
- Advise sexual abstinence during course of treatment
- Provide condoms, educate on correct and consistent use
- Refer for voluntary counseling and testing for HIV, syphilis and Hepatitis B
- Schedule return visit after 7 days and 21 days

Management of pregnant/lactating partner:

- Erythromycin base or ethylsuccinate (never estolate) 500 mg qid × 21 days and refer to higher center.
- Quinolones (like ofloxacin, ciprofloxacin), doxycycline, sulphonamides are contraindicated in pregnant women.
- Consider adding parenteral aminoglycoside (e.g. gentamicin)

Syndrome of lower abdominal pain

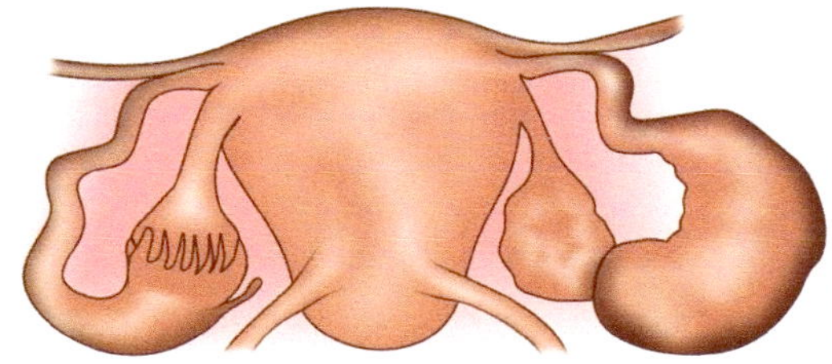

Pelvic inflammatory disease

Causative Organisms:
- *Neisseria gonorrheae*
- *Chlamydia trachomatis*
- *Mycoplasma, Gardnerella,* anaerobic bacteria (*Bacteroides spp*, gram positive cocci)

History of:
- Lower abdominal pain
- Fever
- Vaginal discharge
- Menstrual irregularities like heavy, irregular vaginal bleeding
- Dysmenorrhoea
- Dyspareunia
- Dysuria, tenesmus
- Low backache
- Contraceptive use like IUD

Examination:
- General examination: temperature, pulse, blood pressure
- Per speculum examination: vaginal/ cervical discharge, congestion or ulcers
- Per abdominal tenderness or guarding
- Pelvic examination: Uterine/adnexal tenderness, cervical movement tenderness,

Note: Urine pregnancy test done in all women suspected of having PID to rule out ectopic pregnancy

Laboratory investigations:
If available
- Wet smear examination
- Gram stain for gonorrhea
- Complete blood count and ESR
- Urine microscopy for pus cells

Differential diagnosis
- Ectopic pregnancy
- Twisted ovarian cyst
- Ovarian tumor
- Appendicitis
- Abdominal tuberculosis

Treatment (Out patient treatment)

In mild or moderate PID (absence of tuboovarian abscess) out patient treatment given.

Therapy required to cover *Neisseria gonorrheae*, *Chlamydia trachomatis* and anaerobes.

- Cefixime 400 mg orally bid × 7 days
  PLUS
  Metronidazole 400 mg orally bid × 14 days
- Doxycylcline 100 mg bid x 14 days (to treat chlamydial infection)
- Ibuprofen 400 mg bid for 3-5 days
- Ranitidine 150 mg orally, to prevent gastritis
- Remove intrauterine device, if present, under antibiotic cover of 24-48 hours
- Advise abstinence during course of treatment and educate on correct and consistent use of condoms
- Observe for 3 days. If no improvement (i.e. absence of fever, reduction in abdominal tenderness, reduction in cervical movement, adnexal and uterine tenderness) or if symptoms worsen, refer for in patient treatment.

Caution: PID a serious condition. So refer client to hospital if she does not respond to treatment within 3 days and even earlier if her condition worsens

Syndrome specific guidelines for partner management
- Treat all partners in past 2 months
- Treat male partners for urethral discharge (gonorrhea and chlamydia)
- Advise sexual abstinence during the course of treatment
- Provide condoms, educate on correct and consistent use
- Refer for voluntary counseling and testing for HIV, syphilis and Hepatitis B
- Schedule return visit after 3 days, 7 days and 14 days to ensure compliance

Hospitalization of clients with acute PID should be seriously considered when:
- The diagnosis is uncertain
- Surgical emergencies e.g. appendicitis or ectopic pregnancy cannot be excluded
- Pelvic abscess is suspected
- Severe illness precludes management on outpatient basis
- Woman is pregnant
- Patient is unable to follow or tolerate an outpatient regimen
- Patient has failed to respond to outpatient therapy

Note: All patients requiring hospitalization should be referred to the district hospital

Syndrome of oral and anal STIs

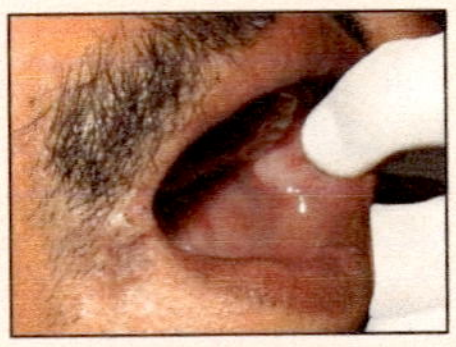

Causative Organisms:
- *Neisseria gonorrhoeae* (gonococcal pharyngitis/proctitis)
- *Chlamydia trachomatis* (chlamydial pharyngitis/proctitis)
- *Treponema pallidum* (syphilis)
- *Haemophilus ducreyi* (chancroid)
- *Klebsiella granulomatis* (donovanosis)
- *Herpes simplex* (labial herpes/herpetic proctitis)

History of:
- Unprotected oral sex patient with pharyngitis.
- Unprotected anal sex patient with anal discharge or tenesmus, diarrhea, blood in stool, abdominal cramping, nausea, bloating

Examination:
- Look for oral ulceration, redness, pharyngeal inflammation
- Genital or anorectal ulcers–single or multiple
- Presence of vesicles
- Rectal pus
- Any other STI syndrome (Do proctoscopy for rectal examination if available)

Laboratory investigations:
- RPR/VDRL for syphilis
- Gram stain examination of rectal swab will show gram negative intracellular diplococcic in case of gonorrhea

Pharyngitis with history of unprotected oral sex **OR** Anal discharge, tenesmus, bloating with history of unprotected anal sex **OR** Rectal pus or bloating with history of unprotected anal sex

→ Yes → Follow flowchart of urethral discharge syndrome and treat accordingly

Genital/anorectal ulcers/vesicles seen **OR** History of recurrent vesicular eruption

→ Yes → Follow flowchart of genital ulcer syndrome

Diarrhea, blood in stools, abdominal cramping, nausea, bloating with history of unprotected anal sex

→ Yes → Azithromycin 1 gm **PLUS** Cefixime 400 mg (follow urethral discharge syndrome flowchart) **PLUS** Anti-diarrheal medicines as needed and Refer to higher facility

Any other STI syndrome → Refer to relevant STI syndromic flowchart

Index

I

J

K

L

M

N

O

P

R

S